NILES PUBLIC LIBRARY

Niles, Illinois

FINE SCHEDULE

Adult Materials . . . . 10 per day
Juvenile Materials . . . . . . .04 per day
Video Tapes . . . . . . $1.50 per day

Suicide and Depression Among Adolescents and Young Adults

Suicide and Depression Among Adolescents and Young Adults

Edited by

Gerald L. Klerman, M.D.

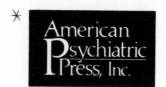

1400 K St. N.W.
Washington, D.C. 20005

Note: The authors have worked to ensure that all information in this book concerning drug dosages, schedules, and routes of administration is accurate as of the time of publication and consistent with standards set by the U.S. Food and Drug Administration and the general medical community. As medical research and practice advance, however, therapeutic standards may change. For this reason and because human and mechanical errors sometimes occur, we recommend that readers follow the advice of a physician who is directly involved in their care or the care of a member of their family.

Books published by American Psychiatric Press, Inc. represent the views and opinions of the individual authors and do not necessarily reflect the policies and opinions of the Press or the American Psychiatric Association.

Library of Congress Cataloging in Publication Data

Suicide and depression among adolescents and young adults.

Based on proceedings of the Conference on Suicide and Depression among Adolescents and Young Adults, held Dec. 3–4, 1982 in Boston, Mass.
Includes bibliographies and index.
1. Youth—United States—Suicidal behavior—Congresses.
2. Depression, mental—United States—Congresses.
3. Adolescent psychology—United States—Congresses.
I. Klerman, Gerald L., 1928–   II. Conference on Suicide and Depression among Adolescents and Young Adults (1982: Boston, Mass.) [DNLM: 1. Adolescent Behavior—congresses.
2. Depression—in adolescence—congresses.   3. Suicide—in adolescence—congresses. HV 6546 S9478 1982]
HV6546.S832   1986   362.2   86–1201
ISBN 0-88048-049-1

Contents

Contributors

Robert L. Arnstein, M.D.
Chief Psychiatrist
Yale University Health Services;
Clinical Professor of Psychiatry
Yale University School of Medicine
New Haven, Connecticut

Susan J. Blumenthal, M.D., M.P.A.
Director
Suicide Research Unit
Center for Study of Affective Disorders
Clinical Research Branch
Division of Extramural Research Programs
National Institute of Mental Health
Rockville, Maryland

Tim Brennan, Ph.D.
Director
Human Systems Institute
Boulder, Colorado;
Instructor
University of Colorado
Graduate School of Public Affairs
Boulder, Colorado

C. Hendricks Brown, Ph.D.
Assistant Professor
Department of Biostatistics
The Johns Hopkins University
School of Hygiene and Public Health
Baltimore, Maryland

W. Edward Craighead, Ph.D.
Visiting Professor
Department of Psychiatry
Duke University Medical Center
Durham, North Carolina

Eva Y. Deykin, D.P.H.
Assistant Professor of Social Work
Department of Maternal and Child Health
Harvard School of Public Health
Cambridge, Massachusetts

Felton Earls, M.D.
Director
William Greenleaf Eliot
Division of Child Psychiatry;
Associate Professor of Psychiatry (Child)
Washington University School of Medicine
St. Louis, Missouri

Sumru Erkut, Ph.D.
Research Associate
Wellesley College
Center for Research on Women
Wellesley, Massachusetts

Ernest M. Gruenberg, M.D., D.P.H.
Professor
Department of Mental Hygiene;
Professor of Psychiatry
The Johns Hopkins University
School of Hygiene and Public Health
Baltimore, Maryland

Robert M.A. Hirschfeld, M.D.
Chief
Center for Studies of Affective Disorders
Clinical Research Branch
Division of Extramural Research Programs
National Institute of Mental Health
Rockville, Maryland

Ada Jemison, M.D.
Child Psychiatry Fellow
Washington University School of Medicine
St. Louis, Missouri

Sheppard G. Kellam, M.D.
Professor and Chairman
The Johns Hopkins University
School of Hygiene and Public Health;
Professor of Psychiatry and Behavioral Science
The Johns Hopkins Medical School
Baltimore, Maryland

Gerald L. Klerman, M.D.
Associate Chairman (Research)
Cornell University Medical Center
New York Hospital
Payne Whitney Psychiatric Clinic
New York, New York

Daniel J. Levinson, Ph.D.
Professor of Psychology
Department of Psychiatry
Yale University School of Medicine
New Haven, Connecticut

John E. Mack, M.D.
Professor of Psychiatry
Harvard Medical School at The Cambridge Hospital;
Chairman
Executive Committee
Department of Psychiatry
Harvard Medical School
Cambridge, Massachusetts

Joe Mullaney, B.A.
Research Assistant
Department of Psychiatry
Washington University School of Medicine and
The Jewish Hospital of St. Louis
St. Louis, Missouri

Pamela J. Perun, Ph.D.
Boalt Hall School of Law
University of California
Berkeley, California

Anne C. Petersen, Ph.D.
Professor of Human Development;
Head
Department of Individual and Family Studies
The Pennsylvania State University
Philadelphia, Pennsylvania

Theodore Reich, M.D.
Professor of Genetics and Psychiatry
Department of Psychiatry
Washington University School of Medicine and
The Jewish Hospital of St. Louis
St. Louis, Missouri

John Rice, Ph.D.
Department of Psychiatry and Preventive Medicine
Washington University School of Medicine and
The Jewish Hospital of St. Louis
St. Louis, Missouri

Julius Richmond, M.D.
Professor of Health Policy
Division of Health Policy—Research and Education
Harvard University
Cambridge, Massachusetts

Gene M. Smith, Ph.D.
Psychologist
Massachusetts General Hospital;
Associate Professor of Psychology in Psychiatry
Harvard Medical School
Cambridge, Massachusetts

Myrna M. Weissman, Ph.D.
Professor of Psychiatry and Epidemiology
Depression Research Unit
Department of Psychiatry
Yale University School of Medicine
New Haven, Connecticut

Introduction

In *Healthy People*, the Surgeon General's Report on Health Promotion and Disease Prevention (1978), I drew attention to the relation between physical health and mental health, stating that "both are enhanced through the maintenance of strong family ties, the assistance of supportive friends, and the use of community support systems" (p. 10, *Healthy People*).

Nowhere is this connection so obvious, or its importance to the nation so pronounced, as in the case of adolescents and young adults. In the age group of 15 to 24 years, accidents, homicides, and suicides account for about three-quarters of all deaths. These deaths have been attributed to maladaptive behavior patterns characterized by judgmental errors, aggression, and sometimes indecision and doubt about wanting to live or die. Generally greater risk-taking occurs during this period of life than in any other (p. 43, *Healthy People*). So it appears that the deaths during this period are more directly affected by the individual's behavior patterns and personal psychological health than during any previous or subsequent phase of the life cycle.

While suicide remains a major source of mortality, depression is a major source of morbidity. Although epidemiological studies are only recently developing for these age groups, the indications are that depressive symptoms are widespread and significantly impair school performance, interpersonal relations, and occupational role performance. Drug use, alcohol consumption, and an increase in teenage pregnancy have all been related to underlying feelings of low self-esteem, despair, alienation, and depression which occur with moderate frequency among adolescents and young adults, in general, and in selected subgroups (such as minorities, women, and the unemployed). Furthermore, emotional problems in these age groups predispose individuals to later psychiatric difficulties, particularly in middle adulthood. The availability of effective preventive interventions would have desirable consequences not only for the periods of adolescence and young adulthood, but also for the mature adult life, at which time these individuals are most productive in the economy and are involved with family life and childrearing.

Overall, the health of adolescents and young adults is very good. Adolescence and young adulthood are among the healthiest periods of life in modern times. This was not true before the 20th century, when problems of poor sanitation and urban crowding contributed to high death rates from infectious disease, nutritional disorders, and other conditions. However, with the improvements in sanitation, nutrition, and housing in the general society, and with improvements in health care (especially with the development of antibiotics and immunization), many of these earlier causes of death among adolescents and young adults are no longer serious problems in modern urban and industrial societies.

Death rates overall are decreasing for most age groups. The vital statistics for adolescents and young adults indicates that although the death rates for these age groups are still very low, they have not declined as rapidly as have death rates for other age groups. Thus, the potential for disability and death is relatively high during adolescence and young adulthood. These conditions create major social and economic costs for society. Families in which adolescents and young adults have been involved in suicide, homicide, venereal disease, alcohol and substance abuse, or injury-related death suffer immense anguish and pain. In addition, there is the burden on the schools and law enforcement system, as well as the economic costs to society of many lost years of productive life.

The loss of years of productive life through injury in this age group makes this one of our major public health problems. To address this important problem, the Conference on Suicide and Depression among Adolescents and Young Adults brought together experts in the fields of clinical psychiatry, developmental psychology, epidemiology, and public health to review the current state of evidence on these phenomena, their antecedents, and their consequences. During the discussion session of the Conference, we discussed opportunities for preventive interventions and research priorities.

In addition to these general public health concerns, there are several trends which have led us to this Conference. First, there is the long history of the public health concerns of the mental health field in the United States. There were several successful early efforts at preventive approaches to problems in mental health. During the mid-19th century, "The Mad Hatter" syndrome was prevalent among hatters and furriers, among whom mercury poisoning was found to cause mental illness. In the first decade of this century, Goldberger discovered the connection between diet and pellagra, demonstrating the effect of a key nutritional deficiency on mental functioning. One of the best-known preventive accomplishments occurred in the 1950s with the eradication of general paresis following the discovery of the specific cause of syphilis in 1911, and the introduction of penicillin during World War II.

A second trend which led to this Conference was the strong interest in mental health shown by the Carter administration in the late 1970s, which continues to have impact even with changes in federal leadership. At that time, there were great hopes for changes in structure and financing which might be brought about in the sphere of mental health, exemplified by the Report of the President's Commission on Mental Health, issued in 1978. Discussing the positive effects of public health efforts, the Report stated: "The history of public health in the past century provides ample evidence that programs designed to prevent disease and disorder can be effective and reasonably economical. Infectious diseases that can now be prevented include smallpox, malaria, typhus, cholera, yellow fever, polio, and measles" (p. 1830). Diphtheria, tetanus, german measles, and mumps have also been controlled with effective vaccines. It is evident from these few examples that illness in general, and mental illnesses in particular, caused by infection, nutritional deficiency, and some environmental and occupational toxins, have been eradicated through the application of scientific research and public health techniques.

Among the key recommendations of the Report was the concentration of greater effort on prevention of mental illness. It stated:

> The Commission is concerned with preventing mental illness and emotional disturbance and with promoting the strengths, resources, and competencies of individuals, families, and communities. Our working definition of "prevention" embraces a broad range of activities which attempt to help individuals avoid becoming "patients" (Vol. 1, p. 51).

A third and related trend which led to this Conference was

based on my own activities as Surgeon General for the Public Health Service. The report we produced, *Healthy People*, heralded a concern for preventive strategies in mental health. During the time that Dr. Gerald Klerman (as Administrator of ADAMHA) and I were in Washington, we made an effort to create greater awareness about the potentially significant contribution of preventive strategies in coping with mental illness, and to tie that to our overall emphasis on the importance of health promotion and disease prevention in our society. It was not the concept of health promotion or disease prevention that was novel; rather, it was our perception that there were new opportunities and the potential for charting new directions, most notably in the area of mental health.

Prevention of mental disorders is a difficult task, and it is useful to step back and consider the ways in which it might be accomplished. The importance of prevention is clear: from a moral point of view, it has the potential to reduce suffering, and from the economic point of view, it reduces societal expense in terms of both direct (fiscal) and indirect (human) costs (Report of the President's Commission on Mental Health and Mental Illness, p. 1834).

In terms of the method by which these goals might be achieved, inquiry into public health problems in mental health rests on the base of epidemiologic knowledge, and it is this model which has guided the research of most participants in the Conference today. "Epidemiology" refers to "the study of the distribution and determinants of disease frequency in man" (MacMahon and Pugh, p. 1). An epidemiologic approach guides research by asking several basic questions, as cited by the Report of the President's Commission on Mental Health and Mental Illness:

1. What groups of adolescents and young persons are at high risk of developing mental illness or emotional disorder?
2. What factors contribute to the risk? What is the relative importance of each of these factors? Which of these risks are identifiable?
3. Can we effectively reduce the most significant of these risk factors?
4. Will reducing risks effectively lower the rate of emotional disorder or mental illness?

Finally, it is important to consider how the epidemiologic approach can be applied to the specific problem of adolescent suicide.

It seems clear that there is a virtual epidemic of adolescent suicide. The purpose of convening this Conference was to identify the incidence, prevalence, and risk factors for suicide, and to try to establish which factors are modifiable and which are not. The problems and challenges, as well as the successes of this enterprise, are contained in the chapters that follow. We have a much richer knowledge base concerning prevention in mental health than we had two decades ago. The Proceedings of this Conference can help us chart a course for acting constructively on the knowledge we have. The mortality data tell us not only how young people die; they also tell us much about how they live. The nation can ill afford the loss of productive life of these young people—a loss which places these problems among the highest priorities in public health.

Julius Richmond, M.D.

References

MacMahon B, Pugh TF: Epidemiology: Principles and Methods. Boston, Little, Brown, 1970

President's Commission on Mental Health: Report to the President From the President's Commission on Mental Health. Publication No. 040–000–0390–8. Washington DC, U.S. Government Printing Office, 1978

Public Health Service, Office of the Surgeon General: Healthy People: The Surgeon General's Report on Health Promotion and Disease Prevention. Public Health Service Publication No. 79–55071. Washington DC, U.S. Government Printing Office, 1978

Chapter 1

DEVELOPMENT IN THE NOVICE PHASE OF EARLY ADULTHOOD

Daniel J. Levinson, Ph.D.

Chapter 1

DEVELOPMENT IN THE NOVICE PHASE
OF EARLY ADULTHOOD

This volume deals with the years from roughly the late teens to the early thirties—the part of the life cycle generally known as adolescence and youth. In the study of psychopathology and adaptational problems of childhood, a child development perspective provides a framework for our understanding of the specific factors operating at a given age. Likewise, an adult development perspective is important to our understanding of specific illnesses and maladjustments in adulthood. The study of adult development on even a modest scale, is, unfortunately, just beginning.

My assigned task is *not* to provide a broad review of theory and research on adult development. It is, more simply, to offer a brief statement of my own theory, which deals with the development of the individual *life structure* in adulthood. The life structure includes aspects of personality, social roles, and social structure, and it includes life events, but it represents a different level of analysis from any of these and evolves on different terms. The theory of life structure development does, however, connect directly to personality development, career development, and adaptation to life events, and it has major implications for them.

I shall discuss the following in turn: 1) the concept of the individual life structure; 2) the general development of the life structure through an alternative series of structure-building and structure-changing (transitional) periods; 3) the novice phase of early adulthood, which includes the first three developmental periods:

the Early Adult Transition (roughly, age 17 to 22); Building an Entry Life Structure (age 22 to 28); and the Age Thirty Transition (age 28 to 33). For a fuller presentation of concepts and findings, see Levinson (1978, 1980, 1981, 1986) and Levinson and Gooden (1985).

The Concept of the Individual Life Structure

The life structure is the underlying pattern or design of a person's life at a given time. Perhaps I can indicate the meaning more clearly by comparing life structure and personality structure. A theory of personality structure is a way of conceptualizing answers to a concrete question: "What kind of person am I?" Different theories offer numerous ways of thinking about this question and of characterizing oneself or others; for example, one's wishes, conflicts, defenses, traits, skills, and values.

A theory of life structure is a way of conceptualizing answers to a different question: "What is my life like now?" As we begin reflecting on this question, many others come to mind: "What are the most important parts of my life, and how are they interrelated? Where do I invest most of my time and energy? Are there some relationships—to spouse, lover, family, occupation, religion, leisure, or whatever—that I would like to modify, to make more satisfying or meaningful? Are there some things not in my life that I would like to include? Are there interests and relationships, now occupying a minor place, that I would like to make more central?"

In pondering these questions, we begin to identify those aspects of the external world that have the greatest significance for us. We characterize our relationship with each of them and examine the interweaving of the various relationships. We find that our relationships are imperfectly integrated within a single pattern or structure.

The primary components of a life structure are the person's *relationships* with various others in the external world. The other may be a person, a group, an institution or culture, or a particular object or place. A significant relationship involves an investment of self (desires, values, commitment, energy, skill), a reciprocal investment by the other person or entity, and one or more social contexts that contain the relationship, shaping it and becoming part of it. Every relationship shows both stability and change as it evolves over time; and it has different functions in the person's life as the life structure itself changes.

At any given time a life structure may have many and diverse components. Ordinarily, one or two components occupy a central place in the structure—usually marriage–family and occupation. The central components are those that have the greatest significance for the self and the evolving life course. They receive the largest share of one's time and energy, and they strongly influence the character of the other components. The peripheral components are easier to change or detach. They involve less investment of self and can be modified with less effect on the fabric of one's life.

In terms of open systems theory, life structure forms a boundary between personality structure and social structure, and governs the transactions between them. A boundary structure is part of the two adjacent systems it connects, and yet is partially separate or autonomous. It can be understood only if we see it as a link between them. *The life structure mediates the relationship between individual and environment.* It is in part the cause, the vehicle, and the effect of that relationship. A theory of life structure must draw equally upon psychology and the social sciences.

The Evolution of the Life Structure: Developmental Periods in Early and Middle Adulthood

When we used the concept of life structure in analyzing the biographies of our subjects, we found an invariant basic pattern (with infinite manifest variations): *The life structure evolves through a relatively orderly sequence of periods during the adult years.*

The sequence consists of an alternating series of structure-building and structure-changing (transitional) periods. The primary task of a *structure-building* period is to form a life structure and enhance life within it: we must make certain key choices, form a structure around them, and pursue our values and goals within this structure. Even when we succeed in creating a stable structure, life is not necessarily tranquil. The task of making major life choices and building a structure is often stressful, indeed, and may involve many kinds of change. A structure-building period ordinarily lasts five to seven years, 10 years at the most. Then the life structure that has formed the basis for stability comes into question and must be modified.

A *transitional* period terminates the existing life structure and

creates the possibility for a new one. The primary tasks of every
transitional period are to reappraise the existing structure, to explore the possibilities for change in self and world, and to move
toward commitment to the crucial choices that form the basis for
a new life structure in the ensuing period. Transitional periods
ordinarily last about five years. Almost half our adult lives are spent
in developmental transitions. No life structure is permanent—periodic change is a given in the nature of our existence.

As a transition comes to an end, one starts making crucial
choices, giving them meaning and commitment, and building a life
structure around them. The choices are, in a sense, the major products of the transition. When all the efforts of the transition are
done—the struggles to improve work or marriage, to explore alternative possibilities of living, to come more to terms with the
self—choices must be made and bets must be placed. One must
decide, "This I will settle for," and start creating a life structure that
will serve as a vehicle for the next step in the journey.

Within early and middle adulthood the developmental periods
unfold as shown in Figure 1. We have found that each period begins
and ends at a well-defined average age with a variation of ±2 years
around the mean. The finding of age-linked periods in adult life
structure development is surprising. Most evidence suggests that
there are no age-linked periods in *personality* development. In
addition, much research on the adult life course focuses on major
life events, which occur at widely differing ages. The periods in life
structure development provide a framework within which we can
study personality change and development (Campbell, 1971; Erikson, 1950, 1958; Gould, 1978; Kegan, 1982; Kohlberg, 1973; Vaillant,
1977; White, 1972), career and family development, and adaptation
to life events (Lowenthal et al., 1975; Neugarten, 1968).

The first three periods of early adulthood, from roughly age
17 to 33, constitute its *novice phase*. They provide an opportunity
to move beyond adolescence, to build a provisional but necessarily
flawed entry life structure, and to learn the limitations of that structure. The two final periods, from 33 to 45, form the *culminating
phase* in which we bring to fruition the efforts of this era.

A similar sequence exists in middle adulthood. We remain
novices in every era until we have had a chance to try out an entry
life structure and then to question and modify it in the mid-era
transition. Only in the period of the Culminating Life Structure, and
the cross-era transition that follows, do we reach the conclusion of

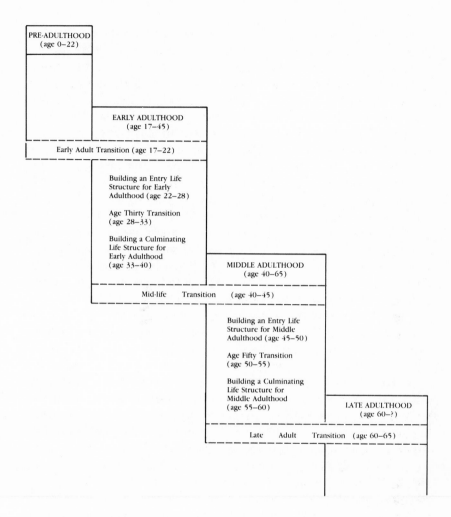

FIGURE 1.   Developmental periods in the eras of early and middle adulthood

that season and begin the shift to the next. During the novice phase we are, to varying degrees, both excited and terrified by the prospects for living in that era. To varying degrees, likewise, we experience the culminating phase as a time of rich satisfactions and of bitter disappointments, discovering as we so often do that the era ultimately gives us much more and much less than we had envisioned.

The Novice Phase of Early Adulthood

My main concern here is with the novice phase of early adulthood. It begins with the start of the Early Adult Transition at about age 17, continues through the period of Building an Entry Life Structure from age 22 to 28, and concludes with the Age Thirty Transition from age 28 to 33. Each of the three developmental periods has its own tasks. Together they form a single phase that serves a crucial developmental function: the process of entry into adulthood.

Clinical problems are often induced by stressful life events such as loss of a loved one, change in social role, geographical moves, problematic personal relationships, economic recession, and discrimination. It is a well established principle in our understanding of childhood and adolescence that *the impact of a stressful life event is mediated by the developmental period in which it occurs*. We know that parental death or divorce will have different meanings for children of different ages, say four or nine or 13. Knowing that a person is in pubescence alerts us to the major developmental issues of this period and leads us to explore the concrete forms they take in this particular person's life.

This developmental principle is equally relevant in adulthood. In dealing with a young adult, it is important to bear in mind that she or he is currently in a specific period within the novice phase. This period creates the opportunity for certain kinds of growth, but it also creates vulnerability to certain kinds of crisis.

The concept of *developmental crisis* provides a useful bridge between normal development and affective disorder. It must be distinguished from a related concept, *adaptive crisis*. The two kinds of crisis may occur simultaneously but they have to be understood and managed differently. An adaptive crisis occurs when a person has great difficulty in finding an even minimally adequate adaptive response to a specific stressful situation.

A developmental crisis can occur in any period, when a person is having great difficulty in meeting the primary developmental tasks of that period. The difficulty may be so great at times that we seem to have no basis for further living. We feel that we can move neither forward nor backward, that we are on the verge of drowning. The integrity of our entire life enterprise is in serious doubt: we experience the imminent danger of chaos, dissolution, the loss of the future. I shall consider the kinds of developmental crisis to which we are most susceptible in each period of the novice phase.

The Early Adult Transition

The Early Adult Transition (age 17 to 22) is a developmental bridge between adolescence and early adulthood. An early adult self is taking shape, containing and to some extent transforming the child and adolescent selves. The boy-man or girl-woman is on the boundary between the childhood world, which was centered in the family of origin, and the early adult world with its new responsibilities, roles, and life choices. We are half-in and half-out of both worlds. We are still very much in adolescence, yet we are also stretching toward the enticing—and forbidding—adult world ahead.

The Early Adult Transition presents three major tasks. One task is to terminate the adolescent life structure and leave the pre-adult world. We have to question the nature of that world and our place in it. We have to modify our pre-adult self and our relationships with important persons and institutions of childhood. Numerous separations and losses are required. A second task is individuation: gaining a stronger sense of one's own identity, values, and goals at that time in the life cycle. Third, it is necessary to make a preliminary step into the adult world: to explore its possibilities, to imagine oneself as a participant in it, to make and test some tentative choices before fully entering it. These three tasks—*termination, individuation, and initiation*—define the essential character of every transitional period in life structure development.

Developmental crises in the Early Adult Transition stem from the particular contradictions, losses, and demands of this place in the life cycle. We are in the full maturity of pre-adulthood, yet barely ready to cross the threshold into early adulthood. The ending of adolescence has both exciting and frightening aspects. We get beyond the heavy constraints of family and school, but lose the protections, supports, and unresponsibilities of childhood. The move into adulthood, too, is a mixed blessing. It offers an abundance of new freedoms, opportunities, and life directions, but the increased independence brings with it the burdens of adult choice and responsibility.

For almost everyone, there are times in this period when the losses and costs of growing up seem much more real than the potential gains. In every transitional period one is suspended, as it were, between past and future. In a cross-era transition, such as this one at around 20 or the Mid-life Transition in the early forties, we are bound to feel some grief over the loss of the outgoing era. We are likely also to have some anxiety about the incoming era— concerns about how much it has to offer and how prepared we are to meet its demands.

Building an Entry Life Structure

The next period I call Building an Entry Life Structure for Early Adulthood (age 22 to 28). Now a young adult has to fashion and test out an initial life structure that provides a viable link between the valued self and the adult society. We must shift the center of gravity of our life from the position of child in the family of origin to the position of novice adult with a new home base that is more truly our own. We have to explore the available possibilities, arrive at a crystallized (though by no means final) definition of ourselves as adults, and build a first adult life structure. For most men, the central components of this structure are usually occupation and family. For most women, work *or* family are central, but not both. We face two major tasks:

1. *Exploration.* We have to discover and generate alternative options for living. The exploratory stance requires us to "hang loose," keeping options open and avoiding strong commitments. Even when we make relatively binding initial choices regarding marriage and occupation, they still have a provisional quality: if they don't work out, change is still possible.
2. *Creating a Stable Structure.* This is a second and contrasting task. A person has to make firm choices, take on adult responsibilities and "make something of my life." The external world expects us to "grow up," get married, enter an occupation, define our goals, and lead a more organized life. The pressures come also from the self: desires for stability and order, roots, membership in the tribe, lasting ties, and fulfillment of core values.

The distinctive character of this developmental period lies in the coexistence of the two tasks of exploration and commitment. Work on one may dominate, but the other is never totally absent. The balance of emphasis on the two tasks varies tremendously.

At one extreme are people who in their early twenties make strong commitments and start building a stable, enduring life structure. They usually make their key choices, especially of spouse and occupation, in the Early Adult Transition and try to maintain great continuity with the pre-adult world. At the other extreme are persons who devote themselves in their twenties primarily to exploration. They go through the entire period on a highly provisional basis with no lasting commitments or goals. They create a structure characterized by flux, superficial ties, and easy movement. They don't invest much of the self in the world or take much of the world into the self.

Most people find a balance of exploration and stable structure. A young adult may opt for stability in one part of life and transiency in another: one person forms a stable marriage but remains occupationally nomadic; another is passionately devoted to an enduring occupational dream while love relationships remain casual or shifting. Still another leads a nomadic life with minimal commitments until perhaps age 25, and only then begins to form a more stable structure. A turning point often occurs at around 25—we "settle down" after an initial transient existence, or we firm up an initial, fragile structure.

Very few of us build our first adult life structure without considerable difficulty and occasional crisis. It is not possible to form an ideally satisfactory life structure the first time around. The tasks of Building an Entry Life Structure are difficult, and we are too young, inexperienced, and torn within ourselves to be able to resolve the contradictions. We do well—as part of normal development—to have only a moderate crisis, to create a fairly satisfactory structure, and to form a basis on which a more adequate structure can be made in the thirties.

The Age Thirty Transition

The Age Thirty Transition, age 28 to 33, is a remarkable gift and burden. It provides an opportunity to work on the flaws of the first adult life structure and to create the basis for the second structure that will be built in the following period.

The main work of fashioning and maintaining an entry life structure is ordinarily done by age 28. The period of Building a Culminating Life Structure for Early Adulthood ordinarily begins at age 33. At that point we must make stronger commitments, form deeper roots and (with whatever mixture of joy, apathy, or resignation) start forming a new life structure that will shape our life until the early forties. The Age Thirty Transition is a bridge between the two life structures. The provisional, exploratory quality of the twenties is ending and we have a sense of greater urgency. Life is becoming more serious, more "for real." One has the feeling: "If I want to change my life—if there are things in it that I don't like, or things missing that I would like to have—this is the time to make a start, for soon it will be too late." The Age Thirty Transition provides a "second chance" to create a more satisfactory life structure within early adulthood.

Some people—clearly a minority—go through the Age Thirty Transition smoothly, without disruption or sense of crisis. They use this period to modify and enrich their lives. An easy transition, without drastic change or turmoil, may occur primarily because one's life is going well and needs only minor adjustments. In some cases, however, the life structure is seriously flawed but one is unable (for various internal and external reasons) to acknowledge the flaws and work at changing them. The illusions and unacknowledged difficulties often surface at a later time, when they exact a heavier cost.

For the great majority—70 to 80 percent of men and women—this transition is a time of moderate to severe crisis. It may take various forms: 1) We may have a relatively stable, organized life, but one that excludes crucially important parts of the self. We question the meaning and value of our work, marriage, and personal relationships. This is a time of increased marital strain, divorce, first marriage, and change in job or occupation. 2) Often, the life structure of the late twenties is relatively incomplete or fragmented. A person may have had a series of jobs and yet have no occupation or clear occupational direction. Although a transient existence was sufficient for a while, the insecurity and rootlessness of this life begin to weigh more heavily. It is more distressing now if we do not have a mate or an occupation or a home base of our own. We become more aware that our life has no center, that it is fragmented into parts we cannot integrate. Or we realize that we have made crucial choices with little commitment and investment of the self. It is time for a change.

While all crises have common features, the character of every crisis is shaped by the period in which it occurs. Thus, a crisis in the Age Thirty Transition is not "merely" a delayed adolescent crisis, though unresolved conflicts of adolescence (and earlier periods) may be reactivated and perhaps more fully resolved in it. Nor is it a "precocious" mid-life crisis, though it has much in common with the transitional problems of persons who, at about 40, feel caught in a life structure that has become intolerable. It is, first of all, a crisis in rebuilding the entry life structure and doing the developmental work of the Age Thirty Transition. In addition, we may use it to work on unresolved conflicts and impairments of earlier periods in adulthood and childhood.

Conclusion

To get a developmental perspective, it is instructive to compare a person's life in the late teens and the early thirties. (For another view, similar in many respects yet different in conceptual focus, see White's (1972) germinal work.) The contrast is remarkable. As the Early Adult Transition begins, our life is still strongly rooted in the family of origin and the pre-adult world; the process of separation is just getting underway. We have a Dream, inchoate or differentiated, and diverse hopes, fears, fantasies, and plans for the future.

Fifteen years later, at the end of the Age Thirty Transition, adolescence seems part of the distant past, far removed from the current world. Changing times have brought change in the fabric of our life. Often, we live in a new geographical locale and a new sociocultural world. By this time one almost certainly has a spouse and family—perhaps has even been divorced and remarried. Our sense of what it means to be a husband or wife and parent has altered dramatically. So too has the meaning of being a son or daughter: One or both parents may have died or, if they are alive, we are becoming a parent to them or losing contact with them. In any case, we are modifying our relationships with them—the parents in our heads and those outside. The character of our occupational life is taking a new shape. The occupation is often different in crucial ways from our earlier expectations. Even if our present occupation is the one we had hoped for, we see in it possibilities and limitations we did not imagine in the Early Adult Transition.

As the Age Thirty Transition ends, we move toward major new choices or recommit ourselves to past choices. A great deal hinges on the choices made at age 32, 33, 34, which provide the groundwork for the culminating life structure. If we choose poorly, the new structure will be badly flawed. Life in the late thirties will become more painful and our attempts to create a better structure will be more difficult and costly. If we choose well—from the viewpoint of our dreams, values, talent, possibilities—we create the foundation for a more satisfactory life structure through which we can work toward the realization of our youthful dreams. Where can we gain what is needed to choose more wisely?

References

Campbell J (Ed.): The Portable Jung. New York, Viking, 1971

Erikson EH: Childhood and Society. New York, Norton, 1950

Erikson EH: Young Man Luther. New York, Norton, 1958

Gould RL: Transformations: Growth and Change in Adult Life. New York, Simon & Schuster, 1978

Kegan R: The Evolving Self. Cambridge, Harvard University Press, 1982

Kohlberg L: Continuities in childhood and adult moral development revisited, in Life Span Developmental Psychology: Personality and Socialization. Edited by Baltes PB, Schaie KW. New York, Academic Press, 1973

Levinson DJ: Toward a conception of the adult life course, in Themes of Love and Work in Adulthood. Edited by Smelser N, Erikson EH. Cambridge, Harvard University Press, 1980

Levinson DJ: Explorations in Biography, in Further Explorations in Personality. Edited by Rabin AI, Aronoff J, Barclay AM, et al. New York, Wiley, 1981

Levinson DJ: The Season's of a Woman's Life. New York, Knopf, in press

Levinson DJ, Gooden WE: The life cycle, in Comprehensive Textbook of Psychiatry, 4th edition. Edited by Kaplan HI, Sadock BJ. Baltimore, Williams and Wilkins, 1985

Levinson DJ with Darrow CN, Klein EB, et al. The Seasons of a Man's Life. New York, Knopf, 1978

Lowenthal MF, Thurnher M, Chiriboga D: Four Stages of Life: A Comparative Study of Women and Men Facing Transitions. San Francisco, Jossey-Bass, 1975

Neugarten BL: Adult personality: toward a psychology of the life cycle, in Middle Age and Aging: Reader in Social Psychology. Edited by Neugarten BL. Chicago, University of Chicago Press, 1968

Vaillant G: Adaptation to Life. Boston, Little, Brown, 1977

White RW: The Enterprise of Living. New York, Holt, Rinehart and Winston, 1972

Chapter 2

EMOTIONAL AND PERSONALITY DEVELOPMENT IN NORMAL ADOLESCENTS AND YOUNG ADULTS

Anne C. Petersen, Ph.D.
W. Edward Craighead, Ph.D.

Chapter 2

EMOTIONAL AND PERSONALITY DEVELOPMENT IN NORMAL ADOLESCENTS AND YOUNG ADULTS

Although development is sometimes thought of as a maturational process of unfolding potential (as in the view of Gesell et al., 1956), most current theorists discuss development as proceeding in interaction with, or as involving a *transaction* with, the social-cultural environment (Sameroff, 1975). An examination of emotional and personality development in adolescence and young adulthood clearly requires consideration of the social context. Important social contexts at this age include the culture, the society, the family, and other social groups, such as peers.

Jessie Bernard, speaking recently about the societal support for families and the care of young children, concluded that the current ambience is a largely negative one (Bernard, 1982). High unemployment, high divorce rates, and the related increase in the number of women in the work force all contribute to the problems of families and developing young people. The lack of support for rearing and educating children is pernicious. Adults who dare to choose to become parents today are expected to raise their families without support from society.

These negative messages about families and children have a double impact upon developing adolescents and young adults. First, as children, they experience the burden of being undervalued and, in some cases, neglected by the society. Second, as emerging adults, they face a rather bleak future. The major social tasks of young adulthood include work and family. With high unemployment and intense competition for available jobs, many young people (particularly if they are black or undereducated) may despair of being able to find any work, much less meaningful employment. With family roles just as difficult, the task of adulthood is likely to be postponed, or engaged in with ambivalence. Since it is believed that identity is developed at least in part through such social roles (Erikson, 1968), the development of identity and personality is likely to be stunted if these social roles cannot be mastered.

With tasks of adulthood becoming more difficult, many young people are working harder. The result, for young people as for the rest of society (Bernard, 1982), is a lack of pleasure in life. This is likely to lead to loneliness and isolation, and both probably contribute to increased depression and suicide.

Depression and suicide among adolescents and young adults are indeed worthy of attention by researchers. The statistics show that suicide has increased 150 percent among youth 15 to 24 years of age over the past 20 years (see Chapter 11 in this volume). It is somewhat ironic that although research evidence (Offer and Offer, 1975) has now refuted earlier theories that adolescence necessarily involved extreme psychological difficulty for all youth, the suicide statistics suggest that in our society we have created an increasingly difficult environment for young people as they pass from childhood to young adulthood.

The earlier theories of normative adolescent turmoil suggested that minimal intervention should occur with adolescents, since it was believed that most young people would "grow out of" their difficulties (Blos, 1962; Freud, 1958; Hall, 1904). The evidence that this is not the case (Rutter et al., 1976; Weiner and Del Gaudio, 1976) has led to revisions in our views about intervention. These results suggest that some kind of intervention ought to take place as soon as problems are identified.

At the same time that we have learned that not all youth experience a tumultuous adolescence (Douvan and Adelson, 1966; Offer and Offer, 1975), and that most of those who do experience extreme difficulty during adolescence fail to "grow out of it" but continue to manifest or develop some sort of disorder, we have also seen evidence of increasing difficulties among youth. Statistics on suicide, accidents, drug abuse, and other problem behavior suggest that adolescents are more prone now than in the past to engage in life-threatening behavior (Green and Horton, 1982). The increased complexity of our society, with the resulting demands upon the adolescents who must learn to live in that society as responsible adults, surely plays a major role in the increased incidence of these various problems (Petersen, 1982; Petersen and Spiga, 1982). Since it is unlikely that we can transform our society into a simpler one, the task is to find ways to help adolescents and their parents to cope more effectively with the demands placed on them. Although these problems are complex and difficult to address, there do seem to be some ways of minimizing difficulties for youth and helping them to live healthier, happier lives.

Theoretical and Methodological Considerations

Before reviewing the state of current knowledge of emotional and personality development in adolescence and young adulthood, we wish to articulate the theoretical and methodological perspectives that have shaped our organization of the issues. We are integrating the developmental and clinical perspectives in considering "normal" development. It is our belief that emotions and personality span a continuum that in the extreme is related to disorder. The theoretical perspectives of clinical and developmental studies have come to be quite distinct, but we feel that this is due, in large part, to their samples rather than to their original conceptions of development or etiology. Developmental studies have generally used nonclinical samples, while clinical studies (that is, studies of mental illness) have generally used patient samples. The views of human development based on these differing samples have led to greater differentiation between health and illness than really exists. Epidemiological studies have begun to bridge this gap and to provide evidence, in general, for the continuity of the various phenomena of interest.

Other kinds of continua are relevant as well. One's status along any continuum is not constant over time. Each person shows variation in moods, for example, from hour to hour, day to day, or week to week. There also appear to be some systematic variations over the life span. For example, one study has found that adolescents do appear to experience more mood fluctuations than do adults (Larson et al., 1980).

In addition to these variations in each phenomenon within the individual, there is also variation in the combinations of emotions that are experienced. Every person experiences some negative emotions at some time. One factor differentiating mentally ill from healthy individuals may be the balance of negative and positive feelings, particularly with a disorder such as depression. Even aspects of schizophrenia, such as thought disorder, are experienced by "normal" individuals at certain times (Harrow and Quinlan, 1977).

What we are leading up to is a conception of normative rather than normal in considering development. Normative development, using statistical concepts of normal distributions, can accommodate shifting means over the life span (and shorter periods of time), and can usefully integrate multiple constructs and measures. In this way, we have more objective information about what is typical or atypical. All too often, developmental researchers assume that everything they observe is normal, while clinical researchers often assume that anything observed in patients is abnormal. A conception integrating these perspectives would seem to be crucial for preventive objectives, since there must be ways of identifying mental health status *before* illness, death, or patienthood are achieved.

Relevant Constructs

More difficult to identify are which phenomena are of greatest importance to understanding outcomes such as suicide. We will focus here on psychological phenomena, although we assume that biological, social, and cognitive factors are also crucial. Indeed, any psychological phenomenon involves these other aspects of human functioning. For example, any feeling must be transmitted by biochemical substances, often stimulated by social interactions, and usually accompanied by cognitions. Petersen (1980) has previously articulated the importance of considering *biopsychosocial* development for understanding adolescence. We will return to some of these issues later in this chapter.

Our consideration of psychological constructs is influenced largely by what researchers have studied. Although we find this unsatisfactory both theoretically and methodologically, it does provide a beginning for articulating improved models for understanding psychological development at adolescence. We shall consider constructs that presume a structural developmental sequence (for example, ego development, moral development, and identity development) as well as those that are less developmentally based, such as self-esteem. The structural types of constructs come closest to measuring personality; less structural are emotion, mood, and the like.

Unfortunately, relatively little research has focused on psychological development, as it is broadly construed. Indeed, most studies have measured only single constructs, though perhaps with multiple measures. Research integrating several perspectives is more unusual, although such integrations are represented in this volume (see Chapter 7 in this volume).

The Nature of Samples

We shall focus on the age period roughly beginning with puberty and ending when young people take on adult work and family roles. Although some of us have called this period *adolescence*, it often extends into the early twenties, a phase of life typically considered young adulthood. College students, the group most often studied, are considered by some investigators as late adolescents and by others as young adults.

Our goal of making developmental inferences from the existing research is somewhat hampered by the fact that most of the clinical research and even some of the developmental research has focused on subjects who happen to be adolescents or young adults, rather than on adolescence as a period of development. Because of the availability to researchers of college student samples, we have a great deal of information on youth of this age. Whether they are representative of late adolescents or young adults is not known. With younger age groups, we have various kinds of samples. Studies of normative samples of middle adolescents have overwhelmingly focused only on white boys. Studies of early adolescents, only recently undertaken, are more generally representative of the population of young people of that age. Clinical studies have covered the age spectrum, although not in a systematic developmental way.

The fact that so much developmental research has used only male subjects presents a major problem for drawing inferences. This sampling bias is confounded by the theoretical perspectives of male researchers. What we have, at present, is a psychology of male development. Therefore, the inferences that we can draw at this point are possibly limited to only half of human development, less if there are class and ethnic group differences as well. To date, these variations are largely uninvestigated, although many are attempting to redress bias in sampling, methods, and theories.

A similar bias may exist with clinical studies. Inferences are largely based upon patient groups, and therefore cannot be extended to people in general, and perhaps not even to all people with the problems being studied. A typical bias has been the over-reporting in the literature of wealthier private patients.

Personality and Emotional Development

Many major changes in development occur during adolescence and young adulthood (Conger and Petersen, 1984). Adolescence is usually thought to begin with a major biological change: puberty (Petersen and Taylor, 1980). This process, taking an average of at least four years for the visible physical changes, has major implications for psychological development. Cognitive development, particularly the capacity for abstract reasoning, is first seen in some individuals during puberty (Elkind, 1974). This change also has major implications for psychological development. Although we discuss these influences in greater detail later in this chapter, they are so important that they deserve mention as background information here.

Personality Development

As we have already indicated, we will describe the state of knowledge in those areas in which there is a substantial body of research. Two such areas involve structural theories of progressive development to maturity: *moral development* and *ego development*. *Identity development* is considered to be *the* developmental task of adolescence but is more outcome- than process-oriented. *Self-image or self-esteem* is thought to be an essential component of human functioning, although there are no particular theories about its development. *Social development*, although not typically considered psychological, is important for personality development, and will also be discussed briefly.

Moral development.   Piaget (1932) first articulated the theory that children gradually develop a sense of right and wrong. His original conceptions were further developed by Kohlberg (1964, 1976), who elaborated the theory and devised a method for assessing moral development. Further refinements of these methods have occurred subsequently (Rest, 1979).

Kohlberg's elaboration of Piaget's theory involves six stages of moral development ordered into three levels: preconventional, conventional, and postconventional. Preconventional stages, characteristic of young children, involve recognition of societal norms of good and bad, but primarily in terms of personal outcomes, such as punishment. Conventional morality is typically seen in middle childhood and begins to incorporate ideas of mutuality, rules, and a social order. Postconventional stages, first seen in adolescence, involve understanding of individual responsibility, the responsibility of the larger society, and the relation between the two.

The large body of research on moral development, including recent longitudinal data, reveals that there are generally gradual but progressive changes that occur in the development of moral reasoning. Appropriate levels of cognitive development appear to be necessary but not sufficient for corresponding stages of moral development. Young adolescents are typically at the first stage of the conventional level, while older adolescents and young adults generally function at the first stage of the postconventional level.

Moral development is linked to social class, urbanization, and gender, with higher levels seen among youth of higher socioeconomic status, urban residents, and boys. These results have caused some concern that the theory is biased and does not represent a universal characterization of moral development (Haan, 1978). Gilligan (1977) has proposed an alternative model of moral development, which integrates interpersonal moral issues, and is more appropriate for females.

Research has revealed the distinction between moral reasoning—a more cognitive construct—and moral behavior (see Conger and Petersen, 1984). Both concepts are quite complex and are not identical theoretically or empirically. In general, behavior often appears to function at a lower level than reasoning. Gilligan's research (Gilligan and Belenky, 1980) reveals that emotional issues often interfere with the individual's ability to utilize full reasoning capacity. On the other hand, situations demanding decisions related to moral behavior can often stimulate advances in moral reasoning (Murphy and Gilligan, 1980).

Some research has also linked moral behavior to feelings and interpersonal motivation. Hoffman (1980), in particular, has linked empathy and guilt to moral development. His perspective is less structural but, rather, integrates various developmental changes with socialization experiences in adolescence.

Ego Development. Loevinger (1976) has developed a theory
of maturation of ego functioning as well as a method of assessing
it. Her conceptualization relies heavily on interpersonal functioning
as a key aspect of experience that affects the ego and involves several
successive stages: impulsive, self-protective, conformist, self-aware
(a transitional stage), conscientious, autonomous, and integrated
(theoretical only). There has recently been a great deal of work on
this construct, and its validity has been established to a substantial
extent (Loevinger, 1979).

Research, both cross-sectional and longitudinal, reveals gradual
but progressive development over the stages (Loevinger, 1979; Redmore and Loevinger, 1979). The modal level for young people as
they enter adolescence is typically self-protective, while older adolescents and young adults typically function at the self-aware level,
marking the transition from the conformist to conscientious stages.

This construct has been criticized for its heavy reliance on
verbal skills, but research shows that there is developmental change
even when IQ is controlled (Loevinger, 1979). As might be expected,
because of the focus on interpersonal skills, girls typically score
higher than boys.

Identity Development. Erikson (1968) argued that *the* developmental task of adolescence is the achievement of identity.
Adolescents need to establish identities as preparation for the various adult roles. Research on identity has been advanced by the
work of Marcia (1966, 1980), who articulated identity statuses based
on the extent of crisis and commitment in the search for identity.
Evidence of some crisis as well as current commitment to an identity
are required for the status of *identity achievement*. The lack of a
crisis leads to a prematurely *foreclosed identity*. Adolescents without
a commitment to an identity, whether or not they have experienced
identity crisis, are said to have a *diffused identity*. Those in active
crisis and with vague commitment to an identity are said to be in
moratorium.

Marcia also developed an interview method for assessing identity status in relevant areas, including occupation and ideology. Although questions remain to be addressed, there is now a substantial
body of work on identity status, primarily using college students as
subjects. This research (Marcia, 1980) has revealed that identity
status is related to anxiety (moratoriums highest and foreclosures
lowest), self-esteem (achievements and moratoriums highest), au-

thoritarianism (foreclosures highest), moral development (achievements and moratoriums at postconventional levels, with foreclosures and diffusions at preconventional and conventional levels), and autonomy (foreclosures and diffusions lowest). Longitudinal research reveals the relative instability of identity statuses, although the general trend is in the direction of identity achievement (Marcia, 1980; Meilman, 1979).

Again there appears to be gender bias in the areas selected as relevant, leading to fewer achieved identities in areas of occupation and ideology for girls. When identity is assessed in terms of premarital sexuality, however, girls appear to be more advanced than boys. Marcia (1980) concludes his review of this work with a plea for research using female subjects and examining identity development in terms of interpersonal issues.

Self-image. Several constructs focusing on the view of the self have been investigated. In general, self-esteem refers to a general positive (or negative) evaluation of self, whereas self-image and self-concept often refer to specific aspects of self-view, such as the academic self, or the social self. Another construct, self-understanding, has just been articulated; this construct has been integrated with cognitive development (Damon and Hart, 1982).

Although popular conceptions of adolescence as a time of great turmoil would suggest generally negative self-views, the bulk of the empirical work suggests that self-esteem gradually increases over the adolescent and young adult years (Bachman and O'Malley, 1977; McCarthy and Hoge, 1982; O'Malley and Bachman, 1983; Wylie, 1979). Studies that identify specific aspects of self-image find increasing focus on interpersonal relationships and self-understanding as central aspects of self-image (Damon and Hart, 1982; Rosenberg, 1979). One important longitudinal study (Dusek and Flaherty, 1981), however, found that the basic structure of self-concept did not change over adolescence.

There has been some research showing a decline in self-esteem in early adolescence (Simmons et al., 1973), particularly among girls who are experiencing a number of changes simultaneously (Simmons et al., 1979). Although there is evidence that change can be stressful, and particularly that too many changes can overwhelm some young adolescents, other research has not replicated the specific result of a general decline in self-esteem during early adolescence (Demo and Savin-Williams, 1983; Petersen, 1981).

Social Development. Although the study of social development per se has focused primarily on younger children, social relationships are clearly important to adolescents and young adults. It is rather ironic, in fact, that there has been so little work, especially in the past decade or two, on social development given its significance at this age. The primary measure of social development in adolescence is the sociometric peer nomination technique, a measure of popularity. As a young adolescent interviewee taught one of us, however, peer relationships involve more than popularity. Intimacy, reciprocity, and social support are key aspects to relationships. Yet we know almost nothing about these constructs with adolescents, and only somewhat more with young adults.

Despite the paucity of research on interpersonal aspects of adolescent relationships, we do have some information about social functioning at adolescence. Conformity to the peer group peaks in early adolescence (11 to 13 years) (Costanzo and Shaw, 1966). Anxiety about friendship seems to peak in middle adolescence, around ages 15 to 16 (Coleman, 1980). Once again, there are important gender differences, with girls showing more conformity in early adolescence and more anxiety about friends in middle adolescence.

Summary. Current research reveals that there are gradual increases along various dimensions of personality development over adolescence and young adulthood. Young people increase in moral and ego development, begin to establish a stable identity, and increase in self-esteem. This picture of youth stands in distinct contrast to that of the troubled adolescent so prevalent in past years.

Emotional Development

The study of emotion has been inadequately addressed in the investigation of both normal and abnormal development in adolescence. Rather, developmental psychology has focused on cognition, and to a lesser degree social development, primarily in younger children. This "left-hemisphere" view of adolescence has resulted from the prominence of cognitive theories of development. Although there have been recent attempts to integrate cognition with other aspects of development (Flavell and Ross, 1981; Petersen and Taylor, 1980), there have been no similar efforts to link emotion with other aspects of adolescent development. Indeed, extant data and theory regarding emotional development are currently inadequate to warrant such an effort. Except for the study of emotions in infants (Emde, 1979), there is no systematic body of literature on emotional development. Further evidence for the insufficiency of research in this area is apparent from the absence of material on this topic in most of the standard volumes on adolescent development (Adelson, 1980). Clearly, additional theoretical and empirical advances regarding normal emotional development are essential, a point eloquently made by Yarrow (1979).

Clinical psychologists and psychiatrists, in contrast to researchers in these fields, have been more concerned with emotional development in adolescents. The salience of emotional functioning and dysfunctioning cannot escape the attention of one treating adolescent problems. The most extensive discussion of emotional development has been presented by psychodynamically oriented theory, within which "emotions, intensely felt at adolescence, have been somewhat neglected as an object of study.... There has been less attention given to a particularized understanding of the effects, to their sources, their effects, their vicissitudes, the defenses against them, the strategies the social order develops for controlling and channeling them" (Adelson and Doehrman, 1980, p. 103). Since there have been no studies (to our knowledge) on normative development of such emotions as love, anger, joy, and the like, we will focus on the empirical work investigating the epidemiology and psychopathology of the most prevalent adolescent mental-health disorders.

General psychopathology. Since we assume that psychological disorders involve the extreme ends of the emotions continuum, it is important to consider the research on psychopathology for what it reveals about normal development. Information regarding psychopathology in adolescents comes primarily from epidemiological studies and reports of prevalence in clinical settings. These data are limited because epidemiological studies have employed classification criteria which differ from clinical classification criteria; prevalence data from clinical settings, on the other hand, fail to provide information regarding individuals who experience the disorder but do not seek treatment. Clinical data are also biased by the tendency to underdiagnose adolescent problems, and especially by the overuse of the *adjustment* (previously situational) *disorders category*, which presumably has less serious subsequent implications for the adolescent than would an alternative diagnosis.

The findings of Weiner and Del Gaudio (1976) indicate the fallacy of this practice and the potential conceptual confusion generated by it. In their study, adolescents diagnosed as having a situational disorder were just about as likely to have serious psychopathology and seek treatment in young adulthood as were the adolescents diagnosed as neurotic or as having a personality disorder.

Epidemiological studies have provided a number of interesting psychopathology findings, which clinical studies tend to corroborate. Although rates vary considerably from study to study, it appears from the data that somewhere between 10 and 20 percent of adolescents experience severe enough psychopathology to warrant clinical intervention (Graham, 1979). The 1978 President's Commission on Mental Health estimated that 15 percent of U.S. school-aged children need clinical intervention for psychiatric or psychological disorders. The prevalence of disorders varies with a number of factors; for example, it is higher in urban settings (Rutter et al., 1975), higher for disrupted families (Rutter et al., 1976), higher among families in which there is a member with a positive diagnosis of psychiatric or psychological disorder (Hetherington and Martin, 1979), and differs by gender (American Psychiatric Association, 1980; Leslie, 1974). These and other factors, however, combine in different ways in the various adolescent disorders. Therefore, in order to understand their interrelationships and implications for emotional development, they are best considered within the context of specific problem areas. Anxiety, depression, and conduct disorders, as well as the related phenomenon of suicide, appear to be those most clearly associated with emotional dysfunction at this age.

Anxiety. In epidemiological and clinical prevalence studies, anxiety, depression, and conduct disorders are the most frequently occurring problems of adolescents. It is important, but difficult, to distinguish between anxiety and depression. One screening self-report study of late adolescents in our laboratory (unpublished data) found higher correlations between measures of depression and anxiety than those obtained *among* standard depression measures. Although this finding reveals measurement problems, it also points to the overlap of anxiety and depression. Undoubtedly, the disorders are experienced simultaneously by some people and separately by others. It is important to identify what produces this situation, and what its preventive and treatment implications are.

Anxiety is a label for a complex pattern of responses characterized by apprehension and fear. It has been used to refer to an emotional state or trait, to behaviors such as avoidance or failure to perform, to physiological arousal, and to cognitive evaluations. There is no way to determine which response produced a rating of anxiety in the studies to be reviewed in this chapter, but, in general, the studies have produced a consistent set of findings relevant to emotional responding.

Anxiety reactions are more common and take a different form in adolescence than in middle childhood, and their frequency appears to increase in the period between the onset of puberty and young adulthood (Chapman, 1974; Senn and Solnit, 1968). The focus of anxiety in middle childhood tends to be attached to a specific object, such as fear of animals or objects. These types of anxiety are replaced toward mid-adolescence to young adulthood by social situational and more abstract phobias, and the onset of agoraphobia (Marks, 1969; Marks and Gelder, 1966). This change in focus of anxiety across age parallels a change in prevalence in boys and girls. During mid-adolescence, anxiety begins to be reported and observed more frequently in females; in late adolescence and young adulthood, a 2:1 female–male ratio on self-report measures appears.

In early reports of follow-up studies of treated clinical populations, more than 50 percent of those children and adolescents labeled "neurotic" (that is, anxious and depressed) improve as they get older, particularly if they are female (Annesley, 1961; Cunningham et al., 1956; Masterson, 1967; Warren, 1965). These subjects fare better than those with other classifications at follow-up. A frequent conclusion has been that anxiety and depression are transitory phenomena, or are a function of adolescent turmoil, a position which no longer appears tenable (Offer et al., 1981). As has been noted, the focus of anxiety changes over time, so it is not surprising that the relationship between anxiety in middle childhood and in adolescence might be low. The focus of anxiety in mid- to late adolescence is social and abstract in nature, which is more like the focus of anxiety in adulthood. Indeed, in one report in which anxiety was studied in late adolescence and early adulthood, the same people tended to be anxious at both times (Gersten et al., 1976). Pritchard and Graham (1966) also found that patients who had been anxious and depressed, and reported specific somatic complaints when younger, were more likely to be diagnosed as anxious or depressed (though not manic-depressed) as adults. These data suggest: a) that a subset of anxious adolescents remains anxious as adults (perhaps the subset which exhibits those symptoms indicative of anxiety at *both* age levels); and b) that even though not all anxious or depressed adolescents become anxious or depressed adults, many anxious or depressed adults were anxious or depressed as adolescents. The data do not support the presumption that *adolescent* anxiety is a self-curative phenomenon, but rather that it is a debilitative problem in need of prevention and/or treatment, and that it is predictive of adult anxiety, especially when the focus of the anxiety is similar to the focus of anxiety in adulthood.

Depression. Although there has been much debate about the existence of depression in childhood and early adolescence, there is little question as to its prominence among clinical disorders in late adolescence. There has been a virtual explosion of research on depression with this latter age group, for which the rate of severe depression is three to five percent, and the rate for moderate depression is 12 to 15 percent. Historically, depression has been labeled as an affective or mood disorder, but recent research has shown that its cognitive, physiological, and behavioral characteristics are just as important (Craighead et al., 1984).

The recent surge of interest and increase in research on childhood and adolescent depression suggest that either depression is beginning at earlier ages than in the past, or that previous estimates of its occurrence were inaccurately low. It is also likely that the sociology of clinical behavior has been such that depression is now expected to occur more often, clinicians have become more sensitive to its occurrence, and its diagnosis is more professionally acceptable (if not, indeed, reinforced!). This burst of professional enthusiasm has only recently begun to produce significant advances in the assessment of depression in children and adolescents (Kazdin, 1981; Kazdin and Petti, 1982); there has been little progress toward its successful treatment or prevention.

Although marked by methodological difficulties, epidemiological and clinical prevalence research offer some clues regarding depression and its development. For example, the Isle of Wight Study reported a prevalence of clinical depression (with stringent criteria) at only .015 percent when the sample was 10 to 11 years old, but 1.5 percent by age 14 (Graham and Rutter, 1973; Rutter et al., 1976). In this study it was also reported that only one in nine 10-year-olds reported moodiness, misery, depression, or feelings of self-depreciation, but that nearly one-half of the 14- to 15-year-old adolescents reported these feelings. Although the rates for mild to moderate depression are slightly lower (about 25 to 30 percent), fairly similar data have been obtained for "normal" seventh and eighth grade children in both our laboratories. Kandel and Davies (1982) also reported that 19.7 percent of their sample of 14- to 18-year-old subjects in an epidemiological study felt sad or depressed during the preceding year.

It is generally accepted that depression occurs two to three times more often in females than in males. This gender difference appears not to emerge until mid-adolescence (Kandel and Davies, 1982). Depression appears to stabilize in girls a year earlier (seventh grade) than it does in boys; girls tend to develop a depressive attributional style a year earlier (seventh grade) than boys, and that relationship remains stronger for older age levels (Craighead et al., 1981). Item analyses of the Children's Depression Inventory revealed that girls (grades three to nine) tended to endorse *internal* types of items and boys endorsed more *external* types of items (Smucker et al., in press).

It has been suggested (Conger and Petersen, 1984) that females are more likely to manifest depression and related difficulties than are males because of the stresses inherent in the female sex role. If this is true, it makes sense that gender differences in depression would first emerge in mid- to late adolescence, because of the "gender intensification" (Hill and Lynch, 1983)—the narrowing and intensification of sex roles—that tends to occur during early adolescence. Recent findings indicated that both boys and girls who endorsed traditional "feminine" characteristics also reported higher depression and lower self-esteem than those early adolescents who endorsed traditional masculine or androgynous characteristics (Green, 1980). This suggests that in the future, as sex roles shift toward greater flexibility and diversity for females, there may be a decline in the relatively greater incidence of depression among girls and women. Dweck's work in the development of gender-related attributional style is also germane to this point (Dweck, 1977; Dweck and Goetz, 1977). She and her colleagues found that the attributional style characteristic of girls corresponds in many ways to the depressive attributional style outlined in the reformulated learned-helplessness model of depression (Abramson et al., 1978); this is also the attributional style descriptive of adolescent depressives (Craighead et al., 1981). Dweck found that her gender-specific attributional style is related to gender-specific environmental feedback: girls learn that they are responsible for their failures, whereas boys are typically told that they could do better if they would just try harder. Interestingly, subsequent research has shown that these feedback patterns will *produce* the related attributional style regardless of gender. The social, developmental, treatment, and preventive implications of this research are enormous (Craighead et al., 1978).

Suicide. Although suicide is upsetting to survivors, it is especially so with a young person, who generally is healthy and has most of a lifetime ahead. Although cause–effect conclusions are unwarranted from current empirical data, depression is commonly thought to be a major cause of suicide (Weissman, 1974). The most predominant characteristic of suicide in one retrospective study was severe or psychotic depression (Flood and Seager, 1968). There is an unusually high incidence of family conflict and disruption, school and social problems, and suicide among relatives and friends of suicidal individuals (Corder et al., 1974; Toolan, 1962; Weissman, 1974).

Suicide is extremely rare in young children and occurs at a very low rate for young adolescents. However, beginning with age 15 and extending through young adulthood, the rate of suicide increases dramatically. Suicide is among the top 10 causes of death for all age groups in the U.S., and among the top three causes of death among adolescents. From the mid-1950s until the late 1970s, suicide rates among the 15- to 24-year-old group increased well over 200 percent, with the rates for males increasing at least 25 percent more than for females (Frederick, 1985).

A peak for completed suicides was reached in the young adult age group (15 to 24) in 1977 at 13.3 per 100,000 completed suicides, and the rate decreased slightly to 12.1 per 100,000 in 1982 (see Table 1). This decrease, however, is due to a decrease in the 20- to 24-year-old age range as the rate of completed suicides has remained stable in the 15- to 19-year-old range; in the 15- to 19-year-old age range, the 1982 rate of 8.7/100,000 is still equal to the 1977 rate of 8.7 per 100,000. For 15- to 19-year-olds, the rate has remained relatively stable for young women, but has increased slightly for young white males, who are at the greatest risk for suicide completion. It is also alarming that the rate for completed suicides among the 10- to 14-year-old age group has shown a recent increase from 0.8 per 100,000 to 1.1 per 100,000. The gender difference in

Table 1. Suicide Rates per 100,000 Population for 1977 to 1982[1]

	Overall	White Males	All Other Males	White Females	All Other Females
			Ages 15–19		
1977	8.7	15.1	6.0	3.5	2.4
1978	7.9	13.6	5.5	3.3	1.3
1979	8.4	14.3	6.7	3.4	2.1
1980	8.5	15.0	5.6	3.3	1.6
1981	8.7	14.9	5.5	3.8	1.6
1982	8.7	15.5	6.2	3.4	1.5
			Ages 20–24		
1977	18.2	30.2	21.6	7.4	5.3
1978	16.5	27.4	21.9	6.6	4.1
1979	16.4	26.8	22.5	6.5	4.6
1980	16.1	27.8	20.0	5.9	3.1
1981	15.6	26.8	17.1	5.9	3.2
1982	15.1	26.4	16.0	5.4	2.9
			Ages 15–25		
1977	13.3	22.4	13.0	5.4	3.7
1978	12.1	20.4	13.0	4.9	2.7
1979	12.4	20.5	14.0	4.9	3.3
1980	12.3	21.4	12.3	4.6	2.3
1981	12.3	21.1	11.1	4.9	2.4
1982	12.1	21.2	11.0	4.5	2.2

[1]Unless otherwise indicated, the statistics for suicide information were supplied by the National Center for Health Statistics, Washington, D.C.

the increase is even more dramatic in this age group, with the rate for female completers being stable, and the rate for male completers increasing from 1.1/100,000 in 1979 to 1.7/100,000 in 1982. Male adolescents outnumber females in completed suicides about three or four to one, but the rate for suicide attempts is just about reversed and higher for young women (Frederick, 1985), which mirrors the attempts rate for the population in general (Weissman, 1974). These suicide rate data are probably conservative because it is likely that suicides are underreported, especially in adolescents, and often disguised as accidents (Conger and Petersen, 1984). If the figures are accurate, they present a serious problem; if they are underestimates, then the problem is even more serious and extensive than it is believed to be.

A number of hypotheses have been set forth to explain the increase in suicide among adolescents. Common explanations are that the increased rate is a result of increased substance abuse and increased violence in the larger society. These variables appear to interact with psychological dysfunction to produce suicide.

Undoubtedly these factors, with their multiplicity of causes, have contributed to the increased suicide rate. There is also a psychological factor, *related to emotional development*, which warrants greater consideration in both the increasing rate of suicide in adolescents and the decreasing age at which suicide is likely to occur. Research has indicated that *hopelessness* is a major factor in suicide (Beck et al., 1975). This raises the intriguing possibility that mid-adolescence is the time at which the responsibilities of adulthood in our current society confront that adolescent who has just acquired an adult body, mind, and feelings, but has inadequate skills to cope with this critical transition; this may lead to a sense of hopelessness. Furthermore, the age level at which this transition occurs may be decreasing. Data to support this phenomenon would have significant treatment and prevention implications. (A similar unique transition may occur for individuals who have recently retired). Inadequate coping with this transition would be associated with the increase in suicide in older men. If this is true, there may emerge an increase in suicide in 60 to 70-year-old women in the decades ahead.

Conduct Disorders. Although not usually considered an "emotional disorder," several findings regarding conduct disorders will be noted because of their relevance to the general issues addressed here. Conduct disorders are diagnosed about three times more often in males than in females. It is not uncommon for the disorder to be reported in early elementary school years. The diagnosis is consistent across age: early conduct disorder is predictive of delinquency and adult antisocial personality and imprisonment. This consistency is no doubt due, in part, to the existence of comparable age-appropriate forms of the disorder over the course of development. In early years, conduct disorder takes the form of aggression toward peers, stealing in the home, and disobedience in the classroom; in later adolescence, the inappropriate behaviors are directed toward destruction and stealing of others' property and truancy (Kennedy, 1984; Robins, 1979). Although conduct disorders have been viewed as distinct from neurotic disorders, recent data suggest an overlap of subsamples of the disorders. For example, Chiles and colleagues (1980) reported that 23 percent of a group of delinquents met the criteria for a major depressive episode. These adolescents may well be those whom Quay (1964, 1966) has called "disturbed–neurotic" delinquents. Given the higher rate of completed suicides among males, the gender differences in conduct disorders and depression, and the strong relationship between depression and suicide, this raises the intriguing possibility that an inordinate number of suicide completers would have correctly been diagnosed as conduct disorder–depressed (Schaffer, 1982). These individuals, particularly the males, would possess both the aggressive behavioral pattern and the emotional state likely to produce suicide.

Relationship Between Emotional and Personality Development

The unfortunate paucity of information regarding emotional development in adolescence forces one largely to speculate about the interrelationship between emotional and personality development at this time. The psychopathology literature offers some hints about what the interrelationships may be.

Psychopathology Implications

Since emotional disorders become stabilized by middle adolescence, it seems possible that early adolescence is a critical time in emotional development. Further indirect support for this idea may be derived from the finding that the characteristics of these disorders, especially depression, begin to cohere at this age in theoretically meaningful ways. As noted earlier, the dramatic increase in suicide around the age of 15 suggests a strong role by this age for emotional functioning, which may combine with a number of other variables to produce the undesirable outcome of suicide.

Taken together, the combined research on personality development and clinical disorders suggests that emotional development plays a major role in the nature of specific disorders. The following two examples illustrate the potential derived from this kind of synthesis. When one combines delayed moral development with underdifferentiated emotional development, it seems likely that conduct disorders will occur, especially in individuals who are deficient in identifying their own feelings as well as the feelings of others (Kennedy, 1984). Depression and depression with anxiety (especially physiologically labile ones), together with poor self-esteem and emotional overdifferentiation, may combine to produce the over-disclosing verbal behavior characteristic of depression (Coyne, 1976). On the same dimensions and consistent with a nonunitary view of unipolar depression (Craighead, 1980), it has also been observed clinically that there is a subset of emotionally underdifferentiated depressives, that is, individuals who engage in *dichotomous emotionality* experiencing the world only as happy or sad (Craighead, 1983). Could gender differences on these combined dimensions be contributing to gender differences in adolescent suicide rates?

Developmental Dysynchrony

The simultaneous consideration of personality and emotional development also raises questions about the role of uneven development across domains. Psychopathology may occur when one developmentally normal domain becomes overemphasized, as in an overly aggressive adolescent male. In fact, one view of anxiety disorder among adults maintains that anxiety is the experience of incongruities across cognitive, physiological, emotional, and behavioral domains of functioning (Rachman and Hodgson, 1974; Hodgson and Rachman, 1974). Indeed, one reason for Freud's development of the concept of the unconscious was to explain the inconsistency between emotional and cognitive experiences in his clients.

It seems plausible that another type of inconsistency, a developmental one, may also be related to psychopathology and to normal emotional and personality development. The hypothesis is that a developmental dysynchrony across emotional, cognitive, physiological, and emotional development may produce poor adjustment and perhaps psychopathology in the adolescent. This is further complicated by the multifaceted nature of each of the components of the developmental process. This suggests that the greater the discrepancy both within and across developmental domains, the greater the disruption to developmental adaptation. The greatest disruptions are reflected in mental illnesses, and the nature of the specific disorders may be determined by the patterns of the developmental disruptions and the degree of developmental dysynchrony (Craighead et al., 1983).

The Role of Gender

As we have noted at several points in this review of research, there is evidence of gender bias in several psychological theories. This bias in question-asking affects the methods used and the results obtained. An example of this bias is with role of gender in moral development theory and methods, which tend to classify girls as conforming because of their focus on the feelings of others and because of their emphasis on reciprocity of relationships in moral decision making. The paucity of work in social development or on the whole field of normal emotional development may be due to gender-related bias. These areas have been considered "female domains" and may have been neglected because researchers (primarily male) have focused on areas more pertinent to their own development and to instrumental areas thought to be more important for human functioning.

Gender also plays a role in terms of developmental differences in boys and girls in the areas that have been studied. It is clear that development proceeds differently for boys and girls, on the average. Sex-role stereotypes of appropriate behavior, as well as differential experiences and opportunities, create somewhat different environments for boys and girls. In addition, there are clearly inherent differences, such as physical size and some aspects of temperament, that may be important as well. The available data suggest that small biological differences in some areas are magnified by differential environments. With other areas, differences between boys and girls appear to be due solely to different experiences and expectations (Petersen et al., 1982).

Gender Role and Development

It seems likely that the developmental differentiation of sex roles is affected by and affects emotional development. Less adequate identity and ego development and lower self-concept probably combine to encourage individuals into adopting traditional sex-roles. Social behavior and cognitive development within these sex-roles then are likely to lead to greater intrapersonal conflict and

poorer adjustment, or eventually to adopting sex-role specific cognitive styles associated with gender related disorders (for example,
conduct disordered boys and anxious and depressed girls).

Finally, the combination of findings from these areas may relate
to the consistency of disorders over time. For example, delayed
moral development, insensitive emotional development, and inappropriate social behaviors appear to characterize conduct disorders, which are stable from ages six to seven through young
adulthood. The basis for the diagnosis and the combination of cognitive, personality, social, and emotional behaviors is the same over
time. They are also consistent, extreme forms of traditional masculine sex roles; there is an associated predominance of males
classified in this diagnostic category. In contrast, the defining foci
of anxiety and depression shift over time, becoming more like the
foci of adult disorders by late adolescence. This shift not only is
associated with increasingly abstract cognitive abilities, as noted
earlier, but also fit better with traditional female sex role attributes;
there are associated gender differences which develop parallel to
the change in the focus of the disorder from early to late adolescence. These gender differences may be affected to a large degree
by the normal development of emotional functioning interacting
with internal and external variables over the period of adolescent
development.

Other Influences on the Development of Emotion and Personality

We stated earlier that our review would not focus on biological or
cognitive aspects of development. These are clearly, however, key
aspects of development during adolescence, which need to be integrated into our discussion.

Biological Development

Adolescence begins with pubertal change, a process that completes the maturation to adult appearance and reproductive capacity
which is set in motion prenatally (Petersen and Taylor, 1980). The
physical changes of puberty occur over an average of four years,
and for some indicators occur approximately two years earlier for
girls than for boys.

Puberty is popularly thought to be the "cause" of adolescent turmoil, moodiness, and other aspects of adolescent behavior. Although all adolescents go through puberty (unless they have some endocrine defect or illness), we know now that not all adolescents manifest these difficulties. In addition, recent work of Petersen and colleagues (Kavrell and Petersen, 1984; Petersen, 1983b) shows that pubertal change is not related to changes in cognition, mood, or self-image for most young people. Body image and related constructs are affected by pubertal change in different ways for boys and girls (Tobin-Richards et al., 1983). In addition, specific subgroups—such as early maturing girls—do have psychological difficulties related to pubertal change (Petersen, 1983a). Other research suggests that most of these effects do not persist but rather are transient (Petersen and Taylor, 1980).

This research does not address the possibility of specific hormonal effects, particularly on short-term mood changes at puberty. Studies both currently underway and planned will add to our knowledge on this topic.

Cognitive Development

There has been increasing recognition of the effect of cognitive development, particularly the capacity for abstract reasoning, on personality and emotional development during adolescence. It is now clear that, like other aspects of development, cognitive change is gradual. There is no sudden appearance of "formal operations." Rather, this change begins in different areas at different times and rates (Keating, 1980). Furthermore, there is recent evidence that abstract reasoning does not "unfold" maturationally but, rather, that this capacity is stimulated by experiences. For example, higher level moral reasoning is produced in some individuals by situations that require complex decision-making (Gilligan and Belenky, 1980). Some individuals regress in such situations, and the reasons for advancement or regression appear to be the result of a complex interaction among emotion, cognition, and social factors.

Therefore, it is not correct to conclude, as some have done, that psychological development is the *result* of cognitive development. Clearly, that capacity to think abstractly facilitates thinking about concepts such as the self and one's identity. It is equally clear, however, that there is a reciprocal interactive interplay among these aspects of development so that cognitive advance may result from an emotional experience.

Situational Factors

We have mentioned throughout this chapter the effects of experience on development. The kinds of experiences one has are obviously related to social class, gender, community, and age. Family factors, school structure and nature, and the peer group also affect experience. There has been some research in all of these factors demonstrating their effects on development (Petersen, in press). More work is needed to integrate the findings and to test integrated models.

Summary

We have identified several issues in psychological development that point to areas needing further conceptualization and research. We know far too little about emotional development during adolescence and young adulthood. Moreover, we know less about the development of girls than of boys.

The research that does exist suggests that there is progressive moral and ego development, increases in self-esteem, and some tendency toward identity achievement. Research on mental disorders suggests that depression and anxiety increase during adolescence, with conduct disorders more stable between childhood and adulthood. Taken together, these results provide a picture of a steady transition on most measures of personality and emotion from childhood to adult levels during adolescence and young adulthood. This picture stands in sharp contrast to the popular one of terrible troubles during adolescence. The same picture obtains for adolescent health behaviors: adolescents do not use drugs, drink, or become pregnant *more* than adults; they simply begin behaving like adults (Petersen, 1982).

The existing research also provides some clues as to why and when difficulties appear. As for the *when*, early adolescence appears to be the *critical transition* with little change appearing after middle adolescence. A number of stressors converge simultaneously during early adolescence that may overwhelm some youth, particularly those with previous vulnerability (Petersen and Spiga, 1982). This would, therefore, be a key time for prevention *and* intervention efforts.

Why difficulties occur is more complex. It is clear that a number of factors are involved, and we need more research examining their relative importance for various kinds of difficulties. Some of these factors may lead to *developmental dysynchrony* discussed earlier, which then may become a stressor itself.

Finally, it is essential that developmental and clinical research become more integrated. The current development research suggests that most youth traverse the transition from childhood to adulthood relatively smoothly. Yet, suicide is increasing among young people. Who is having difficulty? And why? We can no longer blame adolescent problems on normative adolescent turmoil. We must now identify what factors are involved. This will only happen by integrating these two perspectives.

Implications for Prevention Programs

The discussion of previous findings and their integration provides a number of implications for the development and implementation of prevention programs. First, program developers must have a thorough knowledge of developmental, epidemiological, and clinical research in order to know the appropriate target of intervention. Although the focus may be on intervention during adolescence, there must also be a knowledge of earlier precipitators of the disorder and a knowledge of what the disorder will look like in later years. Although it may be appropriate to *treat* a specific animal phobia in a 10-year-old child, the research on anxiety suggests that a preventive program would be better focused on social and/or anxiety to more abstract stimuli.

Second, preventive programs should be geared to the developmental level of the adolescent. Certainly more data regarding normative development, especially on emotional variables, must still be forthcoming. We already know, however, from the work of Meyers and his colleagues (Schleser et al., 1981) that cognitive therapy offered at a developmental level inconsistent with that of the treated child is minimally effective, whereas treatment taking the developmental level into account is more effective. Furthermore, greater generalization and maintenance of cognitive therapy treatment effects are obtained for children of more advanced cognitive levels (Cohen and Schleser, 1984).

Third, prevention programs must be multifaceted; development occurs on social cognitive, physiological, and emotional domains. If, indeed, poor adjustment and psychopathology are related to an inconsistency in development across domains, then it would be essential for prevention programs to focus on more consistent development. Furthermore, the development of these domains may be interdependent, and a knowledge of a normative developmental pattern would facilitate the development of appropriate intervention programs. Although empirical work has not addressed this question, the conclusion seems intuitively obvious. An adolescent who cannot identify his or her emotions or those of others, cannot express or reflect feelings; likewise, an adolescent with excellent emotional identification and differentiation capabilities cannot express them without a modicum of verbal communication skills.

Fourth, gender differences should be taken into account in the development of prevention programs. This raises a difficult social policy issue for the clinician moving from the treatment to the prevention setting. Who decides what the appropriate targets are and how do they relate to gender differences? What is the appropriate level of emotional differentiation? In the long run, what is the most adaptive cognitive coping style, and is it gender specific? Nonetheless, boys and girls do differ; available activities and social roles change in adolescence and these are gender specific. Previous social developments have contributed to gender specific problems. These need to be mediated in preventive programs.

Of course, we are left with the traditional preventive questions, which were not specially addressed in this paper. In what context (community, school, home, or clinic) should prevention occur, and who is the appropriate target for the program (systems, citizens in general, parents, teachers, or adolescents themselves)? The findings on emotional and personality development have, however, highlighted a number of factors that should influence the development and implementation of prevention programs.

References

Abramson LY, Seligman MEP, Teasdale JD: Learned helplessness in humans: critique and reformulation. J Abnorm Psychol 87:49–74, 1978

Adelson J (Ed.): Handbook of Adolescent Psychology. New York, Wiley, 1980

Adelson J, Doehrman MJ: The psychodynamic approach to adolescence, in Handbook of Adolescent Psychology. Edited by Adelson J. New York, Wiley, 1980

American Psychiatric Association: Diagnostic and Statistical Manual of Mental Disorders, Third Edition (DSM-III). Washington DC, American Psychiatric Association, 1980

Annesley PT: Psychiatric illness in adolescence: presentation and prognosis. Journal of Mental Science 107:268–278, 1961

Bachman JG, O'Malley PM: Self-esteem in young men: a longitudinal analysis of the impact of educational and occupational attainment. J Pers Soc Psychol 35:365–380, 1977

Beck AT, Kovacs M, Weissman A: Hopelessness and suicidal behavior: an overview. JAMA 234:1136–1139, 1975

Bernard J: Needs of families: an overview. Paper presented at a MacArthur Foundation conference, Child Care: Growth Fostering Environments for Young Children, Chicago, December 1982

Blos P: On Adolescence: A Psychoanalytic Interpretation. New York, Free Press, 1962

Blos P: The Adolescent Passage: Developmental Issues. New York, International Universities Press, 1979

Chapman AH: Management of Emotional Problems of Children and Adolescents. Philadelphia, Lippincott, 1974

Chiles JA, Miller ML, Cox GB: Depression in an adolescent delinquent population. Arch Gen Psychiatry 37:1179–1184, 1980

Cohen R, Schleser R: Cognitive development and clinical interventions, in Cognitive Behavior Therapy With Children. Edited by Meyers AW, Craighead WE. New York, Plenum, 1984

Coleman JC: Friendship and the peer group in adolescence, in Handbook of Adolescent Psychology. Edited by Adelson J. New York, Wiley, 1980

Conger JJ, Petersen AC: Adolescence and Youth, third edition. New York, Harper & Row, 1984

Corder BF, Shorr W, Corder RF: A study of social and psychological characteristics of adolescent suicide attempters in an urban, disadvantaged area. Adolescence 9:1–6, 1974

Costanzo PR, Shaw ME: Conformity as a function of age level. Child Dev 37:967–975, 1966

Coyne JC: Toward an interactional description of depression. Psychiatry 39:28–40, 1976

Craighead WE: Away from a unitary model of depression. Behavior Therapy 11:122–128, 1980

Craighead WE: Contemporary behavior therapy: if you think and feel, are you still behavioral? Presidential address, Division 12, Section III, presented at the Annual Meeting of the American Psychological Association, Anaheim, CA, August 1983

Craighead WE, Wilcoxon-Craighead L, Meyers AW: New directions in behavior modification with children, in Progress in Behavior Modification, vol. 6. Edited by Hersen M, Eisler RM, Miller PM. New York, Academic Press, 1978

Craighead WE, Smucker MR, Duchnowski A: Childhood and adolescent depression and attributional style. Paper presented at the Annual Meeting of the American Psychological Association, Los Angeles, August 1981

Craighead WE, Meyers AW, Craighead LW, et al: Issues in cognitive-behavior therapy with children, in Perspectives on Behavior Therapy in the Eighties. Edited by Rosenbaum M, Franks CM, Jaffe Y. New York, Springer, 1983

Craighead WE, Kennedy RE, Raczynski JM, et al: Affective disorders: unipolar, in Adult Psychopathology: A Behavioral Perspective. Edited by Turner SM, Hersen M. New York, Wiley, 1984

Cunningham JM, Westerman HH, Fischhoff J: A follow-up study of patients seen in a psychiatric clinic for children. Am J Orthopsychiatry 26:602–612, 1956

Damon W, Hart D: The development of self-understanding from infancy through adolescence. Child Dev 53:841–864, 1982

Demo DH, Savin-Williams RC: Early adolescent self-esteem as a function of social class: Rosenberg and Pearlin revisited. American Journal of Sociology 88:763–764, 1983

Douvan E, Adelson J: The Adolescent Experience. New York, Wiley, 1966

Dusek JB, Flaherty JF: The development of the self-concept during the adolescent years. Monographs of the Society for Research in Child Development 46(4, Serial No. 191), 1981

Dweck CS: Learned helplessness and negative evaluation, in The Educator: Evaluation and Motivation, vol. 14. Edited by Keislar ER. 1977

Dweck CS, Goetz FE: Attributions and learned helplessness, in New Directions in Attribution Research, vol. 2. Edited by Harvey JH, Ickes W, Kidd RF. Hillsdale, NJ, Lawrence Erlbaum Associates, 1977

Elkind D: Recent research on cognitive development in adolescence, in

Adolescence on the Life Cycle: Psychological Change and Social Context. Edited by Dragastin SE, Elder GH. Washington DC, Hemisphere, 1974

Emde RN: Levels of meaning for infant emotions: a biosocial view, in Minnesota Symposia on Child Psychology, vol. 13. Edited by Collins A. Minneapolis, University of Minnesota Press, 1979

Erikson EH: Identity: Youth and Crisis. New York, Norton, 1968

Flavell JH, Ross L (Eds.): Social Cognitive Development: Frontiers and Possible Futures. Cambridge, Cambridge University Press, 1981

Flood R, Seager C: A retrospective examination of psychiatric case records of patients who subsequently committed suicide. Br J Psychiatry 114:443–450, 1968

Frederick CH: An introduction and overview to youth suicide, in Youth Suicide. Edited by Peck ML, Faberow NL, Litman RE. New York, Springer, 1985

Freud A: Adolescence: Psychoanalytic Study of the Child, vol. 13. New York, International Universities Press, 1958

Gersten JC, Langer TS, Eisenberg JB, et al: Stability and change in types of behavioral disturbance of children and adolescents. J Abnorm Child Psychol 4:111–127, 1976

Gesell A, Ilg FL, Ames LB: Youth: The Years From Ten to Sixteen. New York, Harper & Row, 1956

Gilligan C: In a different voice: women's conceptions of the self and of morality. Harvard Educational Review 47:481–517, 1977

Gilligan C, Belenky MF: A naturalistic study of abortion decisions, in Clinical-Developmental Psychology. Edited by Selman R, Yando R. San Francisco, Jossey-Bass, 1980

Graham P: Epidemiological studies, in Psychopathological Disorders of Childhood, second edition. Edited by Quay HC, Werry JS. New York, Wiley, 1979

Graham R, Rutter M: Psychiatric disorders in the young adolescent: a follow-up study. Proceedings of the Royal Society of Medicine 66:1226–1229, 1973

Green BJ: Depression in Early Adolescence: An Exploratory Investigation of its Frequency, Intensity, and Correlates. Unpublished doctoral dissertation, The Pennsylvania State University, 1980

Green LW, Horton D: Adolescent health: issues and challenges, in Promoting Adolescent Health: A Dialogue on Research and Practice. Edited by Coates TJ, Petersen AC, Perry C. New York, Academic Press, 1982

Haan N: Two moralities in action contexts: relationships to thought, ego, regulation, and development. J Pers Soc Psychol 36:286–305, 1978

Hall GS: Adolescence: Its Psychology and Its Relations to Physiology, Anthropology, Sociology, Sex, Crime, Religion, and Education. New York, Appleton, 1904

Harrow M, Quinlan D: Is disordered thinking unique to schizophrenia? Arch Gen Psychiatry 34:15–21, 1977

Hetherington EM, Martin B: Family interaction, in Psychopathological Disorders of Childhood, second edition. Edited by Quay HC, Werry JS. New York, Wiley, 1979

Hill JP, Lynch ME: The intensification of gender-related role expectancies during early adolescence, in Girls at Puberty: Biological and Psychosocial Perspectives. Edited by Brooks-Gunn J, Petersen AC. New York, Plenum Press, 1983

Hodgson RI, Rachman S: Dysynchrony in measures of fear. Behav Res Ther 12:319–326, 1974

Hoffman ML: Moral development in adolescence, in Handbook of Adolescent Psychology. Edited by Adelson J. New York, Wiley, 1980

Kandel DB, Davies M: Epidemiology of depressive mood in adolescents. Arch Gen Psychiatry 39:1205–1212, 1982

Kavrell SM, Petersen AC: Patterns of achievement in early adolescence, in Women and Science. Edited by Maehr ML, Steinkamp MW. Greenwich, CT, JAI Press, 1984

Kazdin AE: Assessment techniques for childhood depression: a critical appraisal. J Am Acad Child Psychiatry 20:358–375, 1981

Kazdin AE, Petti TA: Self-report and interview measures of childhood and adolescent depression. J Child Psychol Psychiatry 23:437–457, 1982

Keating DP: Thinking processes in adolescence, in Handbook of Adolescent Psychology. Edited by Adelson J. New York, Wiley, 1980

Kennedy RE: Cognitive–behavioral interventions with delinquents, in Cognitive-Behavior Therapy with Children. Edited by Meyers AW, Craighead WE. New York, Plenum Press, 1984

Kohlberg L: Development of moral character and moral ideology, in Review of Child Development Research, vol. 1. Edited by Hoffman ML, Hoffman LW. New York, Russell Sage Foundation, 1964

Kohlberg L: Moral stages and moralization: the cognitive–developmental approach, in Moral Development and Behavior. Edited by Likona T. New York, Henry Holt, 1976

Larson R, Csikszentmihalyi M, Graef R: Mood variability and the psychosocial adjustment of adolescents. Journal of Youth and Adolescence 9:469–490, 1980

Leslie SA: Psychiatric disorder in the young adolescents of an industrial town. Br J Psychiatry 125:113–124, 1974

Loevinger J: Ego development: Conceptions and Theories. San Francisco, Jossey-Bass, 1976

Loevinger J: Construct validity of the Sentence Completion Test of ego development. Applied Psychological Measurement 3:281–311, 1979

Marcia JE: Development and validation of ego identity status. J Pers Soc Psychol 3:551–558, 1966

Marcia JE: Identity in adolescence, in Handbook of Adolescent Psychology. Edited by Adelson J. New York, Wiley, 1980

Marks I: Fears and Phobias. New York, Academic Press, 1969

Marks I, Gelder M: Different ages of onset in varieties of phobia. Am J Psychiatry 123:218–221, 1966

Masterson JF: The symptomatic adolescent five years later: he didn't grow out of it. Am J Psychiatry 123:1338–1345, 1967

McCarthy JD, Hoge DR: Analysis of age effects in longitudinal studies of adolescent self-esteem. Developmental Psychology 18:372–379, 1982

Meilman PW: Cross-sectional age changes in ego identity status during adolescence. Developmental Psychology 15:230–231, 1979

Murphy JM, Gilligan C: Moral development in late adolescence and adulthood: a critique and reconstruction of Kohlberg's theory. Human Development 23:77–104, 1980

Offer D, Offer JB: From Teenage to Young Manhood: A Psychological Study. New York, Basic Books, 1975

Offer D, Ostrov E, Howard KI: The Adolescent: A Psychological Self-Portrait. New York, Basic Books, 1981

O'Malley PM, Bachman JG: Self-esteem: change and stability between ages 13 and 23. Developmental Psychology 19:257–268, 1983

Petersen AC: Biopsychosocial processes in the development of sex-related differences, in The Psychobiology of Sex Differences and Sex Roles. Edited by Parsons JE. New York, Hemisphere, 1980

Petersen AC: The development of self-concept in adolescence, in Self-

Concept: Advances in Theory and Research. Edited by Lynch MD, Norem-Hebeisen AA, Gergen KJ. Cambridge, MA, Ballinger, 1981

Petersen AC: Developmental issues in adolescent health, in Promoting Adolescent Health: A Dialogue on Research and Practice. Edited by Coates TJ, Petersen AC, Perry C. New York, Academic Press, 1982

Petersen AC: Menarche: meaning of measures and measuring meaning, in Menarche. Edited by Golub S. New York, D.C. Heath, 1983a

Petersen AC: Pubertal change and cognition, in Girls at Puberty: Biological and Psychosocial Perspectives. Edited by Brooks-Gunn J, Petersen AC. New York, Plenum Press, 1983b

Petersen AC: Pubertal development as a cause of disturbance: myths, realities, and unanswered questions. J Genet Psychol (in press)

Petersen AC, Spiga R: Adolescence and stress, in Handbook of Stress: Theoretical and Clinical Aspects. Edited by Goldberger L, Breznitz S. New York, The Free Press, 1982

Petersen AC, Taylor BC: The biological approach to adolescence: biological change and psychological adaptation, in Handbook of Adolescent Psychology. Edited by Adelson J. New York, Wiley, 1980

Petersen AC, Tobin-Richards MH, Crockett L: Sex differences, in Encyclopedia of Educational Research, fifth edition. Edited by Mitzel HE. New York, The Free Press, 1982

Piaget J: The Moral Judgment of the Child. New York, Harcourt, 1932

President's Commission on Mental Health: Report to the President. Washington DC, U.S. Government Printing Office, 1978

Pritchard M, Graham P: An investigation of a group of patients who have attended both the child and adult departments of the same psychiatric hospital. Br J Psychiatry 112:603–612, 1966

Quay HC: Dimensions of personality in delinquent boys as inferred from the factor analysis of case history data. Child Dev 35:479–484, 1964

Quay HC: Personality patterns in preadolescent delinquent boys. Educational and Psychological Measurement 16:99–110, 1966

Rachman S, Hodgson RI: Synchrony and dysynchrony in fear and avoidance. Behav Res Ther 12:311–318, 1974

Redmore CD, Loevinger J: Ego development in adolescence: longitudinal studies. Journal of Youth and Adolescence 8:1–20, 1979

Rest J: Development of Judging Moral Issues. Minneapolis, University of Minnesota Press, 1979

Robins LN: Follow-up studies, in Psychopathological Disorders of Childhood, second edition. Edited by Quay HC, Werry JS. New York, Wiley, 1979

Rosenberg M: Conceiving the Self. New York, Basic Books, 1979

Rutter M, Cox A, Tupling C, et al: Attainment and adjustment in two geographical areas, I: prevalence of psychiatric disorder. Br J Psychiatry 126:493–509, 1975

Rutter M, Graham P, Chadwick O, et al: Adolescent turmoil: fact or fiction? J Child Psychol Psychiatry 17:35–36, 1976

Sameroff A: Transactional models in early social relations. Human Development 18:65–79, 1975

Schaffer D: Diagnostic considerations in suicidal behavior in children and adolescents. J Am Acad Child Psychiatry 21:414–416, 1982

Schleser R, Meyers AW, Cohen R: Generalization of self-instruction: effects of general versus specific content, active rehearsal, and cognitive level. Child Dev 52:335–340, 1981

Senn MJE, Solnit AJ: Problems in Child Behavior and Development. Philadelphia, Lea & Febinger, 1968

Simmons RG, Rosenberg F, Rosenberg M: Disturbance in the self-image at adolescence. American Sociological Review 38:553–568, 1973

Simmons RG, Blyth DA, Van Cleave EF, et al: Entry into early adolescence: the impact of school structure, puberty, and early dating on self-esteem. American Sociological Review 44:948–967, 1979

Smucker MR, Craighead WE, Craighead LW, et al: Normative and reliability data for the Children's Depression Inventory. J Abnorm Child Psychology (in press)

Tobin-Richards MH, Boxer AM, Petersen AC: The psychological significance of pubertal change: sex differences in perceptions of self during early adolescence, in Girls at Puberty: Biological and Psychosocial Perspectives. Edited by Brooks-Gunn J, Petersen AC. New York, Plenum Press, 1983

Toolan JM: Suicide and suicidal attempts in children and adolescents. Am J Psychiatry 118:719–724, 1962

Warren WA: A study of adolescent psychiatric inpatients and the outcome six or more years later, II: the follow-up study. J Child Psychol Psychiatry 6:141–160, 1965

Weiner IB, Del Gaudio AC: Psychopathology in adolescence: an epidemiological study. Arch Gen Psychiatry 33:187–193, 1976

Weissman MM: The epidemiology of suicide attempts, 1960–1971. Arch Gen Psychiatry 30:737–746, 1974

Wylie RC: The Self-Concept: Theory and Research on Selected Topics, vol. 2, revised edition. Lincoln, University of Nebraska Press, 1979

Yarrow LJ: Emotional development. Am Psychol 10:951–957, 1979

Chapter 3

ADOLESCENT SUICIDE:
AN ARCHITECTURAL MODEL

John E. Mack, M.D.

Chapter 3

ADOLESCENT SUICIDE:
AN ARCHITECTURAL MODEL

For every human being, the question of whether to live or die presents a profound philosophical choice to be confronted many times in the course of one's life. Camus wrote, "There is but one truly philosophical problem, and that is suicide" (Camus, p. 3). The decision to commit suicide is a statement not only that one's own life is not worth living, but may express as well a view that life itself has no value. As clinicians, in working with individuals who are confronting the choice of whether to live or die, we are most interested in the balance of forces which influence, or may influence, the decision in the direction of life. As physicians we are committed to protecting and enhancing life.

A completed suicide, although generally occurring in the context of psychopathology, can at the same time be a highly elaborate and creative, even artistic phenomenon. In *The Myth of Sisyphus*, Camus wrote, "An act like this is prepared within the silence of the heart, as is a great work of art" (Camus, p. 4). Suicide traverses many human realms. The theme is important in sociology, literature, art, and, of course, in religion. In this chapter, I consider suicide as a major clinical challenge. Although I discuss suicide on the individual level, I have in mind the aggregate nature of the problem as well. There are debates in the scientific literature about the incidence of adolescent suicide, whether its apparent marked statistical increase in recent decades is actual, or is an artifact of naming and reporting (Eisenberg, 1980; Bassuk et al., 1982; Offer et al.,

1981). There does, however, appear to have been an actual two- to threefold increase in the incidence of completed suicides in the 15- to 19-year-old age group in the past quarter of a century (National Center for Health Statistics, 1978). It is possible, as Leon Eisenberg suggests, that when one considers the underreporting of suicide, the incidence may be even higher (Eisenberg, 1980).

I wish to suggest a particular approach to adolescent suicide, a way of looking at the problem. Although this approach was developed in relation to teenagers, and grew out of the intensive study of a single adolescent, Vivienne, it is my hope that it may enhance our understanding of the problem of suicide in adults as well (Mack and Hickler, 1981). Adolescents tend not to be very willing to share their deepest thoughts, feelings, and conflicts with other people, especially adults. For this reason, diaries, journals, letters, and other writings, such as poems and school compositions, represent a particularly rich source for understanding the inner life of teenagers.

In this chapter I describe an architectural model, which might also be looked upon as a contextual, structural, or systems approach. In our effort to provide a complete understanding of adolescent suicide from a clinical point of view, it is not sufficient to consider only the individual teenager's private conflicts, however essential a part these may play in the outcome. The elements or parts which comprise the model can be grouped under the following headings:

1. The macrocosm; the sociopolitical context
2. Biological vulnerability; the genetic predisposition to suicide
3. Earliest developmental influences and experiences
4. Personality structure or organization, especially the regulation of self-esteem
5. The individual's object relationships and the state of those relationships as the suicidal preoccupation developed
6. Clinical depression and other psychopathology
7. The ontogeny or developmental relationship to death
8. The contemporary clinical situation or circumstances of the individual's life at the time of assessment.

Since beginning my study of Vivienne's life and suicide with Holly Hickler, I have applied this model to a number of other adolescent cases.

Vivienne Loomis lived in Melrose, Massachusetts. She was 14 years and four months old when she hung herself in December,

1973, in her mother's silversmithing shop with a rope that she obtained from her mother. She was a bright, sensitive, artistic girl who was an excellent writer. In her voluminous journal entries, letters, compositions, and poetry, she gave us a rare look into the inner world of an adolescent struggling with questions of life and death.

The Macrocosm

The macrocosm is the larger world, or the society as a whole, as it affects the individual adolescent. What, for example, is the impact of events, values, and sociopolitical trends and phenomena on a particular child or adolescent? What effect do societal patterns of drug-taking, alcoholism, and violence in our society, including the constant threat of death in a nuclear war, have on adolescents, especially on those who are vulnerable to suicide for other reasons? What do these cultural phenomena mean to teenagers, and how do they affect the choices of life and death? I was recently consulted by the parents of an 11-year-old girl who was afraid of nuclear war. They said their daughter wanted to know whether she would have time to commit suicide if she knew that nuclear bombs were on the way, before they actually exploded.

There are examples in which several suicides occur in the same school, like small epidemics (New York Times, June 16, 1979; Time, Sept. 1, 1980). What is the role of the school system in promoting or preventing suicide? Freud, as you may recall, once remarked that a school ought to do something more than "not driving its pupils to suicide" (Friedman, 1967, p. 61). There have been epidemics of student suicide in Japan and Germany that seem related to the rigidities of their competitive school systems (Newsweek, March 8, 1976; Aug. 28, 1978). There are also trends concerning suicide within the adolescent culture. My 18-year-old son, during a talk we had several months ago about the fact that there seems to be more suicides among teenagers today, remarked, "It's an option that's opened up." Sociopolitical and economic influences may increase the number that actually do commit suicide out of the pool of those who, for other reasons, may be suicide-prone.

Changing sexual mores, and the breakdown of structure and guidance in relation to sexual choice and behavior, may place particular stress upon those teenagers who are less able to handle the emotional challenges or threat of increased freedom in this area. Vivienne, who was one such child, made this clear in several letters she wrote to an important school teacher, about whom more will be said shortly. She wrote in one letter five months before her death:

> I myself have managed to stay unattached, thanks to my unfailing lack of charm. Only one guy tried to rape me five days ago, and I haven't seen him since. Mommy and Daddy would have a fit if they knew, but I didn't find it as traumatic as everybody seems to make it. The fact is that this particular fellow had already had a few six-packs too many. It had nothing to do with me. Well, so much for the "dirt of the day" (Mack and Hickler, p. 82).

A month later she wrote:

> I don't think that I can follow the nation's trend; now the average girl puts down the last good book in the house and says, Shit. Nothing else to do. I guess I'll go over to the stone wall on the corner and get picked up. I don't know. Three times, three people in the last 2½ weeks, have tried to fuck me. Twice I was good and stiff. But each time, I just thought to myself—God! Is this all there is? Not only is there no true love, no giving—but this is all as routine as taking your vitamins in the morning. I don't see how you get Saturday night fun out of it. So I'll probably keep my ideals for the time being. Of course, I don't have, and never have had, any hang-ups about marriage. I just require a deep and caring love (Mack and Hickler, p. 98).

This passage tells a lot, of course, about Vivienne as an individual, about her personal ideals and conflicts. But it also says something about what is going on in the larger society, that a barely 14-year-old girl, in a middle-class family, could be such an acceptable target, an easy prey for any boy or young man who chooses to approach her. She does not feel that she can turn to her parents, nor do her parents behave as if they have a sanction from the society for setting limits.

Vivienne, it is true, had more than average sensitivity to events in the outside world. Her parents described how upset she would become when she would see something on television, such as the Arab–Israeli War of 1973, or the immoral behavior of political leaders. She would sometimes express her thoughts and feelings in poems. One of them was called "Joys of Living":

The Stock Exchange,
Neon signs,
Traffic jams,
Indo China,
Another exam and the Watergate.
New train tables,
Inflation, highway repairs,
Nixon,
His dog "Checkers,"
Your new Bugged home. . .
It's all too late!

(Mack and Hickler, p. 74)

Vivienne was also troubled about the conditions in prisons. "Wasn't that horrible about the prisons?" she asked in her journal. "A man doesn't have any rights or respect or anything! I knew it was *really* bad in prisons, but I didn't know it was that bad. I guess the general public really doesn't know because they are told stories that they like to hear about, and *not* the truth. What should I do!" (Mack and Hickler, p. 51).

I wonder whether teenagers today are confronted with these disturbing realities in a more overwhelming way than they have been in the past, and what part this confrontation plays in suicide and other adolescent disturbances. Did Emily Dickinson write poems at age 14 about political events and social problems in the America of the 1840s?

For each child there is a specific family and societal context. Vivienne's family was Protestant in a strongly Roman Catholic neighborhood. They were liberals in a politically conservative town. They stood out. Her father, who was a minister in a Universalist church, was being criticized in the community and was losing his ministry. There was a poor "fit" between Vivienne's family and the local community. Her mother would dress Vivienne in clothes that somehow were not right—handmade smocks, for example, and she would be ridiculed by her elementary school classmates.

Biological Vulnerability

The Danish adoption studies by Frank Schulsinger, Seymour Kety, and their colleagues demonstrated 12 suicides among 269 biological relatives of 57 adoptees who had committed suicide (Schulsinger, Kety, Rosenthal & Wender, 1979). Among the group of 148 adopted relatives (nonbiological relations, including the parents who raised the children who had committed suicide) there were no suicides. Recent work on the biochemistry of suicide has shown that there are low cerebrospinal fluid (CSF) levels of the serotonin metabolite 5–hydroxyindoleacetic acid in patients who have tried to kill themselves (Brown et al., 1982). It will be interesting to see whether this finding can be corroborated and will lead to other discoveries.

The question of constitutional sensitivity was brought into focus by the work of Paul Bergman and Sibylle Escalona, published in 1949. They demonstrated that there are children who show unusual sensitivities from the beginning of life. These children react differently to noise, colors, or changes in temperature or light. It is uncertain whether such observations can be correlated with later tendencies to be overwhelmed by everyday stresses, or tied to vulnerability to suicide and depression. Applebaum and Holzman examined Rorschachs of individuals who had made suicide attempts, or who later killed themselves, and found that in the color-shading responses there was a tendency for the suicidal individuals to go beyond the given, to read their own ideas and fantasies into the material (Applebaum and Holzman, 1962). The authors concluded that these individuals would have been "better served if they were buffered by the refuge of greater generality, less involvement, and an increased ability to 'let it go at that' " (Applebaum and Holzman, 1962, p. 160).

Early Developmental Influences and Experiences

After Vivienne's death, her mother wrote a narrative for the family. It was clear that from the time of her birth that Vivienne was special. Even the delivery was unusual. "I was determined," her mother wrote, "to use natural childbirth and I decided to be part of an experiment using music. All the time I was in labor I had on earphones. Vivienne's arrival was watched by as many hospital personnel as could crowd into the delivery room, in their interest in the effects of music heard through earphones in lieu of anesthesia. Vivienne arrived, a chubby, purple baby whose tiny apricot tongue revealed the jaundice she had contracted when our incompatible blood types mixed" (Mack and Hickler, p. 7). Throughout Vivienne's infancy, the mother felt this incompatibility. Vivienne was different. She was quiet. She could be left in the playroom. Mrs. Loomis had two other active, more difficult, children—a son nearly four years old, and a daughter two years old.

Vivienne tended to react to early separations by "tuning out" the family, showing another kind of early sensitivity.

At quite an early age, Vivienne expressed responses to loss that were unusual. When she was five both of her grandfathers died. She demonstrated a special empathy, an intense involvement and identification, especially with her mother's grief at the time of the death of her father. Two months before her death, Vivienne wrote in a composition for school about one of her grandfathers:

> My grandfather comes back to me now, with his intensely gentle eyes and a strangely distorted face. An unconquered mind; I remember he always used to tell me that my dear you must never forget in all your life that eyes are for seeing and *dreams* were for pursuing. He is with me now, and he paints me his pictures of flat-tailed doves that glide purposefully over black and scrawny ravens who fight over death. And he shows me carefully the valley where the two mountains of reason and emotion meet and twine their efforts together in winding streams that quietly defy your logic. But just as I relinquish my power to fight this strange current, and I feel the waters rush through my veins, my grandfather is leaving me. . . to remember.
>
> (Mack and Hickler, p. 103)

Vivienne's sensitivity at age four or five presaged the way she would react all her life to separation and loss.

Personality Structure and Organization

In discussing "personality organization," I have in mind especially the narcissistic dimension, the development of self and self-esteem. Vivienne had a strong sense of identity, which needs to be distinguished from the uncertain or low level of her self-regard. She would write in the seventh grade:

> I am the youngest in my family.
> I am one out of twenty in the seventh grade.
> I am the minister's daughter.
> I am a pretender of moods.
> I am a New Englander.
> I am a person who plays the flute.
> I am very polite.
> I am a girl.
> I am me—because everyone is "me" inside
> Everything else.
>
> (Mack and Hickler, p. 34).

This strong sense of self, of identity, did not protect her from suffering a great deal as a result of disturbances of self-esteem. Interestingly, Vivienne was "on to" the narcissistic sector of development in general, especially the aspect of self-love, even though conflicts in the domain of self-regard played such an important role in her depression and suicide. She wrote the following story, which she called *On Vanity*, when she was in the eighth grade:

> Once upon a time there lived a ravishing princess named Prunelda. Prunelda was an extremely vain creature and very hard to please. She dabbled in the arts a bit, but only to the extent of painting self-portraits. She spent days on end in her rooms, which consisted almost solely of mirrors, and this caused her father, King Kong, to indulge in quite a bit of worrying. Prunelda had to get married off soon, or he'd never be rid of her.
>
> Well, not far off in a near-by kingdom lived a dazzling prince named Prince Hector. He, too, was vain and hard to please. One of the most vain things about him was the fact that he wore mirror glasses—the wrong way 'round. Prince Hector did this because he liked to gaze into his eyes and marvel at their beauty. Hector had heard stories of Prunelda and her room of mirrors, and so he decided that he would be allowed to frequent her rooms as often as he wished, and that meant that he would be able to gaze at himself as frequently as he wished by merely looking into her mirrors.
>
> At 3:50 Tuesday afternoon, Prunelda and Hector could be found sitting back to back gazing into the mirrors, entranced in themselves. Soon the compliments came gushing out for themselves: "Splendid!. . . . Magnificent!. . . . Ah! !" Each thought that the other's compliments were for himself and so they took a great liking to each other (not that they ever actually saw each other!).
>
> King Kong knew a sure thing when he saw one, and so he had them married right away. Hector and Prunelda spent many fun-filled years staring into mirrors and what turned out to be flattering each other. So *everyone* lived happily ever after.
>
> The moral to this story is that if you're extremely vain, what you don't know can only help you.
>
> (Mack and Hickler, pp. 58–59)

Vivienne begins, in her 12th year, to reflect great concern with the problem of self-worth. On April 8th, 1971, when she was 11 years and eight months old, she wrote in her journal:

> Do you understand me? Do you love me? Do you know the things I know? Do you feel the way I feel?. . . I bet nobody knows

the things I know or feels the things I feel. Does anyone admire things the way I do? I don't think so, but maybe, no, it couldn't be. Does anyone experience things the way I do? Does anybody take remarks or words the way I do?

Did anybody ever wonder how close they were to their ideal? I do. Does anybody ever wonder how they looked in the eyes of friends? Do people admire me? Does anybody admire me? I hope so. I care what people say to me and what people think about me. I want to set an example that is good. I wish everybody had a healthy grin and I hope I have one anyway. I don't mean to sound stupid or anything, but that's how I really and truly feel. Anyway no one will ever read this anyway so it's OK.

(Mack and Hickler, p. 15)

Early in adolescence the ego-ideal, which is a crucial agency in the regulation of self-esteem, begins to take form, as can be seen in the above example. In the first volume of her diary, written when she was in her late twenties, Anais Nin wrote, "This image [the ideal] is always a great strain to live up to. Some consider the loss of it a cause for suicide" (Nin, p. 128).

The ego-ideal is a structure in the personality that connects the self with other human beings, and provides a link between self and society. It contains the internalized expectations of the individual. It is distinguished from the superego (in some psychoanalytical writings it is part of the "superego system") by being more deeply tied to narcissism and early hurts, representing the projecting forward into the future of the possibility of a kind of "second chance." For we may repair or redeem early hurts and disappointments if we can create a world for ourselves which approximates a model of the visions contained in the ego-ideal. Vivienne's ego-ideal was so exalted and rigid as to be incompatible with daily reality, close to what Edith Jacobsen has called "the wishful ego-ideal" (Jacobson, 1964). Vivienne already gave evidence of this rigidity before she was 12. In June, 1971, she wrote in her journal:

I don't love life, I just love the little bit of life that touches my ideal one. It's my ideal life I love and try to live and introduce into the lives of others. All I can do is hold my stand and not give up until I've accomplished what I want to and not give up or out with exhaustion or with depression and disappointment. I just won't. I'll just stick with it. I will. No matter how hopeless it seems right now. I'll be persistent.

(Mack and Hickler, pp. 27–28)

The ability to "bounce back" from disappointment or injury is an important aspect of personality strength. Vivienne identified this quality and wrote about it. She would say that she *would* bounce back. At times she did. But she did not work through the meaning of major losses and disappointments, the impact of which seemed to accumulate.

Another dimension of personality strength, which is difficult to categorize but is closely connected to the vulnerability to suicide, might be called "the management of affect and disappointment," the ability to bear pain (Zetzel, 1970). Although this capacity seems quite specific to the predisposition to suicide, we understand relatively little about what determines the ability to tolerate depressive or other painful affects. This was clearly a major problem for Vivienne.

Psychoanalytic theorists and clinicians have developed a sophisticated understanding of the mechanisms of internalization and externalization of object representations which seem to characterize the personality organization of suicidal adults (Ash, 1980; Maltsberger and Buie, 1980; Maltsberger, 1983; Meissner, 1977). In particular, the identification with a "victim object," that is, the introjection of the victim aspect of a parent or other figure to whom the patient is closely attached, seems to be a frequent finding in suicide-prone individuals (Meissner, 1983; Orgell, 1974).

Finally, when we speak of personality structure in relation to suicide, we need to include a broader matrix than individual personality. We have to consider also the availability of family and community supports, since these contribute an important element in the ongoing capacities of the self, what I have called elsewhere "self-governance" or "the governance of the self" (Mack, 1978; Mack, 1981).

Object Relations

In considering the individual's object relationships I include those ties which complete the sense of self (self-objects [Kohut, 1971; 1977]), as well as more autonomous relationships with others. We are concerned here, for example, with relationships with parents, the degree to which separation from them has occurred, the quality of the involvement, identifications with them, ties to other adults, competition and intimacy with siblings, and relationships with and availability of friends. Vivienne was closely tied to her parents. But the relationship with her mother was so conflicted that she could not confide in her and felt burdened by her demands. Her father felt that he could not understand this daughter. With her sister, with whom she was close, Vivienne developed a kind of pact in which Laurel would look away from Vivienne's flirtation with suicide if Vivienne would not betray what Laurel was doing—especially her sexual activities—activities which their parents would not approve. Vivienne had a few intimate friends, but had difficulty making friends with a broad representation of her classmates at school and with neighborhood peers.

Teachers play a critical role at this time of life, and can either protect a child from suicide or contribute to its likelihood. When Vivienne was 11 and in the sixth grade, having had several very difficult years in public schools, she was transferred to The Cambridge Friends School, a private school where she met a teacher, John May, who was very sensitive to her situation. He was a conscientious objector to the Vietnam War. He saw, correctly, that Vivienne suffered from injured self-regard. He brought to her a great deal of caring, warmth, and support—telling her, for example, again and again that she should think better of herself. What he did not realize was the degree to which he was functioning, in Kohut's sense, as a kind of self-object for Vivienne, in that he completed something that was missing in her own sense of self-worth. For this reason, when he finally had to leave, it was devastating for Vivienne. This loss played a major role in the tailspin that culminated in her suicide.

Therapists also need to be sensitive to this aspect of their relationship with teenagers. They too may function, without being aware of it, as a self-completing object. Thus, slights, separations, or losses in relation to the therapist can become highly amplified in meaning for teenagers, particularly for those who have disturbances in the domain of self-esteem.

In one of her diary entries, written when she was 12 years and three months old, Vivienne shows how central Mr. May was for her self-esteem, and reveals the devastating impact of his announced departure and the importance of this loss in precipitating her preoccupation with death and suicide:

I wish Mr. May wouldn't go next year. And I wish Dad and Mummy wouldn't keep reminding me that he is.

A weaker, more immediate wish is that Mr. May would invite us to dinner like he said he would.

An impossible wish, though strongest, is that he would invite *me* (alone). Because I love him.

He is going to leave me.

Forever????

He's going to leave me behind as he goes on his merry way. But if he leaves me what way will I have to go? Why won't he stay? When will I die? It seems like I ought to die now while the going's good. While life has still got some joy. That joy will be gone in a year. Maybe I will be too—Oh, ah, silver tears appearing now. I'm crying, ain't I?

(Mack and Hickler, p. 34)

Clinical Depression and Other Psychopathology

In his study of the last months in the lives of 134 persons who committed suicide, Eli Robins found that at least 47 percent of these persons could be diagnosed as having had a major affective illness (Robins, 1981). A greater percentage may have had serious depressions but were difficult to diagnose. Another major diagnostic category was alcoholism. In many alcoholics, depressive feelings of suicidal intensity may surge up during intoxicated states and upset the precarious balance between life and death.

Vivienne sensed that she suffered from depression. In a poem that she called "Patterns of My Lifetime," she showed her awareness of the connection between her depression and egoism:

Crossing over, then down
Falling over, then under:
Down through egotistical
Patterns made in my lifetime.

Emotional depression
Existing, at first unobserved:
An old forgotten sword . . .
Suddenly glistening and sharp!

Eternal hope alternating
From blind, whimsical dependence
To strong, resounding salvation:
A bright candle in the night.

Sentiment weaving its way
Through hope in depression,
Depression in hope:
An amazing grace in itself.

Crossing over, then down.
Falling over, then under:
Down through egotistical
Patterns made in my lifetime.

(Mack and Hickler, pp. 41–42)

In her writings, Vivienne demonstrated repeatedly the close connection between the loss of important relationships, especially that with John May, and her depression. After he left for California, she wrote in her journal:

April 11, 1973

I am worthless, I am of no use to anyone, and no one is of any use to me. What good to kill myself? How can you kill nothing? A person who has committed suicide has had at least something to end. He must know joy to know misery. I have known nothing. Why live? Why die? One is an equal choice to the other. What do I do? I wonder if love would change anything. I don't know anymore. To know that the future looks worse doesn't help me any. I need people and there aren't any who care. It takes tolerance not to give in to death.

(Mack and Hickler, p. 63)

The Developmental Orientation Toward Death

Robert Lifton, Ernest Becker, Gregory Rochlin, and Irvin Yalom have called to our attention that the relationship with death has its own developmental sequences, or ontogeny, and its own set of meanings for particular individuals (Lifton, 1979; Becker, 1973; Rochlin, 1965; Yalom, 1980). Each person carries his or her own personal relationship to death. A variety of personifications of death exist in Western literature.

It is possible that suicide-prone individuals may have had a particularly intimate relationship with death during their lives. In assessing suicide-proneness or risk, it is important to trace this relationship, especially to discover if it has undergone a recent change in the direction of greater familiarity, intimacy, and acceptability. A tendency to romanticize death may be a dangerous sign

of suicidal risk for a particular adolescent. Some shift in the relationship to death is probably a necessary precondition to suicide,
at least of the premeditated type, which is what I primarily consider
here.

Vivienne showed a strong interest in and relationship with
death throughout her life. Vivienne's writings, especially the essay
she wrote about her grandfather, reveal rich death imagery and her
close relationship to death. In an essay about Elie Wiesel's book,
The Accident, she commented upon how she regarded death:

> I have come to consider death an emotional, deep and poetical fact
> of life... I look forward to dying, but I will live my life to the fullest
> first. Death will befall me; I will not befall death.
>
> (Mack and Hickler, pp. 52–53)

In a revised version of this essay, she wrote:

> ... reading the book made me realize that now, if someone should
> live for death or in it willingly, I would understand them perfectly... I
> have often thought of death as a retreat, myself, but somehow I always
> have had the guts to find the truth in life, along with the bitter... I
> believe that the difference between life and death (by will) is having
> the strength to stand up (again?)
>
> (Mack and Hickler, pp. 53–54)

As her depression deepened, death itself became for Vivienne
a kind of self-object with which she developed a personal relationship. She would personify death in various images. Following her
first serious suicide attempt, five months before she died, Vivienne
wrote in her journal:

> Death comes as in increasingly darkening face and unstrained
> thin breathing, which I am sure would soon die away altogether.
> Your head pounds painfully and in the mirror I had the privilege to
> see for myself what my dead face will look like immediately after
> the killing. Somehow this effect is much less upsetting than the first.
> Perhaps this is a sign that my prayers are being considered.
>
> (Mack and Hickler, p. 72)

This idea of suicide as a kind of self-murder recurs in the
suicidal ideation of other adolescents. The following passage was
written by a 16-year-old girl who made several serious suicide at-

tempts which brought her near to death. She kept a journal and wrote letters to her devoted therapist:

> I am struggling with the thoughts of seeing you again. You see one day I'm afraid that you'll turn me away—I think it will be better to leave good than bad. But I know if I leave now I would surely do murder on myself ... I swear I feel so trapped and I don't know what to do. When I got home today the least little thing put me in tears.
>
> (This example was provided by another adolescent's therapist, Dr. Elinor Weeks)

With the sensitive and heroic work of her therapist, this girl was alive and doing well two years later.

By the end of her life, Vivienne had come to be on intimate terms with suicide. She had transformed death from being a scary, dangerous threat, into an image of something beautiful, with which she was on friendly terms. Through increasingly dangerous suicidal experiments she overcame the fear of death and the natural barriers that most of us have to killing ourselves. The following passages are from a letter she wrote to John May 10 days before her death, which he received too late to save her:

> Even though I have gone over and over suicide in the last three months or so and developed what I would consider a logical and socially acceptable attitude on the matter, it all seemed to leave me in a second. I happened to be standing by my mirror. I looked at myself with a sort of wince, and then, almost mechanically, my hands stretched round my throat and centered in for what seemed a long while. And then the ringing in my ears stopped and everything became soft and hazy and I could just make out my head in the mirror, like a separate, bloated object. I started swaying (with no rhythm to it) and I fell into my bedpost and boxes on the floor etc. Unconsciously, I put out my hand to steady myself, and in so doing, started up my circulation. This in turn started me jolting uncontrollably, while still swaying I caught hold of the mirror and my jolts sent the mirror crashing against the wall. KRSHSH KRSHSH! again and again. As soon as I could I stopped it because it was so loud. Then I went through my sister's drawers til I found a long silk scarf. I tucked it up my sleeve so you couldn't tell that it was there and left a note by my bed that said something like "I didn't want you to think that it was because of you when it was only me all the time..." Then I walked three blocks to a public park.... I took out the scarf and wrapped it tightly around my neck and pulled as hard as I could—

I was standing in the shade in case car headlights should pick me up from the road. The first couple of times were like with the mirror (everything soft and hazy—the traffic would slowly fade away to nothing) and I would eventually fall. It was weird because I could see the glass on the ground, but I couldn't feel it at all. And then I would try to get up, but I would be jerking too spasmodically and it would take me several minutes—while at the time I was afraid somebody would come by.

Finally I got it so I was cutting off the air completely and not just the blood. But then my lungs would just about burst and I would let go. After a while I knew the whole thing was useless and rather despairingly resigned myself to all the many tomorrows looming up ahead of me. I said "goodnight" to the trees and ground around me and walked back home. My father asked me, "How was your walk— feel any better?" "Sure." "Yuh. . . Sometimes a little fresh air helps. . . " I could have screamed if I'd had the energy.

(Mack and Hickler, pp. 115–116)

The Contemporary Clinical Context: Precipitating Factors

In the contemporary clinical context I would include recent disturbing events, such as family moves, disappointments or hurts in relationships, and school failures. Vivienne's family was in the process of moving when she died. Furniture had been taken out and the old house looked empty and barren. Jerry Jacobs writes that some form of school failure or disappointment precedes a suicide in a high percentage of cases, especially in school systems which are harsh and provide a minimum of support (Jacobs, 1971).

The current clinical situation would also include specific biological influences, such as alcohol or drug intake. One 12–year-old boy killed himself after rejection by a girl. He had also been taking unknown amounts of mind-altering drugs under the influence of a group of older children. Viral illnesses can have a strong depression-inducing effect, though the mechanism of this is not well understood.

The balance or status of existing relationships affects the likelihood of suicide. Vivienne wrote often about how she felt under great emotional pressure from her parents, especially her mother, who turned to Vivienne with *her* problems. Several months before her death she wrote in a letter:

Mommy came to me for help. And I really have helped her whenever I could. But it puts a certain pressure on me; I'm not even fourteen yet, and Mommy's forty-eight. All the pressure and tension mounted up and I snapped. I decided that I couldn't be as perfect as I wanted and I had to have some outlet. I've been smoking grass since around January. I've gotten stoned often enough, but I never really enjoyed it. Usually I just get high enough to relax.

(Mack and Hickler, p. 83)

The availability of supports is of crucial importance, as, conversely, are minor hurts, rejections, and slights that occur in the days prior to the suicidal event. Small things can make a difference. Criticisms, or words taken as criticisms in passing encounters, can have a devastating effect, out of proportion to their actual importance. Psychotherapy can, of course, be helpful, but ineffectual treatment can be undermining, especially if the teenager and the family are led to believe that something useful is being done when actually it is not. Vivienne was receiving counseling, but it was a group counseling approach that was not working. She came to feel herself to be friendless. Three weeks before her suicide, she wrote a letter to Mr. May:

We are having counseling for the family. I know that I am probably the most destructive factor, but it's a little late for me to say that. Once you said you were glad I was born. Now I have my doubts about the whole thing. If I didn't have to worry about Mommy and Daddy, I wouldn't bother finishing this letter before I hung myself. But I have to stick with them. Sort of like one burden holding up another, which isn't too stable a thing to begin with. For one thing, I haven't got a single friend nearby. As a matter of fact, I have only one friend to speak of at all, and she lives in Belmont. With the gas shortage I see her solely at school.

(Mack and Hickler, p. 111)

Implications for Evaluation and Treatment

The architectural model described here has implications for the evaluation and treatment of a suicidal adolescent. It would lead us to place particular stress on the current life situation. A recent event, such as a move or a disappointment at school, may affect the balance of the teenager's emotional economy. We look especially for warning signals or clues—changes in the child's behavior, such as withdrawal from familiar interests, somatic complaints, changes in habits, expressions of suicidal ideation, and the other indicators that have been described so often in relation to adolescent suicide.

The psychodynamics of depression and suicide need to be evaluated, especially conflicts relating to self-esteem, which are demonstrated when the teenager focuses upon injuries to self-regard and expresses a feeling of low self-worth. We are learning to recognize a personality organization that may contribute to low self-regard. We look for overly hard superego elements, unrealistically exalted idealization, or ego ideal expectations, and evidence of an unusual degree of sensitivity to hurt and disappointment.

The assessment of available supports has to be made carefully. The most crucial support comes from people who are not only available but sensitive to the teenager's distress. These can include parents, family members, friends, neighbors, and, frequently, teachers. Family dynamics which would disturb the teenager's psychic balance need to be assessed, such as, in Vivienne's case, the burdening of the child with problems that the parents are facing. It is important to assess whether parents are living out psychological needs of their own in relation to the teenager and failing, thereby, to see the child's distress.

The relationship of the family with its community, the "fit" or alienation that is experienced, can play a role in the balance of psychological forces which may lead to suicide. Finally, the degree to which the case is known to the evaluator, or to the clinic or agency undertaking the evaluation, needs to be considered. If a patient is unknown, then greater caution and care should be taken to see that appropriate intervention takes place. If the case is known to the evaluator, or to another physician or mental health professional, assessment should be made of the degree to which a holding relationship exists, and the degree to which the teenager can be relied upon to report changes in his or her emotional state.

The choice of treatment grows out of the evaluation described above. It is important, when prescribing treatment for a suicidal adolescent, to pay attention to the total life context. It is crucial to involve the family, as Edward Shapiro and his group at McLean Hospital have described in a recent paper (Shapiro and Freedman, 1982). The object of therapy should be first to protect the child from the immediate risk of suicide. Sometimes this requires hospitalization, especially if the patient is unknown to the clinic. Outpatient treatment should be focused not only on struggles of the individual teenager. It is important to work with parents and other crucial adults so that distressing or emotionally hurtful forces in the child's key relationships can be offset, and family dynamics that undermine the adolescent's self-esteem can be understood. It is often important to involve the school, and for mental health professionals to work with teachers, so that they can become more sensitive to the distress signals that their pupils communicate.

Whether or not to hospitalize an adolescent is a particularly difficult decision. In addition to its protective function, the hospital environment can provoke regressive responses in teenagers. In the hospital, many weeks or months may be required to discover what is "going on" in a suicidal adolescent, which can be intensely disruptive to the child's on-going life experience. Nevertheless, hospitalization may be necessary in order to protect the teenager's life and to initiate a comprehensive treatment plan. When there are resources available for skilled psychodynamically oriented psychotherapy, work should be aimed at achieving significant personality change—a modification of superego harshness and unrealistic ego-ideal expectations, the development of greater ego capacity to bear emotional pain and disappointment, and an effort to repair, through the therapeutic relationship, the developmental injuries that underly the vulnerability to suicide.

Summary

I have proposed an architectural model comprising the elements to be considered in seeking to understand suicidal individuals. Although derived initially from the biographical study of an adolescent girl who killed herself, the model has been helpful in examining other adolescent and adult suicidal cases, and may have wider utility in the understanding and treating of suicidal patients in the total context of their lives.

The elements of the model or system comprise the macrocosm or sociopolitical context; genetic–biological vulnerability; early developmental influences; personality organization and self-esteem regulation; object relationships, past and current; evidences of clinical depression and other psychopathology; the ontogeny of the relationship to death; and the contemporary situation and circumstances at the time of clinical assessment.

Some of the implications of this model for evaluation and treatment have been discussed. It is hoped, further, that by linking the sociopolitical or broader contextual elements—which affect the incidence of suicide—with the biological and psychological forces that create the vulnerability to suicide, this model may prove to be applicable to the understanding of its epidemiology and to the challenge of its prevention.

References

Applebaum A, Holzman S: The color-shading response and suicide. Journal of Projective Techniques 26:155–161, 1962

Ash S: Suicide and the hidden executioner. International Review of Psychoanalysis 25:51–60, 1980

Bassuk L, Schoonover C, Gill D: Lifelines: Clinical Perspectives on Suicide. New York, Plenum Press, 1982

Becker E: The Denial of Death. New York, The Free Press, 1973

Bergman P, Escalona SK: Unusual sensitivities in very young children. Psychoanal Study Child 34:333–352, 1949

Brown L, Ebert MH, Goyer TS, et al: Aggression, suicide and serotonin: relationships to cerebrospinal fluid amine metabolites. Am J Psychiatry 139:741–746, 1982

Camus A: The Myth of Sisyphus: And Other Essays. New York, Alfred A. Knopf, 1955

Eisenberg L: Adolescent suicide: on taking arms against a sea of troubles. Pediatrics 66:315–320, 1980

Friedman P (Ed.): On Suicide: Discussions of the Vienna Psychoanalytic Society—1910. New York, International Universities Press, 1967

Jacobs J: Adolescent Suicide. New York, Wiley, 1971

Jacobson E: The Self and the Object World. New York, International Universities Press, 1964

Kohut H: The Analysis of the Self. New York, International Universities Press, 1971

Kohut H: The Restoration of the Self. New York, International Universities Press, 1977

Lifton RJ: The Broken Connection: On Death and the Continuity of Life. New York, Simon & Schuster, 1979

Mack JE: Psychoanalysis and biography: a narrowing gap. Journal of the Philadelphia Association for Psychoanalysis 5:97–109, 1978

Mack JE: Alcoholism, A.A., and the governance of the self, in Dynamic Approaches to the Understanding and Treatment of Alcoholism. Edited by Bean MH, Zinberg NE. New York, The Free Press, 1981

Mack JE, Hickler H: Vivienne: The Life and Suicide of an Adolescent Girl. Boston, Little, Brown, 1981

Maltsberger JT: Certain disturbances of reality sense in suicidal patients. Paper presented at course on suicide, The Essence of Dynamic Clinical Work. Cambridge MA, Department of Psychiatry, Harvard Medical School, January 28, 1983

Maltsberger JT, Buie DH: The devices of suicide: revenge, riddance, and rebirth. International Review of Psychoanalysis 7:61–72, 1980

Meissner WW: Psychoanalytic notes on suicide. Int J Psychoanal Psychother 6:415–447, 1977

Meissner WW: Suicide and the paranoid process. Paper presented at course on Suicide: The Essence of Dynamic Clinical Work. Cambridge MA, Department of Psychiatry, Harvard Medical School, January 28, 1983

National Center for Health Statistics: Deaths and death rates for suicide. Mortality Statistics Branch, Division of Vital Statistics, 1978

Newsweek: West Germany: suicidal course. March 8, 1976

Newsweek: Teenage Suicide. August 28, 1978

New York Times: Series of Mendham student deaths troubles classmates. June 16, 1979

Nin A: The Diary of Anais Nin, vol. 1 (1931–1934). New York, Harcourt, Brace and World, 1966

Offer D, Ostrov E, Howard KI: The Adolescent: A Psychological Self-Portrait. New York, Basic Books, 1981

Orgell S: Fusion with the victim and suicide. Int J Psychoanal 55:531–538, 1974

Robins E: The Final Months. New York, Oxford Universities Press, 1981

Rochlin G: Griefs and Discontents: The Forces of Change. Boston, Little, Brown, 1965

Schulsinger F, Kety SS, Rosenthal D, et al: A family study of suicide, in Origin, Prevention and Treatment of Affective Disorders. Edited by Schou M, Stromgren E. London and New York, Academic Press, 1979

Shapiro ER, Freedman J: Family dynamics of adolescent suicide. Paper presented at the Annual Meeting of the American Psychoanalytic Association, December, 1982

Time: Suicide belt: rates up for affluent teenagers. September 1, 1980

Yalom ID: Existential Psychotherapy. New York, Basic Books, 1980

Zetzel ER: On the incapacity to bear depression, in The Capacity for Emotional Growth. Edited by Zetzel ER. New York, International Universities Press, 1970

Chapter 4

GENETIC RISK FACTORS FOR THE AFFECTIVE DISORDERS

Theodore Reich, M.D.
John Rice, Ph.D.
Joe Mullaney, B.A.

Chapter 4

GENETIC RISK FACTORS FOR THE AFFECTIVE DISORDERS

The tendency of the affective disorders to aggregate in families has been viewed as an important characteristic by many classical and modern authors. Attempts to measure the frequency of these disorders in the relatives of affected individuals, however, has produced extremely variable results. Generally, a prominent family effect has been reported, especially for severe forms in younger individuals, but the frequency, distribution, and polarity of secondary cases has fluctuated greatly. This is not surprising since diagnostic criteria, methods of ascertainment, and survey techniques of different studies have seldom been comparable, and it has never been clear whether variable results were a consequence of disparate research techniques or a property of the populations being surveyed (Reich et al., 1982).

For the past two decades, family and population studies have become increasingly standardized. Explicit, unambigious criteria for

This study was supported in part by grants MH–25430, AA-03539(ARC), MH–31302(CRC), and MH–37685.

This work was completed with the participation of the collaborative program investigators: G.L. Klerman, M.D. (Chairperson) (Boston); R.M.A. Hirshfeld, M.D. (Project Director and Co-Chairperson), and B.H. Larkin, B.A. (Coordinating Protocol Monitor) (NIMH); M.B. Keller, M.D. and P. Lavori, Ph.D. (Boston); J. Fawcett, M.D. and W.A. Scheftner, M.D. (Chicago); N.C. Andreasen, M.D., W. Coryell, M.D., G. Winokur, M.D., and P. Wasek, B.A. (Iowa City); J. Endicott, Ph.D. and P. McDonald-Scott, M.A. (New York); J. Rice, Ph.D., S. Guze, M.D., T. Reich, M.D., and D. Altis, B.A. (St. Louis). Other contributors include: P.J. Clayton, M.D., J. Croughan, M.D., M.M. Katz, Ph.D., E. Robins, M.D., R.W. Shapiro, M.D., and R. Spitzer, M.D.

diagnosis have been developed, carefully calibrated interview schedules have been produced, and uniform methods of ascertainment have been implemented, so that a growing body of data is available for quantitative description and hypothesis testing (Weissman et al., 1982; Coryell et al., 1981). Even at this early stage, some generalizations seem acceptable; for example, relatives of patients with bipolar illness are more likely to be affected with both bipolar and unipolar disorder than relatives of patients with unipolar forms (Reich et al., 1982); relatives of individuals with an early onset of unipolar illness are at greater risk than relatives of patients with a later onset (Weissman et al., 1984); the tendency for females to be more frequently affected is greater for unipolar illness than for the bipolar form (Rice et al., 1984); and, assortative mating is generally present (Merikangas et al., 1983).

The Heterogeneity Problem

Many different affective syndromes have been delineated using clinical and family characteristics. In some cases, the subforms were identified by hypothetical causal factors such as the endogenous, nonendogenous, or reactive subgroups; in other cases, clinical symptoms were used as a criterion (for example, psychotic or incapacitating subgroups). In an unpublished study, Andreasen and colleagues report that familial distributions of secondary cases using subforms as proband diagnoses have not generally supported this separation. Recent research, however, has shown that the immediate relatives of probands with psychotic illness are at greater risk than comparable relatives of nonpsychotic probands, suggesting that psychotic affective disorders are more closely related to familial factors than are nonpsychotic forms (Leckman et al., 1984; Coryell et al., in press).

The observation that unipolar and bipolar forms of affective disorder tend to aggregate in different families led to the hypothesis that they are different disorders (Leonhard et al., 1962). The separation was incomplete, since relatives of bipolar probands also manifested an excess of unipolar disorders. Since bipolar illness also has an earlier age of onset, more frequent episodes, and differential response to lithium salts, its separate categorization was more strongly based than other subdivisions of nonbipolar forms of the illness (Winokur et al., 1969).

Unipolar depression frequently occurs during the course of other nonaffective psychiatric disorders suggesting the category "secondary unipolar depression." Preliminary studies of the distribution of familial affective disorders in probands with primary and secondary nonbipolar affective disorder suggests their unity with respect to familial transmission (Rice et al., 1984).

It seems likely that the affective disorders are groups of conditions rather than a single entity, so that attempts to discover underlying causes may be greatly enhanced by improved nosology. Several excellent strategies for dealing with the "heterogeneity problem" are provided by family studies. If it can be assumed that the underlying mechanisms in closely related individuals are similar, then affected relatives should be more alike with respect to psychosocial or biological variables responsible for the familial aggregation. Similarly, different subforms of the illness that tend to aggregate in the same families are more likely to be caused by similar combinations of factors than forms which aggregate in different families. Family studies may therefore help to discover increasingly homogeneous clinical entities. Using multiple "thresholds" to model diagnosis, Gershon and colleagues (1982) concluded that schizoaffective disorder, bipolar affective disorder (I and II), and unipolar depression are all parts of the same normally distributed liability vector; that is, they are different degrees of the same underlying process. Their conclusions were based on a large study, conducted over many years, of the families of affected and unaffected subjects. In reviewing these results, the data are most supportive of the unity of the bipolar and schizoaffective forms of the illness. The number of families of probands with unipolar illness is relatively small, and the unity of the unipolar with the bipolar form is therefore less certain (Gershon et al., 1982).

Genetic Factors

Mendelwicz and colleagues studied adult bipolar patients who had been given up for adoption early in life. Personal interviews with the biological and adoptive parents of these probands was compared with interviews of the parents of several control groups. This study conclusively showed that bipolar illness could be transmitted from parent to offspring even if they had been separated early in life by extrafamilial adoption, offering strong support for genetic transmission (Mendelwicz and Rainer, 1977). A similar conclusion was reported by Cadoret in a small sample that also included subjects with unipolar depressive illness (Cadoret, 1978). Further support for the presence of genetic factors has been reported by Kety, who studied a Danish population of adoptees. These data indicate an excess of suicide in the biological relatives of adoptees with affective disorder or other psychiatric disorders leading to suicide (Kety, 1979).

Von Knorring and colleagues conducted a full cross-fostering study of parents and offspring who had been separated by extra-familial adoption in a Swedish population. This study showed that genetic factors played some role in the familial transmission of unipolar depression, but these factors were weak and relatively nonspecific (Van Knorring et al., 1983).

Goodwin and his associates studied the adopted-away sons and daughters of Danish alcoholics. Information was available about the prevalence of affective disorder in the adoptees as well as their adoptive parents. A sample of nonadopted daughters of alcoholic biological parents was also studied. In these studies, the affective disorder that occurred in adopted and nonadopted offspring seemed unrelated to having a biological alcoholic parent. This suggests that nongenetic factors are responsible for the increased frequency of affective disorder in the daughters of alcoholic parents (Goodwin, 1985).

Taken together, the adoption studies support the view that genetic as well as nongenetic factors can be responsible for the familial aggregation of the affective disorders. The way in which these factors interact with individual nonfamilial variables is unknown.

Additional support for the presence of genetic factors is available from studies of monozygotic and dizygotic twins. These studies have generally found that concordance for the affected disorders was greater in monozygotic than in same sex dizygotic twin pairs, suggesting the presence of genetic factors. The recent study of Bertleson also included polarity. These data suggest that genetic factors are most prominent in bipolar affective disorders and that a bipolar genotype sometimes manifests as unipolar depressive illness (Bertleson et al., 1977).

The relationship between bipolar and unipolar disorder is complicated by the observation that patients with unipolar affective disorder may switch polarity, developing the bipolar form of illness.

In patient samples, the rate of switch in polarity has been quite variable, but is approximately 20 percent within approximately six years after the onset of a depressive disorder (Akiskal et al., 1983). It should be noted that bipolar and unipolar probands and their relatives ought to be followed prospectively to determine whether switches in polarity make the families increasingly homogeneous or increasingly different as time passes.

Genetic Linkage

The discovery of close segregation, within a pedigree, of a well characterized genetic marker and a disorder of unknown etiology such as affective disorder would provide powerful evidence for the presence of a genetic factor. Furthermore, a major genetic locus for the disease, situated on a chromosome close to the gene for the genetic marker, would be established. The discovery of genetic linkage is most likely to occur in large pedigrees with many ill members, where cosegregation can be most easily detected.

Several large pedigrees supporting genetic linkage of bipolar illness with color blindness have been reported, but these results have not been adequately confirmed (Reich et al., 1982). Similarly, recent reports of genetic linkage between HLA (histocompatibility antigen) and affective disorder have been reported, but these reports have not been confirmed after careful study. As with other attempts to clarify the familial transmission of these disorders, careful attention to diagnosis may ultimately explain contradictory results. Improved estimates of age of onset, secular trends, and penetrance factors may also clarify seemingly contradictory results (Suarez and Reich, 1984).

Recently, Kidd and colleagues have reported genetic linkage among several markers on the short arm of chromosome 11 and affective disorders in a large Amish kindred. Although not statistically confirmed, the results are suggestive and further research is necessary (Egeland et al., 1984).

Biological Correlates

The identification of specific genetic mechanisms would be greatly enhanced if biological correlates of individual vulnerability could be found. These biological markers would be extremely useful,

whether or not they were a measure of an underlying genetic diathesis, since they could be used to more carefully subdivide affected
and unaffected individuals and their relatives. New phenotypes could
be defined, which include both clinical as well as biological information, and the possibility of demonstrating a unitary etiology would
be advanced. Several neuroendocrine variables distinguish individuals with affective disorders from controls. In addition, neuroendocrine studies have suggested the separation of endogenomorphic
from other types of unipolar depression. These findings, however,
seem to be state dependent, and their relationship to familial illness
is not well characterized (Carroll et al., 1976; Carroll et al., 1981;
Rush et al., 1982).

Neurophysiological approaches to patients with the major affective disorders have shown characteristic sleep pattern disturbances in subjects with affective disorders. Reduced amounts of slow
wave sleep and reduction in REM latency are present in individuals
with severe depression. The extent to which these variables define
an underlying specific familial defect is unknown (Kupfer, 1976;
Kupfer et al., 1976; Kupfer et al., 1980).

Abnormalities of lithium transport across red blood cell membranes have been described in the families of bipolar patients, and
this abnormality may reflect a biological marker for the genetic
diathesis of bipolar illness. Severe affective disorder in the families
of patients with bipolar illness were most closely associated with
this biological finding (Dorus et al., 1983).

Nadi and colleagues has recently reported that fibroblasts taken
from bipolar patients and their affected and unaffected relatives
could be studied in tissue culture, and that the frequency of muscarinic receptors on these cells is increased in a majority of probands and their ill relatives. Since the tissue is several generations
of cells removed from subjects, it is less likely to be influenced by
treatment and other experimental bias which may occur when biological studies are conducted in affected individuals (Nadi et al.,
1984).

Wright and colleagues have also studied biological material
from bipolar patients and their relatives in tissue culture. These
workers used lymphoblastoid cell lines produced using Epstein-
Barr virus to transform lymphocytes. The beta–2–adrenoceptors
were studied on the lymphoblastoid cell membranes. They reported
that a subgroup of bipolar probands and their ill relatives had a
decreased density of these receptors when compared with controls

(Wright et al., 1984). Both of the receptor studies include a relatively small number of informative families, and they require replication.

Psychosocial Correlates

The identification of psychosocial correlates of the affective disorders presents an opportunity for studying important familial and nonfamilial risk factors. As with biological markers, family studies can be used to study the relationship between psychosocial factors and familial transmission. On the one hand, for example, personality characteristics such as introversion, neuroticism, and obsessionality may be correlated with preclinical vulnerability; and on the other hand, life events may provide a clue to factors that lead to the onset of an episode (Hirshfeld and Klerman, 1979). Alternatively, reactivity to life events may define a separate familial disorder, perhaps different from a nonreactive form. Similarly, personal resources may define a threshold beyond which symptomatology manifests. To date, scant data are available that attempt to relate psychosocial variables and the familial distribution of the affective disorders. Not only can studies of psychosocial stressors compliment biological marker studies, but they may well delineate nosologically important subcategories for biological study.

Pollitt (1972) and Akiskal and McKinney (1975) have advanced diathesis-stress models for the affective disorders, which include specific types of organic and psychological precipitating factors in susceptible individuals. Pollitt found that severe viral or bacterial infections and, to a lesser extent, severe psychological stress, were associated with a lower morbidity risk for depression in relatives compared with patients with either no psychological stress or with doubtful psychological stress. Postpartum cases were most like those whose onset seemed spontaneous. The kind of affective disorder that occurred in the relatives was not specified. These studies suggest a greater genetic vulnerability for individuals whose illness does not follow a major stressor. It is hoped that future studies of biological and psychosocial markers will be conducted on the same families, so that important interactions can be detected.

Secular Trends

Using carefully standardized interview schedules and standard diagnostic criteria, several large-scale epidemiological and family studies have reported that the population and familial distribution of the affective disorders has been changing during the past 40 or 50 years. It appears that the age of onset of major depressive disorder is decreasing, especially in persons born since World War II. Furthermore, the frequency of illness in younger persons has been increasing, so that the rate of affective disorder in the general population of individuals currently 20 to 30 years old is far greater than the rate in individuals who are 50 to 60 years old (Weissman et al., 1984). In addition, the sex ratio of affected individuals has been changing so that, among most recently born cohorts, the excess of affected females is diminished. The magnitude of the secular trend is very large, and although it may be due to some unappreciated artifact of experimental design, similar trends in suicide rates suggest that the "cohort effect" is real (Klerman et al., in press; Robins et al., 1984; Weissman and Myers, 1978). Since the effect is observed in general populations and in families of affected individuals, it seems likely that the increase is occurring in susceptible individuals rather than randomly in the general population.

Models of Transmission

In order to test hypotheses about the familial transmission of affective disorders, individual variation must be taken into account. Variable age of onset, severity, and sex-specific frequencies all must be included along with prominent secular trends. The presence of assortative mating and maternal effects further complicates the endeavor.

Models of transmission should include these individual and population variables, so that the distribution of cases in families and comparable populations can be realistically characterized and its elements understood.

The field of "genetic epidemiology" is a rapidly developing branch of clinical genetics, which studies the familial transmission of common illnesses such as the affective disorders. Models are being developed that include polygenic background variation, cultural transmission, and environmental effects common to siblings. Transmission from parent to offspring can include both genetic and nongenetic mechanisms, so that predictions about the risk to an offspring can be made without unwarranted or premature assumptions about the cause of familial aggregation. The way in which major genes behave against a complex background of polygenic and cultural factors is also being studied, so that the conditions under which a major gene could be detected may be found. Informative studies could then be optimally designed. The hope of researchers involved in this work is to provide an organizing structure for the integration of clinical, biological, and psychosocial data in a framework that permits hypotheses to be tested (Morton, 1982).

Genetic epidemiologists are also developing several novel approaches to the heterogeneity problem. Included among these is the "extended pedigree method," in which studies about mode of transmission are conducted on single large kindreds where unitary transmission is more likely. Nonparametric methods, which do not require presumptions about underlying distributions are also being used to minimize the dependence of transmission models on untestable assumptions (Karlin et al., 1981). Finally, several groups are developing methods for combining multiple measurements into an index which can then be used as a measure of underlying genetic or nongenetic variation. The construction of indices may prove to be most useful in studying psychiatric disorders where many complex correlated measurements are often made (Morton et al., 1983).

Prediction of Risk in Susceptible Individuals

Family studies offer an excellent opportunity for combining measurements on related individuals so that the vulnerability of unaffected family members who have not passed the age of risk can be quantified. The types of measurements suitable for this purpose include diagnosis with or without a correlated biological or psychosocial variable. More than one measurement may be made per individual, and categorical as well as quantitative measures can be combined. The vulnerability of young, unaffected family members based on pedigree information can then be used to predict an age-specific risk for the onset of a disorder. This type of analysis serves to define high and low risk individuals who can then be studied prospectively. The prediction of risk must take into account the total number of relatives studied, the number of ill relatives, and the degree of relationship of these relatives to the person at risk. Appropriate corrections for family size and composition must be made, so that risk figures to junior members of different families can be compared.

Several transmission models have been developed in genetic epidemiology; in this chapter an example is given, illustrating one approach to the projection of risk. Only a single diagnosis per individual is included, and the method is being extended to include multiple measurements.

Estimating risk to an unaffected individual requires the fitting of a "transmission model" to a body of family data. First, we are required to measure the various parameters of the model, and then the model can be used to make predictions about the risk to a specific individual in a subsequent study. Usually risks are projected for siblings or offspring who are then studied prospectively. The method is validated by determining whether the risks are realized at follow-up.

The Multifactorial Model of Disease Transmission

The multifactorial model of disease transmission is appropriate for computing correlations among groups of related individuals when assumptions cannot be made about the extent to which familial transmission is caused by genetic factors. This model assumes that all genetic and environmental influences can be combined additively into a single variable termed "the liability to develop the disorder." The liability is assumed to be normally distributed, or can be transformed into a normal distribution, and is truncated by one or more thresholds that divide individuals into affected and unaffected classes (Reich et al., 1972). In the model presented here, the liability of a family of size n is assumed to be distributed as an n–variate normal. Separate liability distributions are assumed for males and females, and age specific population frequencies define the position of the thresholds. More deviant thresholds are used to model age groups in which the disorder is less common.

Typically, data is collected from the study of affected individuals (probands) and their relatives. Probands and relatives are grouped according to their sex and relationship as displayed in Table 1. Traditionally, this grouped data was used along with separate estimates of population prevalences to determine correlations among relatives.

Currently, a method for computing correlations, "segregation analysis," is used to estimate correlations among related individuals (Reich et al., 1979). In this case, the distribution of families rather than groups of related individuals are used as data. Variable family size is taken into account and each family is treated as a separate data point. Correlations estimated by segregation analysis have smaller standard errors, and this method does not require a separate estimate of the population prevalence.

Construction of Transmission Model

In order to make an inference about the risk to an unaffected individual, measurements on many classes of related individuals must be combined; hence, a transmission model is required. The TAU model of disease transmission (Rice et al., 1978; Rice et al., 1980a; Rice et al., 1980b; Rice et al., 1981) constructed with "path analysis" is used here. A path diagram of the model is displayed in Figure 1.

In this model, the sex-specific liability of each individual (X) is divided into a transmissible (T) and a nontransmissible (E) portions. The transmissible portion includes both genetic and cultural factors. The nontransmissible portion includes nonfamilial and environmental sources of variation as well as measurement error. The correlation between mates (m) is the consequence of assortative mating for the phenotypic liability score (X). The portion of the liability which is due to transmissible factors is (t^2). The extent to which transmissible elements are transmitted from parent to offspring is labelled τ in the diagram. In Figure 1, two offspring are shown, and nonfamilial and environmental effects common to siblings (c) are included. If the transmissible factors were entirely polygenic, then the value of τ would be one-half, since parents and offspring share one-half of their genes. If transmission is also due to cultural factors, then τ may take on other values. In the analysis which follows, the value of τ is fixed at one-half for computational simplicity. Likewise, sex-specific common environmental factors may be included; however, in this preliminary analysis, it was assumed that the environmental factors common to siblings were equal for male, female, and opposite sex siblings.

The TAU model just described includes only six parameters that must be estimated. These are (t) for each sex, (m)(c), and the male and female prevalences. In segregation analysis an attempt is made to find the value of these six parameters, which provide the closest fit of the model to the data. An optimization procedure,

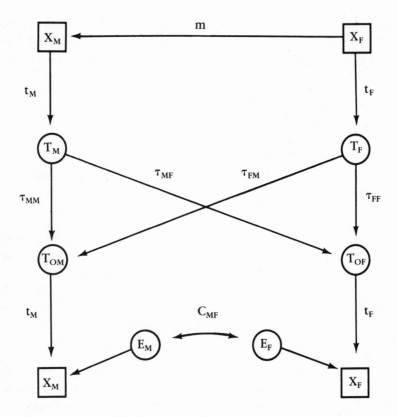

Figure 1. Path diagram of the transmission of complex (genetic and nongenetic) factors from parents to offspring when a sex-dimorphism is present. The subscripts M and F refer to sex of each individual; the subscript O refers to offspring; other subscripts are defined in the text.

which uses maximum likelihood statistics, produces the values of the underlying model that most closely resembles the data.

The Prediction of Risk

In order to predict the risk to a junior member of a particular family, age, sex, and relationship specific correlations must be computed among all members. In large families, the number of such correlations increases rapidly, since each individual family member must be correlated with all the others. Fortunately, the value of these correlations can be computed quickly from the TAU model, and the unique correlational structure represented by each family can then be used to calculate the risk to a junior member. This method does not require that all members of the pedigree be included, and missing observations present no problems. In the application described here, only relatives who had been personally interviewed were used to estimate the parameters of the TAU model. However, computer programs are being developed that combine family history and interview data, taking into account the relative inefficiency of family history information.

The Familial Transmission of Major Depressive Disorder

The National Collaborative Study of Depression–Clinical is a large multicenter family and follow-up study of a stratified random sample of probands with major depressive disorder, their spouses, and first degree relatives. The study includes approximately 1,000 probands who are being followed biannually. An extensive battery of personal interview and psychological test schedules were given at intake. A single personal interview was conducted on available first degree relatives and spouses of approximately 600 probands (Katz et al., 1979). This report is based on diagnostic information from the Schedule for the Affective Disorders and Schizophrenias interview (SADS–L) personally administered to probands, relatives, and spouses. Research Diagnostic Criteria (RDC) were used in the diagnosis of major depressive disorder (Spitzer et al., 1978). Relatives younger than 18 years were not interviewed. This report is based on personal interviews of 475 probands with a diagnosis of major depressive disorder, and 1,735 first degree relatives and spouses. The data are preliminary and the full sample may be somewhat different.

The lifetime frequency of major depressive disorder in relatives and spouses of probands with major depressive disorder is displayed in Table 1. There is a prominent sex effect in that female relatives are more frequently affected than male relatives, and the number of female probands is greater. The frequency of illness in the relatives of male and female probands is similar.

All probands, by definition, were ill at intake; however, most affected relatives had been ill prior to their interview and were then in remission.

In keeping with other studies, the rates of illness were lower in older relatives than in their younger counterparts. Because of

Table 1. Illness in Relatives of Probands with Major Depressive Disorder (Percent)

	Male Probands N = 184				Female Probands N = 291			
	N	Major Depressive Disorder	Other Diagnosis	Never Ill	N	Major Depressive Disorder	Other Diagnosis	Never Ill
Father	88	21.6	25.0	53.4	89	15.7	42.7	41.6
Mother	112	33.9	21.4	44.6	149	31.5	21.5	47.0
Brother	121	26.4	32.2	41.3	223	25.1	28.2	46.6
Sister	150	41.3	21.3	37.3	294	42.5	19.4	38.1
Son	30	33.3	23.3	43.3	103	27.2	31.1	41.7
Daughter	43	25.6	34.9	39.5	100	35.0	26.0	39.0
Spouse	95	46.3	17.9	35.8	138	19.6	35.5	44.9

Table 2. Parameters of the Tau Model of Disease Transmission for Major Depressive Disorder

R_{mate}	.18
t_{male}	.58
t_{female}	.74
τ^*	.50
c	.06

*Parameter fixed at .50

this strong secular trend, a complex age-specific population prevalence function was defined during segregation analysis. That is, we used the distribution of families in our data to estimate the population frequency of illness for individuals of different ages. For males, the expected lifetime population frequency for persons 18 to 19 years old was approximately one percent; 11 percent for persons between 19 and 63 years old; and for persons older than 63 years, approximately two percent. For females, the rate was approximately 11 percent for persons younger than 23 years, 28 percent for persons between 23 and 46, and 18 percent for persons older than 46 years. The age-specific rate in males under age 19 and over age 63 was based on very few observations; however, the other estimates are based on large numbers.

In the segregation analysis reported here, age of onset was not used. The reason for omitting this important variable was that the relationship between age of onset and familial distribution of illness has not yet been successfully modeled in the presence of strong secular trends. Instead, age-specific lifetime frequencies are used to "age adjust" the data.

The parameters of the TAU model of disease transmission, which were found by segregation analysis, are displayed in Table 2. It can be seen that the transmissibility of the disorder is less in males than in females, and that assortative mating is present. Environmental effects common to siblings are present, but the value of this correlation (c) is small and not significantly different from zero. The parameter τ was fixed at the value of one-half and was not searched on during segregation analysis.

Using path analysis of the segregation distribution in our data, the proportion of the variance accounted for by transmissible factors in females is 0.55 and in males is 0.34; a significant difference. The

Table 3.   Lifetime Risk for Major Depressive Disorder to an Unaffected Son
or Daughter Who is Early in the Period of Risk

Affectational Status of		Risk to	
Father	Mother	Son	Daughter
+	+	.35	.64
−	+	.24	.47
+	−	.23	.45
−	−	.13	.27

+ or − indicates an affected or unaffected parent.

assortative mating parameter (m) was significantly different from
zero.

Risk Prediction For Small and Large Pedigrees

The lifetime risk for affective disorder to a young unaffected member of a family was computed as a function of the affectional status,
age, and sex of each individual in the family. For computational
purposes it was assumed that the prediction was made when offspring were early in the period of risk, and it was also assumed
that the population prevalence for the lifetime risk of illness to these
junior individuals was 35 percent in females and 17.5 percent in
males.

The lifetime risk to a son or daughter is computed as a function
of the affectional status of each parent, without information on
other members of the family (Table 3). Even this simple family—
that is, two parents and either a son or daughter—requires five sex-
specific correlations to compute the risks in Table 3. The correlations are calculated as a function of the parameters of the TAU model
displayed in Table 2.

In Table 3, it can be seen that the risk to sons is less than the
risk to daughters when the affectional status of the parents is the
same. Subdividing families in this fashion provides a wide range of
risks that can be used in prospective studies. When only data is
available on parents, however, the number of risk classes is small,
reducing the utility of these small families.

When taking a family history, information may be available from
the extended maternal and paternal sides of a family. Usually, interviewing several family members yields good information about
the presence or absence of illness in the nuclear family of a proband

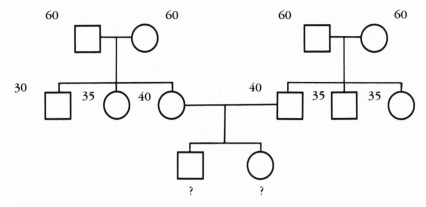

Figure 2. Hypothetical two generation pedigree used to predict lifetime risk to junior members of a third generation. Numbers refer to current ages of family members. Affectational status is given in Table 4.

and the nuclear family of the proband's spouse. In Figure 2, two small nuclear families, each consisting of five members related by marriage, are included. The risk to either a son or daughter has been calculated. In this hypothetical pedigree, the father and mother were assumed to have one brother and sister, although in many families, larger pedigree structures are available.

In order to calculate the risks to the son or daughter in Figure 2, 44 predicted correlations were calculated using the parameters of the TAU model. These include correlations among remote inlaws as well as nuclear family members. Sex-specific grandparent–grandchild correlations are also required. The risk for major depression is displayed in Table 4 as a function of the affectational status and age of family members. For computational simplicity the pedigree structure was kept constant, but the presence or absence of illness was changed to illustrate the full range of risks that may occur.

Only a small sample of the total number of possible risks are displayed. The range of risks for sons is between 0.1 and 0.57, and for daughters is between 0.21 and 0.86. The risk is maximal when all family members are affected and minimal when all are unaffected. As before, the risk to sons is less than the risk to daughters, and the large number of risk classes provides a wide range of high and low risk subjects. Comparing Table 4 with Table 3, it can be seen that the range of risks is greater in the larger pedigree than in the smaller. In addition, the larger pedigree provides more classes of risk. Accordingly, the addition of information about other members

Table 4. Lifetime Risk for Major Depressive Disorder to a Young Unaffected Son or Daughter Who is Early in the Period of Risk

Maternal					Paternal					Risk to	
Grandfather	Grandmother	Aunt	Uncle	Mother	Grandfather	Grandmother	Aunt	Uncle	Father	Son	Daughter
+	+	+	+	+	+	+	+	+	+	.57	.86
−	+	+	+	+	−	+	+	+	+	.49	.80
−	+	+	−	+	−	+	−	−	+	.42	.72
−	+	−	+	+	−	+	+	−	+	.36	.65
+	+	+	−	+	−	+	+	−	−	.35	.65
−	+	+	−	+	−	−	−	−	−	.27	.52
−	−	−	−	+	−	+	+	−	−	.24	.47
−	+	+	+	−	−	+	+	−	−	.22	.44
−	−	+	−	−	−	−	−	−	−	.15	.31
−	−	−	−	−	−	−	−	−	−	.10	.21

+ or − refers to the affectional status of relatives.

Lifetime population prevalence for major affective disorder for junior members is assumed to be 0.35 for family and 0.175 for mates.

of the pedigree has increased the specificity of the predictions.

Using the risk figures displayed in Tables 3 and 4, as well as many which are not displayed, some general conclusions can be drawn about the relationship between the status of family members and risk. The status of female family members has a greater effect on the risk to offspring than male members of equal relationship. Having affected relatives on maternal and paternal sides amplifies the risk when compared with families in which affected members occur only on one side. The sex effect in the risk to the offspring is most prominent for families that include many affected relatives. Finally, more closely related family members have a greater impact on the prediction of risk than more remote relatives.

Comment

The prediction of risk in susceptible individuals based on the status, age, and sex of first and second degree family members requires many assumptions. In the analysis described here, it was assumed that age-specific lifetime frequencies determined the threshold in an underlying liability distribution. Follow-up studies, however, would be required to test the accuracy of the risks, providing validation for the approach. Several interview studies of the offspring and siblings of probands with affective disorder are underway so that validation of this approach will be available.

The identification of high and low risk subjects based on pedigree information offers an excellent opportunity for studying the influence of psychosocial and biological correlates. To the extent that the subjects are young and unaffected, initial measurements can be made prior to the onset of illness. The relationship between such measurements and the later development of an affective disorder may well be definitive in identifying etiological variables. It should be noted that the risks to siblings of affected individuals in high density families are the consequence of both transmissible factors (including genetic factors) and nontransmissible factors that amplify the correlation among siblings (common sibling environment). Accordingly, variables that are predictive of the onset in siblings may be different from variables that are predictive of the onset in offspring.

The major drawback of a follow-up of high and low risk offspring is the long duration required to realize the predicted risk.

Fortunately, the risks themselves can be used as the correlates with biological and psychosocial variables. This may be accomplished in several ways. The risks may either be graded as quantitative liability scores so that a mean and variance could be attached to each class of high or low risk subjects. Or, susceptible subjects could be ranked accordingly to the risks, and these ranks used as "risk scores." In either case, the estimate of risk might be correlated with other measurements, and the discovery of a strong relationship between a particular psychosocial or biological measure and risk of illness would be an important first step in the direct measurement of underlying transmissible factors.

The use of ranks as correlates rather than as quantitative scores has the advantage of being robust if some of the assumptions of the underlying model are not met. Gene environment interactions may thus be detected even if they have a nonlinear relationship to risk. An added advantage of the use of ranks is that the outcome is less dependent on prior estimates of the population frequency, which are often most difficult to obtain and least accurate when compared with the frequency of illness in family members.

It should be remembered that biological and psychosocial correlates may predict the onset of an episode even if they are not correlated with the vulnerability score of an individual based on the status of family members. This can occur when these correlates are a measure of individual nonfamilial variation (that is, random individual environment), which also accounts for a large measure of variability in male as well as female subjects. Genetic epidemiologists have developed methods for combining several measures into indices that may well improve the assessment of underlying familial and nonfamilial variables.

Contemporary models of the familial transmission of complex disorders, such as major depressive disorder, do not usually include secular trends. Furthermore, variable age of onset usually represents nonfamilial random variation, so that affected individuals of the same age whose ages of onset differ have the same average liability score (Thompson and Weissman, 1981; Heinbuch et al., 1980; Risch, 1983). Recent analyses published by Weissman et al. (1984) indicate that the risk for affective disorder to a relative is a function of the age of onset of the proband. In these data, onset prior to the age of 20 greatly increased the risk to relatives, suggesting that the liability of early onset cases was greater than late onset forms. Models of familial transmission, which include secular trends and age of onset functions that may or may not be correlated with liability, are being explored. In addition, transmission parameters themselves may be a function of the age or cohort of birth of family members, and new approaches to these complex time dependent variables are being devised. A deeper understanding of the relationship between cohort of birth, age of onset, and familial transmission will modify the prediction of risk using pedigree data.

The correlational structure described here was based on a single diagnosis per individual. Computer programs are being developed so that several correlated diagnoses can be included for each individual; and, to the extent that they share underlying transmissible factors, the risk to relatives may be further specified. An example of the combined approach might be the joint use of information about alcoholism and major depressive disorder to predict the risk for major depressive disorder, alcoholism, or both in susceptible offspring. Similarly, complex pedigrees, which include nondiagnostic information such as personality or biological variables, could be used along with diagnosis to increase the accuracy of prediction.

Summary

A method has been described for combining diagnostic information on immediate and more remote relatives of affected individuals to produce a measure of their susceptibility. The multifactorial model of disease transmission and the TAU model derived from path analysis were used, along with segregation analysis to determine a set of underlying transmission variables for major depressive disorder. Small and large pedigrees of varying density were then constructed to illustrate the prediction of risk of major depressive disorder in susceptible individuals. Age- and sex-specific variation was taken into account and assortative mating was included. The age-specific population frequency of illness was used to age-adjust the data so that secular trends could be accommodated.

Data for this report was drawn from a preliminary subsample of families participating in the National Collaborative Study of Depression. Personal interviews were used throughout.

References

Akiskal HS, McKinney WT Jr: Overview of recent research in depression: integration of ten conceptual models into a comprehensive clinical frame. Arch Gen Psychiatry 32:285–305, 1975

Akiskal HS, Walker P, Puzantian VR, et al: Bipolar outcome in the course of depressive illness. J Affect Dis 5:115–128, 1983

Bertleson A, Harvald B, Hauge M: A Danish twin study of manic-depressive disorders. Br J Psychiatry 130:330–351, 1977

Cadoret RJ: Evidence for genetic inheritance of primary affective disorder in adoptees. Am J Psychiatry 135:463–466, 1978

Carroll BJ, Curtis GC, Mendels J: Neuroendocrine regulation and depression, II: discrimination of depressed from nondepressed controls. Arch Gen Psychiatry 33:1051–1057, 1976

Carroll BJ, Feinberg M, Greden JF, et al: A specific laboratory test for the diagnosis of melancholia. Arch Gen Psychiatry 38:15–22, 1981

Coryell W, Winokur G, Andreasen N: Effect of case definition on affective disorder rates. Am J Psychiatry 138:1106–1110, 1981

Coryell W, Endicott J, Keller MB, et al: The validity of *DSM-III* in psychotic depression, 1984. Am J Psychiatry (in press)

Dorus E, Cox NJ, Gibbons RD, et al: Lithium ion transport and affective disorders within families of bipolar disorder. Arch Gen Psychiatry 40:545–552, 1983

Egeland JA, Pauls DL, Kidd JR, et al: Is a gene for affective disorder located on the short arm of Chromosome II? Am J Hum Genet 36:3S, 1984

Gershon ES, Hamovit S, Guroff JJ, et al: A family study of schizoaffective, bipolar I, bipolar II, unipolar and normal control probands. Arch Gen Psychiatry 39:1157–1167, 1982

Goodwin DJ: Alcoholism and genetics. Arch Gen Psychiatry 42:171–174, 1985

Heinbuch RC, Matthysee S, Kidd KK: Estimating age-of-onset distributions for disorders with variable onset. Am J Hum Genet 32:564–574, 1980

Hirschfeld RMA, Klerman GL: Personality attributes and affective disorder. Am J Psychiatry 136:67–70, 1979

Leckman JF, Weissman MM, Prusoff BA: Subtypes of depression: family study perspective. Arch Gen Psychiatry 41:833–838, 1984

Leonhard K, Korff I, Shulz H: Die Temperamente in der familien der monopolaren und bipolaren phasichen psychosen. Psychiatrie, Neurologie und Medizinische Psychologie 145:416, 1962

Karlin S, Williams PT, Jensen S, et al: Genetic analysis of the Stanford LRC data, I: structured exploratory analysis of height and weight measurement. Am J Epidemiol 113:307–324, 1981

Katz MM, Secunda SK, Hirschfeld RMA, et al: NIMH–Clinical Research Branch Collaborative Program on the Psychobiology of Depression. Arch Gen Psychiatry 36:765–771, 1979

Kety S: Disorders of the human brain. Scientific American 202–214, Sept. 8, 1979

Klerman GL, Lavori PW, Rice J, et al: Birth cohort trends in rates of major depressive disorder among relatives of patients with affective disorder. Arch Gen Psychiatry 42:689–693, 1985

Kupfer DJ: REM latency: a psychobiological marker for primary depressive disease. Biol Psychiatry 11:159–174, 1976

Kupfer DJ, Foster FC, Reich L, et al: EEG sleep changes as predictors in depression. Am J Psychiatry 133:622–626, 1976

Kupfer DJ, Broody A, Coble PA, et al: EEG sleep and affective psychosis. J Affect Dis 2:17–25, 1980

Merikangas KR, Bromet EJ, Spiker DG: Assortative mating, social adjustment and course of illness in primary affective disorder. Arch Gen Psychiatry 40:795–800, 1983

Mendelwicz J, Rainer JD: Adoption study supporting genetic transmission in manic depressive illness. Nature 268:327–329, 1977

Morton NE: Outline of genetic epidemiology. Basel, S. Karger, 1982

Morton NE, Rao DC, Lalouel JM: Methods in Genetic Epidemiology. Basel, S. Karger, 1983

Nadi NS, Nurnberger JI, Gershon ES: Muscarinic cholinergic receptors on skin fibroblasts in affective disorder. N Engl J Med 311:225–230, 1984

Politt J: The relationship between genetic and precipitating factors in depressive illness. Br J Psychiatry 121:67–70, 1972

Reich T, James J, Morris CA: The use of multiple thresholds in determining the mode of transmission of semi-continuous traits. Ann Hum Gen 36:163–184, 1972

Reich T, Rice J, Cloninger CR, et al: The use of multiple thresholds and segregation analysis in analysing the phenotype heterogeneity of multifactorial traits. Ann Hum Genet 42:371–390, 1979

Reich T, Cloninger CR, Suarez BK, et al: Genetics of the affective psychoses, in Handbook of Psychiatry 3: Psychoses of Uncertain Aetiology. Edited by Wing JK, Wing L. New York, Cambridge University Press, 1982

Rice J, Cloninger CR, Reich T: Multifactorial inheritance with cultural transmission and assortative mating, I: description and basic properties of the unitary models. Am J Hum Genet 30:618–643, 1978

Rice J, Cloninger CR, Reich T: The analysis of behavioral traits in the presence of cultural transmission and assortative mating: applications to IQ and SES. Behav Genet 10:73–92, 1980a

Rice J, Cloninger CR, Reich T: General causal models for sex differences in the familial transmission of multifactorial traits: an application to human spatial visualizing ability. Social Biology 27:36–47, 1980b

Rice J, Nichols P, Gottesman II: Assessment of sex differences for qualitative multifactorial traits using path analysis. Psychiatr Res 4:301–312, 1981

Rice J, Reich T, Andreasen NC, et al: Sex-related differences in depression: familial evidence. J Affect Dis 71:199–210, 1984

Risch N: Estimating morbidity risks with variable age of onset: review of methods and a maximum likelihood approach. Biometrics 39:929–939, 1983

Robins LN, Helzer JE, Weissman MM, et al: Lifetime prevalence of specific psychiatric disorders in three sites. Arch Gen Psychiatry 41:949–958, 1984

Rush AJ, Giles DE, Roffwarg HP, et al: Sleep EEG and dexamethasone suppression test findings in outpatients with unipolar affective disorders. Biol Psychiatry 17:327–341, 1982

Spitzer RL, Endicott J, Robins E: Research diagnostic criteria: rationale and reliability. Arch Gen Psychiatry 35:773–782, 1978

Suarez BK, Reich T: HLA and major affective disorders. Arch Gen Psychiatry 41:22–27, 1984

Thompson WD, Weissman MM: Quantifying lifetime risk of psychiatric disorder. J Psychiatr Res 16:113–126, 1981

Van Knorring AL, Cloninger CR, Bohman M, et al: An adoption study of depressive disorders and substance abuse. Arch Gen Psychiatry 40:943–950, 1983

Weissman MM, Myers JK: Affective disorders in a United States urban community: the use of research diagnostic criteria in an epidemiologic survey. Arch Gen Psychiatry 35:1304–1311, 1978

Weissman MM, Kidd KK, Presoff BA: Variability in rates of affective disorder in relatives of depressed and normal probands. Arch Gen Psychiatry 39:1397–1404, 1982

Weissman MM, Wickramaratne P, Merikangas KR, et al: Onset of major depression in early adulthood. Arch Gen Psychiatry 41:1136–1143, 1984

Winokur G, Clayton P, Reich T: Manic Depressive Illness. St. Louis, C.V. Mosby, 1969

Wright AF, Crichton DN, Loudon JB, et al: β-adrenoceptor binding defects in cell lines from families with manic-depressive disorder. Ann Hum Genet 48:201–214, 1984

Chapter 5

BEING YOUNG AND FEMALE: RISK FACTORS FOR MAJOR DEPRESSION

Myrna M. Weissman, Ph.D.

Chapter 5

BEING YOUNG AND FEMALE: RISK FACTORS FOR MAJOR DEPRESSION

Depression is a significant health problem for young women. Although the increased risk of depression among women has been noted for more than 200 years, the emphasis on depression in young women is more recent. In a review of the epidemiologic data on depression, covering 30 countries over a period of more than 40 years, we found that, with few exceptions, depression had a high prevalence and was consistently more common in women than men, both as a symptom and as a clinical disorder (Weissman and Klerman, 1977). Depression was the psychiatric complaint most often reported by women in physicians' offices and in outpatient psychiatric clinics, as well as among women in the community who were not receiving any medical or psychiatric treatment (Weissman and Myers, 1978). Moreover, the incidence of depression seems to be increasing. Today, the typically depressed patient is apt to be a young woman under age 40, in her most productive years, often married and rearing children. Depression is no longer confined to middle-aged and elderly women, and seldom leads to hospitalization. Moreover, depression has a serious impact on the younger woman's

This work was supported in part by Alcohol, Drug Abuse, and Mental Health Administration (ADAMHA) research grants MH–28274 from the Center for Epidemiologic Studies and the Center for Studies of Affective Disorders: by MH–36197, also from the Center for Studies of Affective Disorders, National Institute of Mental Health, Rockville, MD; and by the Network on Risk and Protective Factors in the Major Mental Disorders, funded by the John D. and Catherine T. MacArthur Foundation.

capacity to enjoy life, to sustain intimate and enduring relationships, and to realize her full capacities (Weissman and Paykel, 1974).

Suicide attempts and depression are highly related disorders. Many suicide attempters are depressed, and a substantial minority of depressives have made suicide attempts. Therefore, attempted suicide, which also has a high prevalence, is, albeit indirect, another reflection of depression in women at an earlier stage of their life cycle. Whereas the typical depressed woman is a married person between 25 and 40 years of age, the typical suicide attempter is a single woman under the age of 25, often as young as 15. In a comprehensive review of studies of suicide attempters covering six countries and a period of more than 10 years, we consistently found that the typical suicide attempter was a young single woman (Weissman, 1974; Wexler et al., 1978). Rates of suicide attempts have increased dramatically over the past two decades in Western industrialized countries. This increase was found even after correcting for population growth or for changes in methods of reporting. The sex ratio for suicide attempts is about two females for every male and, for depression, two to three females for every male.

The increase in rates of major depression among women has sparked the curiosity of biologists, sociologists, and feminists, and many hypotheses have been put forth. The various explanations to account for the finding and the available data were reviewed by Dr. Klerman and me in 1977. We concluded that the increased rates among women were real, and not an artifact of differences in help-seeking or in reporting stress or distress. We proposed various theories for the increased risk to women and reviewed the available evidence to explain them (Weissman and Klerman, 1977).

This chapter reviews the new evidence since 1977, reports what we know about rates and risk factors for depression in young women, and discusses possible preventive intervention trials in light of these risk factors.

What is Depression?

In any discussion of depression in women, we must first clarify the definition of depression, since the rates and risk factors will vary by the definition used. In considering the epidemiology of depression it is useful to differentiate between depressive symptoms, the syndrome of major depression, and bipolar disorder. Depressive symptoms usually include dysphoric mood; appetite and sleep disturbance; loss of interest or pleasure; loss of energy; feelings of worthlessness, hopelessness, or guilt; difficulty thinking; and thoughts of death. These symptoms can occur in a variety of medical as well as psychiatric disorders, and usually have been measured in epidemiologic studies by self-report scales.

The syndrome of major depression, as defined by the Diagnostic and Statistical Manual of Mental Disorders, Third Edition (*DSM-III*) (American Psychiatric Association, 1980), includes similar symptoms, but also includes criteria of persistence and impairment. The symptoms must persist for at least one to two weeks, resulting in impairment in social functioning. There are exclusion criteria as well. The symptoms must occur in the absence of other disorders (such as schizophrenia) that may better explain the condition.

Bipolar disorder, as defined by the *DSM-III*, is differentiated from major depression in that the patient with bipolar disorder has experienced sometime in the past a manic or hypomanic episode (that is, an episode of affective disturbance characterized by increased activity and talking, elevated, irritable and/or expansive mood, flight of ideas, grandiosity, and decreased need for sleep). The person with major depression experiences only depressive episodes.

Major depression and bipolar disorder differ by age of onset, treatment response, prevalence, and risk factors (Hirshfeld and Cross, 1982). Most important for this discussion, the sex ratios for bipolar disorder are about equal, so that being female is not specifically a risk factor for bipolar disorder. Depressive symptoms are also more common in women than in men. However, they are heterogeneous and probably include a variety of psychiatric and medical conditions (Boyd et al., 1982). Therefore, this chapter will focus on major depression, unless otherwise indicated.

How Common is Depression in Women?

There is little doubt that major depression is a common disorder. Community surveys show that from 20 to 30 percent of adult women experience a major depression at some point in their lives (Boyd et al., 1982; Weissman et al., 1982), although the exact rate varies. In a 1975 survey of more than 500 persons over the age of 25 living in New Haven, Connecticut, we found that on the day of the interview nearly four percent of the women were in the midst of a major depressive episode, and only about one-third had received any treatment for their depression (Weissman et al., 1981). These findings were replicated in the 1981 Epidemiologic Catchment Area (EAC) Study that included nearly 15,000 persons 18 years and older, living in three urban areas (New Haven, Connecticut, Baltimore, Maryland, St. Louis, Missouri), and based on *DSM-III* criteria for major depression (Myers et al., 1984; Regier et al., 1984). In one of the few community surveys that focused exclusively on adolescents, it was found that 19.7 percent of adolescents (aged 14 to 18) were bothered by feeling sad or depressed in the past year. The rates of symptoms were higher in females (Kandel and Davies, 1982). Currently in the United States there are no community studies on the syndromes of depression in adolescents. Suicide attempts, another reflection of depression in young women, also have a high prevalence, estimated annually at 100/100,000 among men and women of all ages. Although specific age and sex rates have not been presented (Weissman, 1974; Wexler et al., 1978) the rates for younger women would be much higher.

Risk Factors

How Does Age Affect the Risk for Females?

Recent community surveys of rates of depression, as well as the indirect evidence from the rates of suicide attempts, suggest that younger women have the highest rates of depression.

Hirschfeld and Cross (1982) noted a higher prevalence of depressive symptoms in young adults (aged 18 to 44 years) than in older adults. The highest rates of depressive symptoms were found in women younger than 35 years of age, while the peak prevalence in men occurred during the 55- to 70-year-old age range. Kandel and Davies (1982) found that adolescent females had more often reported feeling sad and depressed than did their mothers. The rates were lowest in adolescent boys and their fathers.

Consistent with the findings from community studies, evidence available from clinical studies also suggests higher prevalences of the depressive syndrome in younger populations than in older groups. In an ongoing study of a heterogenous group of depressed and manic patients, 61 percent of the 902 patients sampled were younger than 40 years of age (Hirschfeld and Cross, 1982).

The Weissman and Myers (1978) survey of New Haven found considerably higher lifetime rates of major depression in persons aged 26 to 45 where the lifetime rate was 23.8/100, as compared to persons aged 65 and older where the lifetime rate was 14.4/100. At all ages, women had higher rates than did men.

The higher lifetime rates in the younger age group that had been at risk for shorter periods of time suggest an increasing incidence of depression in younger age cohorts. Explanations, including memory or acknowledgment problems, or selective survival of the elderly, are also possible. The higher lifetime rates of depression in younger persons is a consistent finding and has been replicated in a study of families of depressives (Weissman et al., 1984a), in the ECA Study (Weissman et al., 1984b), and in a large family study of birth cohort trends among relatives of patients with affective illness (Klerman et al., 1985).

Physiological Events in a Woman's Life Cycle

It is useful to consider common recurring physiological events in a woman's life cycle, which may explain the increased risk of depression in families.

Premenstrual period. Premenstrual tension (PMT) includes feeling irritated, bloated, tense, and blue during the 3 to 5 days before the onset of menses. Although reported by many women, these feelings usually do not occur with regularity in all women, and recent studies suggest that they do not seem to change a woman's actual performance at home or work, nor to be particularly apparent to others.

There is no conclusive evidence, thus far, to suggest that women are more vulnerable to the depressive syndrome during the premenstrual period (Weissman and Klerman, 1977). It is unclear whether the blue feelings reported by some women in the premenstrual phase are related to major depression, or whether they have a physiological basis. Investigations relating mood changes to the phases in the menstrual cycle by use of modern endocrinological methods and sensitive quantitative hormonal assays have been under way at Columbia University in New York and at Massachusetts General Hospital in Boston. The clinical studies thus far completed at Columbia University point out the complexity of the problem;

for example, that there are some subtypes of PMT that resemble some subtypes of affective disorders (Endicott et al., 1981; Halbreich et al., 1982, 1983).

Contraceptive medication. While there is widespread suspicion that oral contraceptives "cause depression," it is unclear from the studies thus far whether there is a physiological basis for any association (Weissman and Klerman, 1977). If a relationship exists between the use of oral contraceptives and the onset of depression, the relationship could just as well be associated with the psychological conflicts over preventing pregnancy or unwanted exposure to sexual relationships, as it could be to the pharmacologic ingredients of "the pill." A small number of women may be sensitive to steroid hormones in oral contraceptives. However, scientists have not been able to determine whether oral contraceptives increase the risk of depression on a pharmacological basis.

Postpartum period. The "new baby blues," mild and transitory feelings of sadness and tearfulness, are so common in the first few weeks following childbirth that they are considered "normal," rarely require treatment (Cox et al., 1982; Nott, 1982; Weissman and Klerman, 1977), and usually are self-limited. However, for a small number of women, a longer postpartum period of up to six months does carry a risk of more serious clinical depression (Nott, 1982, Pitt, 1982). Moreover, women who have previously become clinically depressed (not just mildly blue) in the postpartum period are at much greater risk for another recurrence with subsequent pregnancies and deliveries. The postpartum period does increase the risk of depression, but we do not know whether this is due to biological reasons such as hormonal changes, to the psychological reasons such as fear of responsibilities for the care of a child, or to changes in the marital relations.

The menopause. Despite conventional wisdom and popular folklore, the current data from several excellent epidemiologic studies in the United Kingdom, the United States, and Scandinavia show that women in the menopausal period are not at an increased risk for depression (Weissman, 1979). While the menopause is not directly relevant to a study of depression in younger women, there is an indirect relevance. Although there appears to be a decrease in depression among older women, the increase in the overall rates of depression suggests that it is the younger women who are contributing to the increase.

The decrease in the occurrence of menopausal depression, called "involutional melancholia," may be a recent trend in the United States, the United Kingdom, and Scandinavia. The decrease in the rates of depression in the menopausal years seems to be counterbalanced by an increase in rates among the younger age groups.

Is the Sex Difference Due to Genetic Transmission?

There is little question that major depression is a family affair. Persons who have a family history of major depression in their first degree relatives are at an increased risk (about two- to threefold) themselves for developing a major depression, minor affective disorder, or both (Gershon et al., 1982; Weissman et al., 1982).

A parent who is depressed dramatically increases the risk that his or her children (under the age of 18) will be depressed. The effect on the children is nearly doubled if both parents are depressed (Weissman et al., 1984b). Moreover, the onset of depression can begin at quite a young age in the children. The data on sex differences in the rates of depression among prepubertal children are unclear.

Alternatively, if a child has a depressed parent, there is a high probability that both parents will be depressed, since there is a high degree of assortative mating for depression (Merikangas, 1982). It is unclear whether depressed persons are attracted to and marry other depressed persons or persons vulnerable to depression, or whether being married to a depressed person is depressing; that is, the time sequence of the onset of the depression—pre- and post-marriage—and the family history and personality characteristics of depressed mates have not been fully studied, although such research is currently under way. It is also unclear whether the gender of the person first depressed increases the probability that the mate will later become depressed.

A major unresolved issue is whether this increased risk of depression in biological relatives of depressed probands is genetic and, if so, whether it can explain the sex differences. A greater frequency of a disorder in one sex is a genetically interesting phenomenon. One possible explanation is X-linkage; that is, the location of the relevant locus on the X chromosome. For an X-linked locus, if the trait is dominant, females (with two X chromosomes) will be affected more commonly. A rare X-linked recessive trait will seldom appear in the parents of children of an affective male, but will always be found in both the father and all sons of an affected female. A rare X-linked dominant trait will usually appear in the mother and all of the daughters of an affected male, and will occur in at least one parent and at least one-half of the children of an affected female. The exact frequency with which first-degree relatives are affected is also a function of the allele frequency in the population and of the mating pattern. Based on assumptions of random mating and an X-linked dominant trait, for every affected male sibling of an affected female, there would be three affected female siblings.

The results of family studies investigating X-linkage are conflicting. Perris has reported data consistent with X-linked transmission for major depression but not for bipolar disorder. However, Helzer, Winokur, Reich, and others found data suggesting X-linkage for bipolar disorder but not for major depression. The inconsistency of the findings has continued into recent studies as well. Gershon and his co-workers have found no evidence for X-linkage of bipolar affective disorder in a study in Jerusalem (Weissman and Klerman, 1977).

Another possible explanation for the different incidences in the two sexes is a differential interaction of genotype and environment depending on gender. A sex effect can be seen as evidence for a differential threshold, with the less commonly affected gender having a higher threshold (Weissman and Klerman, 1977). The underlying liability is determined by a combination of genetic and environmental factors.

Possible genetic transmission as an explanation of the increased risk of major depression in women has been investigated by Merikangas and colleagues (1985). If the sex difference is related to the genetic transmission of a disorder, in family studies, relatives of the less prevalent sex of the proband would have higher rates of the disorder. Thus, if the sex difference in major depression were related to genetic factors, it would be expected that relatives of male probands would have higher rates of depression than would relatives of female probands. This principle has been demonstrated for several other complex human disorders with a genetic component and an increased prevalence in one sex, such as stuttering and Tourette's Syndrome.

If rates do not differ among relatives of male and female probands, one can conclude that the sex difference in prevalence of the trait is not due to genetic transmission of that trait. This explanation is true for the majority of multifactorial genetic models that have been applied to complex human disorders.

Examining data on over 1,000 first degree relatives of 133 probands with major depression and 82 matched normal controls, Merikangas and colleagues (1985) found that the sex of the proband was not involved in the transmission of depression, because relatives of male and female probands had equal rates of depression. The results suggested that the increased prevalence of depression in women cannot be attributed to genetic factors responsible for the transmission of depression. Sex of the proband was not associated with different risks for relatives.

The sex difference can therefore be attributed to nontransmissible factors. Major depression, however, is probably heterogeneous as to etiology. These results may not apply to all subtypes of the disorder. Furthermore, genetic factors may be involved in other factors (such as endocrine), which may be related to the penetrance of the disorder.

Rice and colleagues (1984) reached similar conclusions. In a study of 523 families of affectively ill probands, they found equal sex ratios of bipolar disorder in relatives and increased rates of major depression in females, which persisted when relatives were classified by a variety of subtypes of major depression. There was a maternal effect for primary major depression, which applied equally to both sisters and brothers of probands. These findings on sex differences are compatible with a cultural or a nongenetic biological mechanism in transmission. While the findings suggest that genetic factors cannot explain the preponderance of women in rates of depression, genetic factors are likely to be important in the transmission of some form of major depression for both sexes.

Marriage

Being married.   In a few attempts to test the hypothesis that the high rates of depression are related to the disadvantages of the woman's social status, particular attention has been given to differential rates of mental illness among married and unmarried women. If this hypothesis is correct, marriage should be of greater disadvantage to the woman than to the man, since married women are likely to embody the traditional roles and therefore should have higher rates of depression. Gove, in particular, has focused his research on examining rates of mental illness among married women and married men. Gove and his associates (see Weissman and Klerman, 1977) found that the higher overall rates of many mental illnesses among females are largely accounted for by the higher rates for married women. In each marital status category, single, divorced, and widowed women have lower rates of mental illness than men. He concluded that being married has a protective effect for males but a detrimental effect for females. In a community study of adults in upstate New York, Ensel (1982) found that only one group of married women was at high risk for depression. These were young women aged 17 to 24. One out of every three young married females suffered from depression. However, unmarried women in general had the highest rates of depression, suggesting that it was not marriage per se but the age of the married women that was contributing to their increased rates of depression.

The Gove hypothesis about married women was not replicated by Weissman and Myers in their 1975 survey of New Haven, nor in the New Haven 1980 ECA study (Leaf et al., in press). The discrepancy here may have to do with the definition of depression. When depressive symptoms in the 1975 survey are studied—irrespective of diagnosis—the rates of symptoms, ranked lowest to highest, are for married men; married women; single and widowed women; single, widowed, and divorced men; and separated and divorced women (Hirschfeld and Cross, 1982). However, for major depression, rates are somewhat lower for married persons and for those with an intimate heterosexual relationship.

Marital status, marital relationships, and sex differences in rates continue to be an important area of investigation. The data that unmarried women have lower rates of mental illness than unmarried men, but that married women have higher rates than married men, while not replicated in all studies, are cited as evidence that the excess of depressive symptoms in women are not due entirely to biological factors intrinsic to being female but, rather, are contributed to by the conflicts generated by the traditional female role. However, the fact that younger aged women seem to be at greater risk for depression is a provocative finding that should be pursued.

The quality of the marriage. The fact of a marriage per se may not be as important in contributing to depression as is its quality. Lack of an intimate and confiding heterosexual relationship and marital disputes have been shown to be related to depression in women. Brown and Harris (1978) studied the relationship between life events and depression in a sample of women in the community, and found that lack of an intimate and confiding heterosexual relationship increased the risk for depression in the face of life events. Confidants other than spouse or boyfriend did not have as protective an effect. Rather, the general levels of satisfaction and intimacy in the heterosexual relationship, and the amount of emotional support that her partner gave the woman in her role, were the important factors in preventing depression in the face of life stress. Employment outside the home also was a protective factor, although much less so. As interpreted by Brown and Harris, employment provided a protective effect by alleviating boredom, increasing self-esteem, improving economic circumstances, and increasing social contacts.

The association between poor interpersonal relations within the marriage and clinical depression is further supported by studies of depressed women during psychiatric treatment (Roy, 1978). Rounsaville and colleagues (1979) found that depressed patients, more often than nondepressed patients, reported marital discord to be the most common event in the previous six months. Weissman and Paykel (1974) found that acutely depressed women, as compared to matched normal controls, reported considerably more problems in marital intimacy, especially in the ability to communicate with the spouse. Moreover, these marital problems were enduring and did not completely subside with the women's symptomatic remission of the acute depression.

Leaf and colleagues (in press) found that the six-month rates of major depression were 45/100 among women who said they were not getting along with their spouse. When married women aged 18 to 44 were interviewed, the rates were even higher. It is impossible to interpret the direction of causality between marital problems and depression in a cross-sectional study, and either may be the cause. Merikangas and colleagues (1983) found that there was a high degree of assortative mating in the depressed women. While assortative mating did not impact on the course of the symptomatic illness, it did relate to the course of social functioning of the patient. Depressed women with an affectively ill spouse had much poorer social functioning over a two-year period following the index episode, and a much higher divorce rate. The divorce and separation rate was higher for all depressed patients, and it was even higher (27 percent) among the couples concordant for depression in comparison to the discordant couples (four percent). It is unclear whether assortative mating impacts differently on men and women.

The breakup of the marriage. There is no question that separation and divorce increase the risk of depression in both men and women, and this can occur even in the person who initiated the separation or divorce (Bloom et al., 1978). Interestingly, however, we have found that women are more likely to come for treatment of depression during the marital breakdown and dispute period, whereas men rarely seek treatment until after the dissolution of the marriage by separation or divorce, when they become aware of the lost nurturance of the marriage. This suggests that marital disruption impacts differently on men and women (Rounsaville et al., 1979).

For many persons, however, divorce represents one of the more serious disruptions of personal-bond attachments, even if those attachments were negative. For women, divorce also means the loss of the role of wife to that of being a single woman, usually accompanied by a change in financial status, perhaps assumption of outside work, new friends, and the complications of raising children as a single parent, (Kessler and McRae, 1982).

Small Children

Several studies have suggested that the presence of small children may contribute to depression in young women (Brown and Harris, 1978; Hare and Shaw, 1965; Richman, 1978; Roy, 1978). In their London survey, Brown and Harris (1978) found the following: loss of a mother in childhood; three or more children under the age of 14 living at home; the already noted absence of an intimate and confiding relationship with husband or boyfriend; and lack of full-time employment outside of the home, were highly predictive of depression in women in the face of life stress. Taken together, these results suggest that an intimate supportive marriage can be protective and serve as a buffer for a woman, but that chronic marital problems and lack of intimacy may be more considerably detrimental than being single or being married with many small children. Unclear is the role of personality and how much it may predispose to marital and parental problems and divorce (Briscoe and Smith, 1973; Brugha et al., 1982; Henderson et al., 1981).

Death of a Loved One

Grief is a normal reaction to the death of a loved one, and usually resolves within two to four months. Abnormal grief is a specific problem arising from an inability to go through the usual process of mourning. Persons at increased risk for depression are those who have lost a loved one and do not go through a normal grieving reaction, or allow themselves an opportunity for recovery and reconstitution of their lives. Women, therefore, are at increased risk to depression to unresolved grief because, demographically, they are at much higher risk for grief. Despite the recent decrease in mortality in men, there is still a considerable differential in life expectancy between men and women. Today, women live an average of four to seven years longer than men. Compounding the life expectancy differential between men and women is the fact that most women are younger than the men they marry. Therefore, the majority of women who marry, even if the marriage does not end in divorce, can expect to spend nearly 10 years alone as a widow. Fortunately, grief is not a common experience among young women, but studies by Clayton (1981), Kraus and Lilienfeld (1979), and Parkes and Brown (1972) have shown that the experience of widowhood is much more difficult for younger women than for older women.

Moving

Moving has always been a strong characteristic of the American way of life. Throughout our history, changing patterns of agriculture and industry have encouraged the enterprising and the courageous to pull up stakes. Today, approximately 18 percent of our population–40 million people—makes at least one move each year. Americans of every class and income constantly move in larger numbers, and moving is much more common among the young under the age of 25. For young professionals, particularly, frequent and distant moves may be necessary to insure progress in their careers.

Only in recent years, however, have the psychological effects of mobility on family life been noted. The impact can be compounded if the woman is educated and wishes to pursue an independent career, and especially during the years when her children are young.

Moving can increase the risk of depression, especially for women, even if the move is voluntary and results in greater financial rewards and better standards of living (Hull, 1979). Since moving occurs more frequently among younger persons, young women are at increased risk.

The Changing Role of Women

Rising expectations, access to new opportunities, and efforts to redress the social inequalities of women have been suggested as risks for depression. Depressions may occur not when things are at their worst but when there is a possibility for improvement and a discrepancy between one's rising aspirations and the likelihood of fulfilling them. The Women's Movement, government legislation, and efforts to improve educational and employment opportunities for women have created higher expectations. Social and economic achievements often have not kept pace with the promises, especially in a tightening job market, and in situations in which longstanding discriminatory practices perpetuate unequal opportunities.

New career expectations for women may also create internal personal conflicts, particularly among those women who want traditional families as well as employment and recognition outside the home. While the Women's Movement has mainly involved middle- and upper-class educated women, the Movement has had an impact on women from other social classes where opportunities for work outside the home, management of money, dominance in the marriage, and so forth, may be difficult. Even among educated and economically comfortable women there continues to be ambivalence and conflict about careers not conventionally seen as feminine. Clayton et al. (1980), Pitts et al. (1979), Welner et al. (1979), and others have found very high rates of depression in female M.D. and Ph.D. professionals, which were related to prejudice and conflict in their training and employment.

There have been several studies on the impact of women's employment on their own and on their spouse's mental health (Cochrane and Stopes-Roe, 1981; Ensel, 1982; Kessler and McRae, 1982; Warr and Parry, 1982). The results are conflicting. They show that working wives and housewives do not differ in type or prevalence of psychiatric disorders (Newberry et al., 1979); that paid employment and the woman's well-being depend on the quality of her job and her nonoccupational involvement (Warr and Parry, 1982); that paid employment increases the woman's well-being, but not necessarily that of her spouse (Kessler and McRae, 1982); and that age and/or cohort of the working woman may be important factors in the impact of work on the woman's emotional health (Ensel, 1982).

The changing role of women and the present socioeconomic situation may have an impact on a number of areas. The Women's Movement increased the opportunities and expectations for women in employment and in education. These increased expectations came at a time of constraints in real opportunities for both men and women. Easterlin (1982), an economist, relates the constraints in opportunities to demographic changes. He notes that more people were born between 1946 and 1957 than were born in the previous 30 years. Thus, this generation—now young adults—is encountering more competition for everything—jobs, education, housing, and the like. There is greater economic pressure, and therefore a whole series of psychological strains, as a consequence of this pressure. The strain is particularly intensified as women have also entered the labor and career forces at the same time that opportunities are more competitive for everyone.

The data here are inconclusive. Srole and Fischer (1980), in a 20-year follow-up study of the overall mental health and impairment of a cohort of over 1,000 men and women living in midtown Manhattan in 1954, found no significant deterioration in the mental health of either the men or the women over the 20-year period. When different birth cohorts were examined by comparing the mental health of men and women aged 40 to 59 in 1954 (that is, born 1895–1914) with the mental health of men and women aged 40 to 59 in 1974 (born 1915–1934), they found that the younger women (those born in the latter birth cohort) experienced an improvement in their mental health. The authors attributed this improvement to the enhanced social and economic conditions of women.

Recent research on the specific mental disorders does not replicate Srole and Fischer's findings of a decrease in psychiatric disorders among the more recent birth cohorts. When lifetime rates of psychiatric disorders were obtained retrospectively, an *increase*, not a decrease, in the lifetime rates of both the men and the women in the younger age group has been found, suggesting that there may be an increasing, not decreasing, incidence of psychiatric disorder in young people (Klerman et al., 1985). We also found a decreasing age of onset for depression (Weissman et al., 1984a). The measure of psychiatric illness used in the Srole and Fischer work differs from that used in the recent studies, and the retro-spective nature of the recent studies may be obscuring changes in rates. Studies of the changing incidence of psychiatric disorder over time, using population samples, is a fruitful area of pursuit. Support for the hypothesis that the women's movement is associated with psychological distress is unclear and contradictory. It is unlikely that it is the major factor for the excess of depression in women, since the high rates of depression among women substantially antedate the Women's Movement.

Implications for Prevention

Definitions of Prevention

There are at least three levels of prevention: primary, second-ary, and tertiary (Mausner and Bahn, 1974). *Primary* prevention is prevention of a disorder by altering susceptibility or by reducing exposure in individuals who are susceptible but not yet ill. Primary prevention requires an understanding of the risk factors that render a person susceptible or exposed. For chronic nonpsychiatric dis-eases, this often requires modification of deeply rooted behaviors associated with diet, smoking, physical activity, and the like. *Secondary* prevention is the early detection and treatment of a disorder, in which its progression is slowed or its complications and disability are reduced. Tertiary prevention consists of limiting the disability and rehabilitation in those cases in which a disorder has already occurred and left residual damage. This discussion focuses only on primary and secondary prevention.

Risk Factor Research

Preventive intervention strategies should be based on a solid foundation of research that has isolated and identified the persons, periods, and situations or risks for depression. The salient areas include:

1. broad community-based epidemiologic studies that use consis-tent and operationalized diagnostic criteria to overcome the problem of reporting and response set, that are longitudinal to detect changes in incidence and prevalence and associated risk

factors, and that include younger age groups

2. cross-cultural epidemiologic studies, using consistent and similar diagnostic criteria, to determine whether depression is less frequent in females in nonindustrialized countries, or in countries where women have had consistently longer periods of equal access to the labor market

3. longitudinal studies of the help-seeking patterns and rates of depression of women who do not assume the traditional female roles, especially in countries where women have achieved increased emancipation

4. further research on the genetics of major depression, including the less severe forms of the disorder, and examination of the rates of depression in first degree relatives of depressed patients, to determine whether they fit frequencies and patterns consistent with a particular mode of inheritance

5. endocrine studies of the relationship between hormonal changes and mood, particularly during the menstrual cycle and during use of oral contraceptives

6. close surveillance of changes in rates by sex, marital, and women's occupational status as they relate to changing demographic and economic factors

7. epidemiologic community-based studies of children and adolescents, to determine the incidence and prevalence rates of depression and the sex ratios of depression in children, and to relate the rates to risk factors at an early age

8. studies of children at risk, particularly the young children of depressed parents (including nonpsychiatrically ill parents and parents with a chronic physical illness), to determine the early signs of disorder in children; to determine when and how the sex differences in rates of depression become manifest; and to determine whether there are differentiated risk factors by sex (such studies are currently underway at several university centers)

9. longitudinal studies of young couples considering marriage, to determine the prevalence, sequence, and factors contributing to assortative mating.

Education of Professionals Seeing Young Women

The risk factors for depression in women are childbirth and child-rearing, marital problems, separation and divorce, and moving. There are many excellent treatments for depression, both pharmacologic and psychotherapeutic, whose efficacy has been established through controlled clinical trials. However, epidemiologic studies show that most depressions are untreated (Shapiro et al., 1984; Weissman et al., 1981). Women are treated in the health care system with great frequency and are mostly seen by professionals who are not psychiatrists. Therefore, general and family practitioners, college health personnel, pediatricians, obstetricians/gynecologists, and nonmedical mental health personnel—particularly those who see young women during periods of risk—should be educated in the recognition of depression, the available treatments, and the timing of referrals. The increased awareness might provide early detection of cases and appropriate intervention (that is, secondary prevention for persons already symptomatic, and primary prevention for those who are not).

Appropriate and early treatment might also reduce chronicity, as clinical follow-up studies indicate that untreated depressions have high rates of chronicity (Keller et al., 1982a). Education of the medical professional should also include training in the methods of taking a detailed family history. There is little question that depression is familial. Depressed women have increased frequency of a depressed spouse, parents, siblings, and children, especially young children. Alternately, depressed children often have one or more parents who are depressed. This finding has implications for persons treating adults and children. The familial nature of depression should be considered and inquired about when the patient is depressed. This information could lead to primary prevention for unaffected family members, and secondary prevention through early case finding for affected family members.

There are now several simple systematic interviewing methods to detect depression in adults and in children. After brief training, these methods can readily be administered by nonmedical personnel and could become part of standard medical and mental health practice. The training could be incorporated into medical and nonmedical professional (such as social workers and nurses) education, or as part of CME programs for physicians or other professionals.

Preventive Intervention Trials

In discussing intervention trials, it is useful to differentiate between primary and secondary prevention. Several specific pre-

ventive intervention trials are suggested by the data thus far. These
are:

1. *Separation/divorce.* A study to test out the efficacy of various
   psychological treatments during the separation/divorce period.
   This would be primary prevention.
2. *Family therapy for depression.* A study to test the efficacy of
   family therapy for depressed patients, especially where there is
   evidence of assortative mating. This would provide secondary
   prevention for the patient and ill family members and, possibly,
   primary prevention for the family members who are not symptomatic.
3. *Moving.* A study to test the efficacy of brief psychological preparation of families that are about to move. This would be primary prevention.
4. *Marital disputes.* A study to test the efficacy of conjoint marital
   therapy versus individual therapy in depressed patients with
   marital disputes. This would be secondary prevention for the
   spouse who is depressed and primary prevention for the spouse
   who is well.
5. *Distressed at-risk individuals.* A study to identify women at high-
   risk periods in apparent preclinical distress, and to determine
   the efficacy of early identification and supportive intervention.
   The populations could include young women during periods
   of transition, such as when entering the labor force or when
   entering or leaving college, young women with more than three
   children, women in marital crisis, or women in prolonged periods of new-baby blues. The detection of these women at risk
   might best be conducted in high schools and colleges, and in
   pediatric, obstetric, or primary care settings, but not in psychiatric settings.
6. *Bereavement.* A study to test the efficacy of widow-to-widow
   programs, versus individual counseling of young widows, in
   enhancing social functioning and preventing unresolved grief.
   This would be primary prevention.

Summary

There is little question that being young and female increases the
risk of being depressed. The increased rates of depression in women

have been documented over many years. The gradual increase in the rates among young women seems to be a more recent phenomenon. While periods of increased risk can be documented, the precise nature of the risk, whether it is related to biological vulnerability or changes in social conditions, is quite unclear. The changing incidence of depression in young women, if documented by properly designed longitudinal studies (none are currently available), would argue against a strictly biological hypothesis. However, the consistency of the findings on rates in women across Western cultures and different educational groups would argue against a strictly environmental hypothesis.

This chapter has outlined some of the diagnostic problems and the gaps in evidence, as well as suggested areas of possible fruitful research. There is little doubt, however, that the sex difference found in depression is a promising lead. It is highly unlikely that any one of the explanations already described will be the sole factor accounting for the phenomenon, or that all types of depressions will be associated with the same risk factors. As was shown, the explanations cross such a wide variety of disciplines that rarely are all interactions entertained by any one group of investigators. There has been an unfortunate tendency for fragmentation, so that the investigators in genetics, social psychology, or endocrinology are not specifically aware of attempts by their scientific colleagues to deal with similar phenomena. While there is a gap in understanding the reasons for the increased rates of depression in women, there is considerably less gap in understanding periods and persons at risk. Given the considerable advances in the detection and treatment of depression over the last two decades, there are now many fruitful opportunities for preventive intervention at several levels.

References

American Psychiatric Association: Diagnostic and Statistical Manual of Mental Disorders, Third Edition (DSM-III). Washington DC, American Psychiatric Association, 1980

Bloom B, Asher SJ, White SW: Marital disruption as a stressor: a review and analysis. Psychol Bull 85:867–894, 1978

Boyd JH, Weissman MM: The epidemiology of affective disorders: a reexamination and future directions. Arch Gen Psychiatry 38:1039–1046, 1981

Boyd JH, Weissman MM, Thompson WD, et al: Screening for depression in a community sample. Arch Gen Psychiatry 39:1195–1204, 1982

Briscoe BW, Smith J: Depression and marital turmoil. Arch Gen Psychiatry 29:811–817, 1973

Brown GW, Harris T: Social Origins of Depression. London, Tavistock, 1978

Brugha T, Conroy R, Walsh N, et al: Social networks, attachments and support in minor affective disorders: a replication. Br J Psychiatry 141:249–255, 1982

Clayton PJ: Bereavement, in Handbook of Affective Disorders. Edited by Paykel ES. London, Churchill Livingston, 1981

Clayton PJ, Marten S, Davis MA, et al: Mood disorders in women professionals. J Affect Dis 2:37–46, 1980

Cochrane R, Stopes-Roe M: Women, marriage, employment and mental health. Br J Psychiatry 139:373–381, 1981

Cox JL, Connor Y, Kendell RE: Prospective study of the psychiatric disorders of childbirth. Br J Psychiatry 140:111–117, 1982

Easterlin RA: Birth and Fortune: The Impact of Numbers on Personal Welfare. New York, Basic Books, 1980

Endicott J, Halbreich U, Schacht S, et al: Premenstrual changes and affective disorders. Psychosom Med 43:519–529, 1981

Ensel WM: The role of age in the relationship of gender and marital status to depression. J Nerv Ment Dis 170:536–543, 1982

Gershon ES, Hamovit J, Guroff JJ, et al: A family study of schizoaffective, bipolar I, bipolar II, unipolar, and normal control probands. Arch Gen Psychiatry 39:1157–1172, 1982

Halbreich U, Endicott J, Schacht S, et al: The diversity of premenstrual changes as reflected in the Premenstrual Assessment Form. Acta Psychiatr Scand 65:46–65, 1982

Halbreich U, Endicott J, Nee J: Premenstrual depressive changes: value of differentiation. Arch Gen Psychiatry 40:535–542, 1983

Hare EH, Shaw GK: Mental Health in a New Housing Estate. Maudsley Monograph 12. London, Oxford University Press, 1965

Henderson S, Byrne DG, Duncan-Jones P: Neurosis and The Social Environment. London, Academic Press, 1981

Hirschfeld RMA, Cross CK: Epidemiology of affective disorders: psychosocial risk factors. Arch Gen Psychiatry 39:35–46, 1982

Hull D: Migration, adaption, and illness: a review. Soc Sci Med 13A:25–36, 1979

Kandel DB, Davies M: The epidemiology of depressive mood in adolescents. Arch Gen Psychiatry 39:1205–1216, 1982

Keller MB, Shapiro RW, Lavori PW, et al: Recovery in major depressive disorder. Arch Gen Psychiatry 39:905–910, 1982a

Keller MB, Shapiro RW, Lavori PW, et al: Relapse in major depressive disorder. Arch Gen Psychiatry 39:911–920, 1982b

Kessler RC: Marital status and depression: the role of coping resources. Social Forces (in press)

Kessler RC, McRae JA: The effect of wives' employment on the mental health of married men and women. American Sociological Review 47:216–227, 1982

Klerman GL, Lavori PW, Rice J, et al: Birth cohort trends in rates of major depressive disorder among relatives of patients with affective disorder. Arch Gen Psychiatry 42:689–693, 1985

Kraus AM, Lilienfeld AM: Some epidemiologic aspects of the high mortality rate in the young widowed group. J Chron Dis 10:207–217, 1979

Leaf PJ, Weissman MM, Myers, JK, et al: Psychosocial risks and correlates of major depression in one United States urban community, in Mental Disorder in the Community: Progress and Challenge. Edited by Barrett J. New York, Guilford Press (in press)

Mausner J, Bahn A: Epidemiology. Philadelphia, WB Saunders, 1974

Merikangas KR: Assortative mating for psychiatric disorders and psychological traits. Arch Gen Psychiatry 39:1173–1180, 1982

Merikangas KR, Spiker DG: Assortative mating among inpatients with primary affective disorder. Psychol Med 12:753–764, 1982

Merikangas KR, Bromet EJ, Spiker DG: The relationship of assortative mating to social adjustment and course of illness in primary affective disorder. Arch Gen Psychiatry 40:795–800, 1983

Merikangas KR, Weissman MM, Pauls DL: Genetic factors in the sex ratio of major depression. Psychol Med 15:63–69, 1985

Myers JK, Weissman MM, Tischler GL, et al: Six-month prevalence of psychiatric disorders in three communities: 1980–1982. Arch Gen Psychiatry 41:959–967, 1984

Newberry P, Weissman MM, Myers JK: Working wives and housewives: do they differ in mental status and social adjustment? Am J Orthopsychiatry 49:282–291, 1979

Nott PN: Psychiatric illness following childbirth in Southampton: a case register study. Psychol Med 12:557–561, 1982

Parks CM, Brown R: Health after bereavement: a controlled study of young widows and widowers. Psychosom Med 34:449–461, 1972

Pitt B: Depression and childbirth, in Handbook of Affective Disorders. Edited by Paykel ES. London, Churchill Livingstone, 1982

Pitts FN, Schuller B, Rich CL, et al: Suicide among U.S. women physicians. Am J Psychiatry 136:694–696, 1979

Regier DA, Myers JK, Kramer M, et al: the NIMH Epidemiologic Catchment Area program: historical context, major objectives, and study population characteristics. Arch Gen Psychiatry 41:934–941, 1984

Richman N: Depression in mothers of young children. J Royal Soc Med 71:489–493, 1978

Rice J, Reich T, Andreasen NC, et al: Sex-related differences in depression: familial evidence. J Affect Dis 71:199–210, 1984

Rounsaville BJ, Weissman MM, Prusoff BA, et al: Marital disputes and treatment outcome in depressed women. Compr Psychiatry 20:483–490, 1979

Roy A: Vulnerability factors and depression in women. Br J Psychiatry 133:106–110, 1978

Shapiro S, Skinner EA, Kessler LG, et al: Utilization of health and mental health services: three epidemiologic catchment area sites. Arch Gen Psychiatry 41:971–978, 1984

Srole L, Fischer AK: The midtown Manhattan longitudinal study vs. 'the mental paradise lost' doctrine. Arch Gen Psychiatry 37:209–221, 1980

Warr P, Parry G: Paid employment and women's psychological well-being. Psychol Bull 92:498–516, 1982

Weissman MM: The epidemiology of suicide attempts, 1960 to 1971. Arch Gen Psychiatry 30:737–746, 1974

Weissman MM: The myth of involutional melancholia. JAMA 242:742–744, 1979

Weissman MM, Klerman GL: Sex differences and the epidemiology of depression. Arch Gen Psychiatry 34:98–111, 1977

Weissman MM, Myers JK: Affective disorders in a United States community: the use of research diagnostic criteria in an epidemiologic survey. Arch Gen Psychiatry 34:1304–1311, 1978

130

Weissman MM, Paykel ES: The Depressed Woman: A Study of Social Relationships. Chicago, University of Chicago Press, 1974

Weissman MM, Myers JK, Thompson WD: Depression and its treatment in a U.S. urban community, 1975–76. Arch Gen Psychiatry 38:417–421, 1981

Weissman MM, Kidd KK, Prusoff BA: Variability in the rates of affective disorders in the relatives of severe and mild major nonbipolar depressives and normals. Arch Gen Psychiatry 39:1397–1403, 1982

Weissman MM, Leaf PJ, Holzer CE, et al: The epidemiology of depression: an update on sex differences in rates. J Affect Dis 7:179–188, 1984a

Weissman MM, Prusoff BA, Gammon DG, et al: Psychopathology in the children (ages 6–18) of depressed and normal parents. J Am Acad Child Psychiatry 23:78–84, 1984b

Welner A, Martin, S, Wochnik E, et al: Psychiatric disorders among professional women. Arch Gen Psychiatry 36:169–172, 1979

Wexler L, Weissman MM, Kasl SV: Suicide attempts 1970–75: updating a United States study and comparisons with international trends. Br J Psychiatry 132:180–185, 1978

Chapter 6

SUICIDAL BEHAVIOR IN AMERICAN BLACKS

Felton Earls, M.D.
Ada Jemison, M.D.

Chapter 6

SUICIDAL BEHAVIOR IN AMERICAN BLACKS

The purpose of this chapter is to formulate a series of research questions and methodological concerns that will ultimately increase knowledge of self-destructiveness in blacks and lead to effective preventative strategies. Two basic assumptions underlie this discussion:

1. There exists a continuum of depressed mood, depressive illness, aggressivity, self-destructive behavior, and suicide. This continuum may be more readily defined in the black population than in the white population as a result of social contextual variables. Self-destructive behavior, and antisocial behavior with its attendant involvement with the police, frequently result in violent death among blacks, which is not readily distinguishable from suicide.

2. The significance and severity of these problems often go unrecognized due to a lack of clinical acumen in realizing the contribution that social, economic, historical, and cultural factors play in the development of these problems. An extensive review of this issue is already available (Adebimpe, 1981).

As reflected in U.S. mortality statistics for the past 20 to 30 years, suicide rates in children, adolescents, and young adults have doubled; and for males in the age groups 15 to 19, 20 to 24, and 25 to 29, these rates have tripled. Vital statistical data also point to an

133

increase in homicide rates over the same period, a problem that is particularly dramatic for adolescent and young adult black males. While life expectancy for all other groups increased during the 1960s, life expectancy for young, black males decreased. Although this trend has begun to reverse itself, the life expectancy for young black males in the 15- to 29-year-old age group still lags behind.

Historical Overview

Prudhomme's essay on suicide in the "American Negro" represents one of the most substantial efforts during the first half of this century to understand the unique aspects of depression and suicidal behavior in black Americans (Prudhomme, 1938). Essentially psychoanalytic in viewpoint, his essay examined the historical, cultural, and economic contexts of black American life in the 1930s as a means of explaining the relatively low rate of suicide and depression in this group. He described a pattern of emotions and motivations that curiously seemed to protect blacks from depression and suicidal behavior, while raising the probability of assaultive behavior and homicide:

> Surrounded on all sides by inimical forces, the Negro is always in a state of tension. One might almost say that this reaction is not only instinctive but even hereditary, but that is only because the environment breeds it into the Negro child, from his earliest days when he is made to discern color differences. A constant stream of stimuli bombarding the personality with feelings of humiliation, must inevitably produce among others a state of continuously existing hatred. . . . Any group of people similarly situated socially, would respond in the same manner. . . . (p. 200)
>
> Now, if it be true that one of the most significant mechanisms in suicide is hatred turned inwardly, it is evident that such turning in of hatred is not probably in the Negro except in a minimal number of cases, for the constant presence of stimuli for hatred, necessitates the immediate discharge of hatred outwardly. (p. 200)

Prudhomme, like many of his contemporaries, did not believe that black Americans were civilized enough to become depressed or seriously suicidal, because they had been denied access to what he termed the "cumulative effects" of education (meaning the occurrence of several generations of higher educational experience in a family). This "cumulative effect," he suggested, was a necessary condition to being dissatisfied with one's lot, dissatisfaction which increases the vulnerability toward depression and suicidal behavior. Prudhomme had the vision to forecast that, with increasing educational status, the combined effects of external and internal sources of self-hatred and the "cumulative effects" of education would lead to increasing rates of self-destructive behavior in black Americans. He warned that: ". . . the lower suicide rate is . . . traceable to the peculiar, and psychologically vicious, environment which the majority group has imposed on the minority group. As the environment approximates that of the majority, the suicide rate becomes higher" (Prudhomme, p. 391).

Some 30 years later, Hendin (1969) confirmed the prophecy of Prudhomme. In a series of case studies on successful suicides, he contended that the rage and frustration engendered by impoverished urban existence played a significant role in the depression and suicides of black patients. Using New York City mortality data, Hendin showed that both homicide and suicide reached peak prevalence in black males in the 20- to 35-year-old age group. This finding was qualitatively different from the findings in the population of white males studied. Suicidal and homicidal behavior reflected the noxious pressures and social disadvantage of big city life much more directly in blacks than in whites.

What had changed between Prudhomme's analysis and the current era that Hendin was first to describe? Through the Civil Rights Movement, blacks had been seeking social, economic, and educational equality; a massive migration from rural South to the urban North and Northeast United States had occurred; and the particular zones that blacks settled in cities of the North and Northeast were rapidly decaying. It was not the simple absorption of knowledge and awareness about the world in general that, as Prudhomme had contended, was responsible for the increase in black suicide—but a very complex, multifaceted, and extreme environmental change (Seiden, 1972).

The Present Scene as Reflected in Vital Statistics

Since the early 1970s it has been thought that suicide and homicide may have a common ground. Holinger (1981), using 1961-1975 U.S. mortality data showing that suicides, accidents, and homicides were the leading causes of mortality in the 15- to 29-year-old age group, proposes that they might be grouped together as "violent deaths." Homicides and accidents in young people may "to some extent represent suicidal tendencies through self-imposed risks and self-destructiveness" (p. 280). Though he does not separately examine this category by race, implications for blacks, as will be shown, are alarming.

Dennis (1979) addresses specifically the phenomenon of homicide in the young black male. She points out that life expectancy for this group is less than that for any other age group, reflecting an increased mortality from accidents, suicides, and homicides. It is significant that homicide as a cause of mortality is far greater in the nonwhite male group than any other. The age-adjusted death rate for homicide for all nonwhite males in the U.S. 20 to 29 years old in 1960 was 41.9 per 100,000, and increased to 72.8 per 100,000 by 1970. Reporting data from the state of Michigan, Dennis shows that life expectancy decreased from 64.3 to 61.1 in the years between 1960 and 1970 for nonwhite males. This reversed the narrowing of the difference in life expectancy between nonwhite and white males that had been the trend since the beginning of the century.

Holinger and Offer (1982) suggest that as the proportion of adolescents and young adults in the total population declines, suicide rates will also decline. However, the latest available vital statistics for the U.S. show that the suicide rate for young black males was continuing to climb in 1976, and, in fact, had slightly exceeded the rate for white males in the same age group. Though the rate for black females continues to be the lowest of all groups, the rate of increase for this group is greater than any other. These data, combined with other highly visible factors that are known to interfere with health (such as high unemployment rates, high rates of drug abuse, and high homicide rates in central cities) suggest that the suicide rate among blacks may continue to increase over the next decade.

The current mortality rates of nonwhites (a vital statistical category consisting of blacks predominantly) indicates that the peak age of death due to suicide occurs in the young adult population for both males and females. As shown in Tables 1 and 2, this is in contrast to peak ages of death in the white population. For white females, the peak age is over 40; for white males, the peak age is 80 to 84. Though the overall suicide rates for white males exceed that of black males (the same is true for white females and black

Table 1. Peak Death Rates by Age, Race, and Sex for Suicide (1969)

Race and Sex	Age in Years	Peak Death Rate per 100,000
White male	80–84	50.6
White female	40–44, 50–54	13.4
All other male	30–34	18.6
All other female	25–29	6.4

Reprinted from U.S. Bureau of the Census, Bureau of Vital Statistics. Washington DC, U.S. Government Printing Office, 1978.

Table 2. Peak Death Rates by Age, Race, and Sex for Suicide (1976)

Race and Sex	Age in Years	Peak Death Rate per 100,000
White male	J 85	49.9
White female	50–54	13.9
All other male	25–29; J 85	24.4; 27.9
All other female	30–34	6.7

Reprinted from U.S. Bureau of the Census: Vital Statistics of the U.S. Washington DC, U.S. Government Printing Office, 1978.

females), the differential is narrowing. More pertinent is the fact that for the young adult population, the rates are now comparable. In 1976, the death rate from suicide in nonwhite males 25 to 29 years old was 24.4 per 100,000, compared to 24.1 per 100,000 in white males.

A dramatically different picture is represented for homicide, and these data are shown in Tables 3 and 4. In this instance, the peak death rates occur in the 25- to 34-year-old age range for all four groups. But the rate for nonwhite males is nearly 12 times the rate for white males (138.4/100,000 as compared to 11.6/100,000), and the rate for nonwhite females is eight times the rate for white females (27.4/100,000 as compared to 3.2/100,000). The loss in life expectancy due to violent deaths, already shown by Holinger (1981) to exceed all other causes of death for the population as a whole, becomes an even more pressing problem for young blacks. The rates for homicide alone justify use of the term "epidemic" when the numbers of lives lost in otherwise physically healthy persons is considered.

Table 3.   Peak Death Rates by Age, Race, and Sex for Homicide (1969)

Race and Sex	Age in Years	Peak Death Rate per 100,000
White male	25–34	11.6
White female	25–34	3.2
All other male	25–34	138.4
All other female	25–34	27.4

Reprinted from U.S. Bureau of the Census: Vital Statistics of the U.S. Washington DC, U.S. Government Printing Office, 1978.

Table 4.   Peak Death Rates by Age, Race, and Sex for Homicide (1976)

Race and Sex	Age in Years	Peak Death Rate per 100,000
White male	35–39	14.7
White female	20–24	4.2
All other male	25–29	132.7
All other female	25–29	25.1

Reprinted from U.S. Bureau of the Census: Vital Statistics of the U.S. Washington DC, U.S. Government Printing Office, 1978.

Epidemiological and Clinical Studies

Epidemiological and clinical studies of affective illness, depressive symptomatology, and suicidal behavior in nonwhite groups complete the picture presented by vital statistics data. Examining over 200,000 consecutive emergency visits to the Strong Memorial Hospital in Rochester, New York, Pedersen et al. (1973) calculated the rate of suicide attempts in Monroe County (the Monroe County register serving as the population base). The rate for suicide attempts was five times the suicide rate, 57.3 as compared to 10.4/ 100,000. Confirming previous findings in black populations, they found no instances of suicide attempts in black males over the age of 45, although more than 20 percent of all attempts in white males occurred in the older population. A similar finding was reported for black versus white females. At the youngest ages (15 to 24 years), black males had nearly twice the rate of suicide attempts as white males—153 as compared to 90/100,000—and black females had over three times the rate of white females, 803 as compared to 238/ 100,000. Interestingly, over 84 percent of black suicide attempters were from the lowest socioeconomic classes, compared to 27 percent of whites.

Studies of affective illness show that hospitalized blacks tend to be younger and poorer than hospitalized whites (Powell, 1982; Raskin et al., 1975). They are more likely to be misdiagnosed as schizophrenic, and also present a somewhat different clinical picture (Liss et al., 1973; Welner et al., 1973). The illnesses of hospitalized blacks tend to have a more rapid onset and tend to be characterized by a greater degree of hostility, irritability, and assaultiveness than illnesses of hospitalized whites (Jones et al., 1981; Raskin et al., 1975). In one study, 70 percent of depressed black males were reported to have made a suicide attempt prior to hospitalization (Raskin et al., 1975).

A recent study of suicidal behavior in hospitalized children and adolescents (aged 6 to 16 years) is important in completing the clinical picture of this phenomenon at the youngest ages (Cohen-Sandler et al., 1982). Unlike nonsuicidal depressed children and psychiatric controls, children with suicidal behavior experienced an escalating number of life events as they entered the preadolescent and adolescent years. These children were reported to threaten other people more often and to be less withdrawn than the two control groups. The investigators did not report their data in terms of racial differences, but because the sample was composed of one-half black children and demographic factors were not significant, a tentative conclusion can be drawn that racial differences were not discriminating in the sample. This study is unique because it represents a satisfactorily controlled study in which differences in symptomatology and social experiences antedating hospitalization were examined. An important finding is the absolute increase in the number of life events with age, which, if replicated, will correct a common clinical assumption that both early environmental deprivation (representing distal or vulnerability factors) and adolescent life crises (as proximal or precipitating factors) are necessary conditions for suicidal behavior to occur. There is a need to clarify this issue separately for black and white children, since the early environmental disadvantage of minority groups is commonly presumed to place them at higher risk than white children for a variety of negative outcomes.

In a study of the general population, Goldberg (1981) has shown that 10 to 12 percent of 16- to 24-year-olds in Kansas City report suicidal ideation, and that the majority of young adults with suicidal ideation also report high levels of depression. No differences were found for whites and blacks.

In a study of adolescents in New York State, using selected depression items from the Sympton Checklist (SCL–90), Kandel and Davies (1982) also show no differences in depressive symptoms among whites, blacks, Puerto Ricans, and other Hispanic groups. Socioeconomic factors became important only when the family income was less than $3,000 per year.

Two other general population studies are important because they allow comparison of two minority groups with a white group. Frerichs and colleagues' (1981) Los Angeles study found that the prevalence of depressive symptoms increased with age among Hispanics, while the inverse was true for blacks and whites. When socioeconomic status was controlled, it became clear that membership in a minority group had little or no influence on the prevalence of depressive symptoms. Vernon and Roberts (1982) report higher rates of lifetime major depression in whites (19.2 percent) and Mexican-Americans (18.9 percent) than in blacks (9.6 percent) in an Alameda County study in which the Schedule for Affective Disorders and Schizophrenia–Lifetime Version (SADS–L) was used. Rates for current major depression were higher in Mexican-Americans (2.5 percent) and blacks (2.1 percent) than in whites. It is of some interest that educational status was directly related to depression in whites, and indirectly related in Mexican-Americans; blacks represented an inconsistent pattern of association between these variables.

Based on the available current data, the following conclusions can be reached:

1. At younger ages, blacks experience suicide and suicide attempts at rates that are either the same or greater than the rates experienced by whites. Rates of affective illness and depressive symptoms, however, appear to be either the same or less for blacks than for whites.
2. If one looks at the category of "violent deaths," including both suicide and homicide, then the loss of expected life in young blacks, especially young black males, becomes alarmingly high.
3. Evidence from case histories actually supports the contention that there is a continuum of depressive symptomatology, depressive illness, self-destructive behavior, suicide attempts, and

suicide. The consequences of this continuum for American blacks are cause for concern.

4. The clinical presentation of affective illness in minorities, and especially those in the adolescent and young adult population, may be characterized by greater degrees of anger, hostility, denial, and self-destructive behavior (such as drug abuse and antisocial acts); more rapid onset; and increased frequency of suicidal behavior than the clinical presentation of affective illness in whites.

5. Socioeconomic and historical factors play influential roles in determining rates of depressive symptomatology, suicide, and homicide in blacks. The historical trend in rates of homicide is somewhat less dramatic than rates of suicide, since homicide rates have been high since the beginning of the century.

On examining these statements, it can be asserted that the spectrum of affective illness and suicidal behavior may be substantially different for American minorities than for the majority culture. Moreover, different minority groups experience unique social, economic, political, and educational stresses that interact and result in distinct clinical profiles of depressive illness and suicidal behavior. To facilitate understanding and enhance treatment effectiveness, it is necessary to examine not just the symptomatology of minority patients, but the context that gives rise to such symptoms. Studies that are restricted to comparative descriptions of symptoms fail to capture the unique circumstances that produce pathological behavior of the sort discussed here.

Research Directions

We recommend that seven areas of research activity be given high priority over the next 10 years. First, it is important to conduct clinical studies to examine in detail the association among depressive symptoms, aggressive behavior, and suicidal or homicidal behavior. Standardized interviewing methods and rigorous diagnostic criteria should be used. Efforts should be made to match race of interviewer and patient, so that the effects of interviewer bias and patient resistance will be minimized (Hanson and Klerman, 1974). There is also a distinct advantage in carrying out some of these studies in institutions and clinics that are administered by blacks.

Because many unexplained deaths in black youth are associated with drug abuse and police involvement, the significance of these factors and their association with depression in young minorities must be carefully delineated. Methods for psychological "autopsies" and "biopsies" should be adopted to uncover *motivations* and *methods* used in suicides and suicide attempts among minority youth.

Second, jail and prison populations should be examined not only because they are "captive" and, therefore, eminently researchable, but because blacks are markedly overrepresented in such institutions. This group might be compared to samples of black college students, to provide an interesting within-race contrast of persons within the same age range. The logic of such a comparison is supported by the common experience that blacks with markedly different educational and occupational status frequently come from the same neighborhoods, and in some cases even from the same families. A research design that examines such within-category differences would add immeasurably to our understanding of the particular psychosocial circumstances that lead to violent deaths in some, but not all, who are at similar risk when only demographic and shared environmental variables are evaluated.

Third, depression, suicidal ideation, suicide attempts, and suicide may all occur at different rates in blacks attending segregated as opposed to desegregated schools and colleges. Powell (1982) has demonstrated lower levels of self-esteem in black junior high school students attending desegregated as opposed to segregated schools. Strayhorn (1980) has also reported that black medical students view themselves as under more psychosocial stress than their white classmates in a desegregated medical school. The finding suggests that social contexts and prevailing racial attitudes may be important risk factors in the vulnerability of blacks to develop depressive illnesses, suicidal behavior, and suicide.

Fourth, the influences that education, mobility, employment status, and residence in urban centers has on the social support system of blacks should be closely examined. The historically important role of religion in black culture, representing an important source of social support and institutionalized coping, may be giving way to such influences. From a mental health perspective, increased educational opportunity through the desegregation of schools may be a mixed blessing. As Prudhomme suggested a half-century ago, increased achievement of blacks may occur at the cost of increased rates of depression and self-destructiveness. The relationship between unemployment in young black males and the development of depressive illness or aggressive behavior warrants systematic examination using a combination of clinical and epidemiologic methods. Such studies are needed; it is important to know whether chronic or temporary unemployment heightens the risk for depression, alcoholism, suicidal behavior, and homicide. Since it is likely that our economy will continue to produce high unemployment rates, and because it is also likely that these rates will remain relatively higher among blacks, it is essential to launch research efforts to delineate the relationship between unemployment and mental health.

Fifth, research on the association between physical disease and mental disorder in young blacks must be encouraged. To what extent both types of illnesses may be precipitated or influenced by psychosocial factors warrants careful investigation. For example, the possibility of a linkage between hypertension and depression in blacks should be examined. Although it is feasible that there might be a common pathophysiological mechanism responsible for both disorders, this association may be spurious. If such a relationship were to be firmly established, it could be that both were caused by psychosocial stress.

Sixth, examination of the patterns of health care utilization in blacks may yield valuable clues on the risks of suicide and other forms of violent deaths. Of particular importance is the examination of accidents among young black males. Interviewing these men about their life circumstances and social environments might reveal a subgroup at high risk for experiencing a violent death within a short interval of time.

Finally, examination of geographical trends in suicide and homicide rates among blacks and other minority groups must be made. Preliminary data suggesting that suicide rates among blacks vary inversely with the proportion of blacks living in various states and regions of the country has been reported (Lester, 1980). This kind of demographic analysis needs to be replicated and refined using the latest available population data for clues as to which regions or states need to be given special consideration for prevention efforts. Again, demographic changes in minority groups making up certain regions may also provide valuable clues to predicting changes in suicide and homicide rates.

Obviously, there is much important research to be done. The quality and impact of this work will depend on the degree to which minority mental health professionals and minority institutions influence and/or direct these efforts. Unfortunately, a serious deficiency exists in the number of minority mental health researchers and the resources available in predominantly black colleges and medical schools. Yet persons in these settings have a unique advantage in formulating questions, in gaining access to research populations, and in increasing the likelihood that the results of studies actually lead to decisive and beneficial action. Given the current resources of black institutions, however, it is unlikely that they alone can successfully conduct the range of studies recommended. University departments with advanced skills and a long history of research productivity should be encouraged to develop technical and advisory relationships with black institutions to conduct the kinds of studies that have been outlined in this chapter. These are necessary steps to developing sound prevention strategies and to improving the care and treatment of minority patients.

There is a limited base of existing knowledge on which prevention programs for blacks can be planned. Statistical as well as clinical data suggest that the circumstances that have led to high rates of violent deaths among blacks, particularly over the last 20 years, warrant separate investigation.

References

Adebimpe VR: Overview: white norms and psychiatric diagnosis of black patients. Am J Psychiatry 138:279–285, 1981

Cohen-Sandler R, Berman AL, King RA: Life stress and symptomatology: determinants of suicidal behavior in children. J Am Acad Child Psychiatry 21:178–186, 1982

Dennis RE: The role of homicide in decreasing life expectancy, in Lethal Aspects of Urban Violence. Edited by Rose HM. Lexington, MA, D.C. Heath, 1979

Frerichs RR, Aneshensel CS, Clark VA: Prevalence of depression in Los Angeles County. Am J Epidemiol 113:691–699, 1981

Goldberg EL: Depression and suicide ideation in the young adult. Am J Psychiatry 138:35–40, 1981

Hanson B, Klerman GL: Interracial problems in the assessment of clinical depression: concordance differences between white psychiatrists and black and white patients. Psychopharmacol Bull 10:65–67, 1974

Hendin H: Black suicide. Arch Gen Psychiatry 21:407–422, 1969

Holinger PC: Self-destructiveness among the young: an epidemiological study of violent deaths. Int J Soc Psychiatry 27:277–282, 1981

Holinger PC, Offer D: Prediction of adolescent suicide: a population model. Am J Psychiatry 139:302–307, 1982

Jones BE, Gray BA, Parson EB: Manic-depressive illness among poor urban blacks. Am J Psychiatry 138:654–657, 1981

Kandel DB, Davies M: Epidemiology of depressive mood in adolescents. Arch Gen Psychiatry 39:1205–1212, 1982

Lester D: Letter to the Editor—Regional suicide rates and the hazards of minority status. Am J Psychiatry 137:1469–1470, 1980

Liss JL, Welner A, Robins E, et al: Psychiatric symptoms in white and black inpatients, I: record study. Compr Psychiatry 14:475–481, 1973

Pedersen AM, Awad GA, Kindler AR: Epidemiological differences between white and nonwhite suicide attempters. Am J Psychiatry 130:1071–1076, 1973

Powell GJ: Overview of the epidemiology of mental illness among Afro-Americans, in The Afro-American Family: Assessment, Treatment, and Research Issues. Edited by Bass BA, Wyatt GE, Powell GJ. New York, Grune & Stratton, 1982

Prudhomme C: The problem of suicide in the American Negro. Psychoanal Rev 25:187–204; 372–391, 1938

Raskin A, Crook TH, Herman KD: Psychiatric history and symptom differences in black and white depressed inpatients. J Consult Clin Psychol 43:73–80, 1975

Seiden RH: Why are suicides of young blacks increasing? Public Health Rep 87:3–8, 1972

Strayhorn G: Perceived stress and social supports of black and white medical students. J Med Educ 55:618–620, 1980

Vernon SW, Roberts RC: Use of the SADS–RDC in a tri-ethnic community survey. Arch Gen Psychiatry 39:47–52, 1982

Vital Statistics of the United States, DHEW, 1978

Welner A, Liss JL, Robins E: Psychiatric symptoms in white and black inpatients, II: follow-up study. Compr Psychiatry 14:483–488, 1973

Chapter 7

SOCIAL ADAPTATIONAL AND PSYCHOLOGICAL ANTECEDENTS IN THE FIRST GRADE OF ADOLESCENT PSYCHOPATHOLOGY TEN YEARS LATER

Sheppard G. Kellam, M.D.
C. Hendricks Brown, Ph.D.

Chapter 7

Social Adaptational and Psychological Antecedents in the First Grade of Adolescent Psychopathology Ten Years Later

The developmental paths leading to mental health or mental disorder, and to social adaptation or maladaptation, are of central importance to understanding their causes as well as their enhancement, prevention, or treatment. Community epidemiological studies with a life span developmental perspective are major tools for investigating these matters. The work presented in this chapter stems from such an orientation. We report here on investigations of early psychological and social adaptational antecedents on the paths leading to psychiatric distress in adolescents, 10 years further along the life span. Included for comparison are analyses of the antecedents of adolescent drug, alcohol, and cigarette use as well. These data were gathered prospectively on a total population of first grade children in Woodlawn, an urban black ghetto community on the south side of Chicago, and are part of the large community epidemiological developmental data base gathered on consecutive co-

The authors wish to acknowledge the crucial contributions of the Woodlawn community, its families and children, and the community board members who over the last 20 years have provided support and guidance for this research and service enterprise. Particular thanks are due Mrs. Rose Bates, who continues to instruct us regarding community issues. The faculty and staffs of the Woodlawn Public and Catholic elementary schools and those of the Chicago Public High Schools made crucial contributions. Over the years Dr. Curtis Melnick, former Associate Superintendent of the Chicago Board of Education, has been very important to this project. Jeannette Branch, the former Director of the Woodlawn Mental Health Center, and later during the follow-up with the South Side Youth Program, has

horts of children and families of that community.

The developmental paths leading to psychopathology and other outcomes can be conceptualized as involving biological capacities for adaptation in interaction with characteristics and demands of environment, limited or enhanced by the growing store of experience and information gained by the child as the life span evolves. The social structural characteristics of family, school, work, peers, intimate partner, and community comprise the major immediate social environments that can tax or aid the individual's capacity to respond at different phases along the life cycle.

The mental health status of an individual is influenced not only by biological capacities and social structural characteristics, but also by the nature of the interaction between the individual and the environment. This interaction consists of social task demands made within particular social fields and the individual's behavioral responses. Natural raters, such as teachers, parents, supervisors, spouses, and peers, rate these behavioral responses in regard to adequacy of role performance. We have named this demand/response perspective social adaptation, and the ratings of the individual by natural raters we termed social adaptational status. Social adaptational status, particularly as it evolves over time, is what is commonly judged the level of success or failure of an individual in society. This con-

been involved in all aspects of the research and was responsible for the collection of the teacher ratings of social adaptational status.

We are grateful for the assistance of our colleagues, past and present, at the Social Psychiatry Study Center in many aspects of the study. Margaret Ensminger, Ph.D., has been Co-principal Investigator of the Woodlawn project for many years and continues to supervise, advise, and carry out research on these data. Pamela Hecht, Ph.D., Chief of Data Management at the Social Psychiatry Study Center, was responsible for the organization and preparation of data sets used here. Barnett Rubin, Ph.D., made many of the log-linear runs reported in this paper and participated in their interpretation. George Bohrnstedt, Ph.D., and Kenneth Day, Ph.D., examined the psychometric properties of the teenage psychiatric symptom measures.

These studies have been supported by the following grants: State of Illinois Department of Mental Health Grant Numbers 17-224 and 17-322; National Institute of Mental Health Number MH-15760 and Research Scientist Development Award Grant Number 1K01-MH-47596; the Maurice Falk Medical Fund; for the follow-up, National Institute on Drug Abuse Grant Number DA-00787; Ten Year Prospective Study of Teen Smoking Number PHS-1-R01-DA-02591. Biomedical Research Grants from The Johns Hopkins University School of Hygiene and Public Health also provided support.

In recent years, long-term analyses have been strongly supported by the John D. and Catherine T. MacArthur Foundation.

ceptual framework appears to be applicable across societies, and possibly across species as well.

In the Woodlawn studies, social adaptational status has been regarded as conceptually distinct from the internal psychological status of the individual, called psychological well-being, and these two concepts have been measured independently. In our longitudinal analyses, we have used this distinctness to study developmental paths comprised of SAS and psychological well-being measures, along with social structural characteristics of family, school, and peer group as these evolve over time. We find in social adaptational status important early predictors of outcomes, including psychiatric symptoms, heavy drug, alcohol, and tobacco use, delinquency, and school achievement. Our work has focused on examining similarities and differences in developmental antecedents leading to these and other outcomes, as well as examining developmental sex differences (Kellam et al., 1983a; Ensminger et al., 1982; Ensminger et al., 1983; Kellam et al., 1980; Fleming et al., 1982).

In this chapter we report on a set of these relationships linking social adaptational status and psychological well-being in the first grade to self-reports of psychiatric symptoms by adolescents 10 years later. We also include a contrasting set of outcomes; namely, use of drugs, alcohol, and cigarettes by the adolescents. These contrasting outcomes give us an opportunity to examine the specificity along developmental paths of particular risk factors or predictors for a specific outcome. The only way we can discern the degree to which an early predictor is specific to a particular outcome is by looking at a set of outcomes together. Kohn (1976) made this point in a review of 25 years of social and behavioral research, calling attention to the fact that much work has been done on single outcomes, thus limiting theory building to a great extent. One need only review even such proximal areas of investigation as delinquency and substance use to see how insular scientific literatures often are. The same holds true for psychopathology and substance use.

Studies of Social Adaptational Status and Psychological Well-Being as Predictors of Psychiatric Symptoms and Substance Use

Because of the importance of prospective longitudinal research in the areas this chapter treats, this review will mainly focus on studies

employing such a design. We first summarize findings on antecedents of psychiatric symptoms. We divide the antecedents between
our categories of psychological well-being and social adaptational
status. We then examine studies of antecedents of substance use in
the same way. We have tried to bring out findings on sex differences
since these are extremely important, although they are often not
reported.

Predictors of Teenage and Adult Psychiatric Symptoms

Psychological well-being predictors. A variety of childhood symptoms and syndromes appear to be related to later psychopathology, but few such childhood conditions exhibit either
clear continuity to the same outcome or a clear developmental path
to another specific one. Organic brain dysfunction and brain damage
seem to lead to a variety of later disorders in both sexes (Rutter et
al., 1970; Warren, 1965; Shaffer et al., 1979; Watt, 1974). Hyperactive
children may be more nervous, restless, temperamental, impulsive,
depressed, or lacking in self-esteem than control children at adolescent or adult follow-up (Borland and Heckman, 1976; Milich and
Loney, 1979; Stewart et al., 1973; Hechtman et al., 1981). These
studies did not include enough females in the sample to provide
firm conclusions about sex differences in the later outcome of hyperactivity.

Several studies have found that early neurotic syndromes do
not clearly predict later syndromes (Rutter, 1972); Pritchard and
Graham, 1966; Warren, 1965; Robins, 1966). However, many investigators do report early psychiatric symptoms associated with later
psychiatric symptoms and, in some reports, later psychosis. Two
studies found early feelings of depression to be an antecedent of
schizophrenia for males (Robins, 1966; Watt, 1974). Childhood nail
biting, worrying, and specific fears seem to predict a number of
later outcomes, including adult anxiety in both sexes (Pritchard and
Graham, 1966) and schizophrenia among males (Robins, 1966). In
the Woodlawn population, measures of anxiety and depression and
trouble with feelings in first grade predicted symptom ratings for
the females 10 years later (Kellam et al., 1983b). Emotional instability
in children predicted later schizophrenia in one study (Watt, 1974).
Another linked "lack of malleability" to later psychiatric disorder
in both sexes (Graham et al., 1973). Somatic symptoms and muscular
tension in childhood seem also to be somewhat related to later

psychological problems, both in the Woodlawn population (Kellam et al., 1983b) and elsewhere (Robins, 1966).

Social adaptational status predictors. Early social mal-adaptation strongly appears to predict various psychological outcomes in adolescence and adulthood. Numerous studies, including Woodlawn, have linked early learning difficulties to later psychiatric problems. Learning problems have been shown to be related to later schizophrenia (Watt, 1974) and depressed feelings in males (Kellam et al., 1983; Kellam et al., 1985a), and to paranoid feelings in females (Robins, 1966).

IQ, which we consider to be a quasi-social adaptational status measure when it is tested under loosely controlled conditions in a classroom for institutional purposes, is related to many later psychological problems. Shaffer and colleagues (1979) linked low childhood IQ to later general psychiatric disorder. Rutter and associates (1970) found that early low IQ led to"neurotic disorder" in females but to "antisocial disorder" (a social adaptational rather than psychological problem) in males. One study presented evidence that above-average IQ increased the chances of a positive outcome for autistic children of either sex (Stewart and Gath, 1978). In the Woodlawn population, higher first grade IQ scores were linked to decreased risk of psychiatric symptoms 10 years later (Kellam et al., 1983a; 1983b).

Early aggressive and antisocial behavior strongly predict many later psychological problems, according to many studies. In the Woodlawn studies, however, when we include other concomitant variables (such as learning problems) in the equation, we have found aggression to predict only social adaptational, not psychological, problems. Such behavior, nevertheless, is a reported predictor of later schizophrenia for males (Watt, 1978; Robins, 1966) and of sociopathic personality for both sexes (Robins, 1966).

Predictors of Substance Use

Psychological well-being predictors. A number of researchers have reported that early psychological distress in teenagers predicts substance use (Smith and Fogg, 1978; Paton et al., 1977; Kaplan, 1975). In the Woodlawn population, however, we found no predictive effect in first grade males, and one in the opposite direction for females: psychiatric symptoms in the first grade were weakly associated with less substance use 10 years later (Kellam et al., 1983a; 1983b).

One important set of psychological variables includes the individual's cognitive and affective orientation toward drug use and society's views thereof. Perceived use by others is an important predictor (Jessor and Jessor, 1978; Robins et al., 1977; Kandel et al., 1978). Not too surprisingly, Kandel and colleagues (1978), Sadava (1973), and Smith and Fogg (1978) have established that favorable attitudes toward substance use predict use. In general, attachment to or alienation from the dominant values of society shows a consistent relationship to substance use (Jessor and Jessor, 1978; Sadava, 1973; Smith and Fogg, 1978; Kandel et al., 1978). Ensminger and colleagues (1982) have reported clear replication of this result and have discussed it within the framework of social control theory.

Social adaptational status predictors. One major group of SAS predictors concerns performance in school. The relationship of academic achievement to substance use seems to depend upon the stage of life and the population studied. A number of investigators have reported that poor high school performance is a common antecedent of substance use (Jessor and Jessor, 1978; Kandel et al., 1978; Smith and Fogg, 1978). In contrast, studies by Mellinger et al. (1978) and the Jessors (1978) have indicated that college students who had higher grade point averages smoked marijuana more often than students who had lower grade point averages. Another study reported that high school students who used marijuana and hallucinogens tended to have lower grades, but higher general intelligence (Johnston, 1973). Previous studies of the Woodlawn data found that teacher-rated learning problems in first grade were not related to substance use 10 years later, but results of studies on aggressive behavior in males, and performance on first grade readiness and IQ tests, showed that: 1) aggressive males used substances more often later, but did not start earlier than their cohort; and, independently of this, 2) those first graders with higher test scores developed into adolescents who used substances more often (Kellam et al., 1980; Kellam et al., 1983a). This second relation was true for both sexes, and appears to be due to earlier age at first use (Fleming et al., 1982).

A number of studies have found that various measures of social passivity were related to lower substance use. Smith and Fogg (1978) found that ratings of obedience by both self and peers were among the best criterion variables in a discriminant analysis of nonusers, early users, and late users of marijuana. They also found that peer ratings of "tenderness" were related negatively to the initiation of use. Previous studies of substance use in the Woodlawn population found that males rated shy by first grade teachers were significantly less likely to use cigarettes and marijuana 10 years later (Kellam et al., 1980; 1983a). There were trends in the same direction for hard liquor and beer or wine. None of these results were evident for females.

Aggressive or antisocial behavior may be the most frequently replicated predictor of substance use (Johnston, 1973; Johnston et al., 1978; Kandel et al., 1978). Robins (1978) summarized her consistent findings from three independent investigations, of the relation between childhood and adolescent antisocial behavior on the one hand, and adult outcomes on the other. She reported that, across three studies, there was a reliable association of early fighting, truancy, arrests, and drinking with adult alcoholism and drug abuse (Robins, 1966; Robins and Murphy, 1967; Robins et al., 1977). The Woodlawn studies have supported these findings, and have established the prediction as far back as age six or seven—in first grade—but only for males. Males rated as aggressive by their first grade teachers were significantly more likely to be heavy substance users 10 years later (Kellam et al., 1980; Ensminger et al., 1982; Kellam et al., 1983a; Fleming et al., 1982).

One result of the Woodlawn studies that has not, to our knowledge, been reported elsewhere, is that those males who are both shy and aggressive in the first grade form a special population. Rather than falling between the shy nonaggressives and the aggressive nonshy groups in levels of use, the shy-aggressives appear to have the highest rate of use of all groups studied (Kellam et al., 1983a). We will report further on these data in this chapter.

Community Epidemiology:
The Woodlawn Study Population

For investigating the paths leading to psychopathology, the prospective longitudinal study of total defined populations is a major methodological advance over studies that examine clinic or volunteer populations. Neither of these last two groups can be assumed to represent the full population of interest, since many confounding factors intervene in both help-seeking and volunteering (Kellam et al., 1981). In community-specific epidemiological studies, we can hold constant the broad characteristics of the community while we focus on the effects of variation in families, in classrooms and schools, and in the other local social contexts. Since rates of maladaptation, symptoms, and disorders may vary from one kind of community to another, replication in similar and different kinds of communities also must be part of research strategy.

Woodlawn is a black, poor, urban community on the south side of Chicago. Between 1964 and 1968, we assessed the classroom performance and psychological well-being of all the first graders in this community at several points in each of four consecutive school years. There was a follow-up assessment of those children in the four cohorts who were still in Woodlawn in the third grade. We also conducted interviews in the spring of 1965 and the spring of 1967 with the mothers or surrogate mothers of the children who were in first grade in those two school years. These assessments were coupled with service and evaluation programs (Kellam et al., 1975) and were supported by a community board composed of leaders from the community's larger citizen organizations (Kellam and Branch, 1971; Kellam et al., 1972).

The studies of first-grade measures reported here are based on the 1966-1967 cohort. In 1975-1976, we located and successfully reinterviewed 75 percent of the mothers or surrogate mothers of the original 1,242 families, the total population of children who remained in Woodlawn for that first grade year. The mothers' refusal rate was 5.9 percent. An additional 18.5 percent of mothers were not reinterviewed because we could not find them, because the families had moved from Chicago, or because the study children were deceased.

After the mother was interviewed and had given permission, the teenager was approached for reassessment. The children had been six or seven years old in first grade and were 16 or 17 at the time of follow-up. Of the 939 reinterviewed mothers, 75 percent ($N = 705$) of their teenage study children participated in the reassessments, and constituted the study population for the long-term outcomes. In order to assess possible bias resulting from sample attrition, we compared family, school, and psychological data from the time of first grade among three populations of children: those whose mothers were not reinterviewed, those whose mothers were reinterviewed but who were not themselves reinterviewed, and those whose mothers and themselves were reinterviewed. We found no statistically significant differences in teacher ratings, early test scores, or early clinical ratings among these three groups. We have described the methods of follow-up elsewhere (see, for example, Agrawal et al., 1978; Kellam et al., 1980).

Social Adaptation and Psychological Well-Being: A Two-Dimensional Concept of Mental Health

Mental health has two distinct aspects which can be conceptualized and measured separately: psychological well-being, and social adaptational status. From the standpoint of the individual, mental health is both an internal feeling of psychological well-being related to affective status and self-esteem, as well as a state of cognitive competence. It is measured by behaviors thought to reflect these aspects of the individual's state. Certain behaviors are termed symptoms; certain aggregates of symptoms are termed syndromes or disorders.

From the standpoint of society, however, mental health consists of the adequacy of the individual's role function in the major social fields appropriate to his or her stage in the life cycle. This is the aspect of mental health we call social adaptational status (Kellam et al., 1975; Kellam and Ensminger, 1980). Following the work of Havinghurst (1952), Erikson (1959, 1963), Parsons (1964), Neugarten (1979), and others, we view individuals as passing through vaguely demarcated stages of life and as being involved in one, two, or a few major social fields at each stage. These social fields have "natural raters" who define the social tasks required in that field, and who rate the adequacy of the individual's performance. These ratings constitute the individual's social adaptational status.

The natural rater sometimes assesses individuals formally, as first grade teachers do with grades and tests. Parents may have less formal means of assessment but are equally authoritative. The supervisor on the job and significant others in the peer group are additional examples of natural raters important at different stages of life. Along with psychological first grade predictors, this chapter reports on two social adaptational status measures in the classroom: teacher's ratings, and school administered test scores. Our past findings suggest that specific first grade social adaptational status measures have particularly important long-term predictive and developmental significance for adolescence. Social adaptational status

Table 1.   Representative Maladaptive Behaviors and Social Tasks

Maladaptive Behaviors	Categories of Social Tasks

Shyness
   Shy, timid, alone too much, friendless,
   aloof
	Social contact

Aggressiveness
   Fights too much, lies, resists authority, is
   destructive to others, disobedient
	Authority acceptance

Immaturity
   Acts too young, cries too much, has
   tantrums, seeks too much attention
	Maturation

Underachievement
   Does not learn as well as he or she is able,
   lazy, does not come prepared for work,
   underachieves, lacks effort
	Cognitive achievement

Concentration Problems
   Fidgets, is unable to sit still in classroom,
   restless, does not pay attention
	Concentration

therefore provides a major integrating focus for prevention research—that is, if we can improve specific aspects of social adaptational status, can we thereby improve specific outcomes?

Description of Measures

Social Adaptational Status in the First Grade

Social adaptation can best be measured by asking natural raters to define specific tasks required of the individuals in a particular social field, and then having the relevant natural rater evaluate the individual's performance. In the first year of the study, 57 first grade teachers were asked to define those behaviors which they thought would indicate that the child was having difficulty accomplishing the tasks of the classroom. Two research staff members independently sorted 435 items into five categories that included the kinds of problem behaviors mentioned by the teachers (Kellam et al., 1975). A representative sample of maladaptive behavioral items and the social tasks inferred from them can be seen in Table 1.

A four-point global scale was made for each category of task, ranging from adapting within minimal limits, to mild, moderate, and severe maladapting. Ratings were obtained for each child in the classroom for each task three times in the first grade, and again in the third grade. Structured interviews with the teacher were used in a quiet room in the school by an experienced social worker who had herself been a teacher.

The Metropolitan Readiness Test was administered in the class-room early in the first grade, and an IQ test was also administered in the classroom toward the end of the first grade. We consider these tests quasi-social adaptational status measures, since they are school task demands made of the students by the school, and are administered to large groups of children with only modest stan-dardization. The reliability and validity of both the test scores and the teacher ratings have been extensively described in earlier pub-lications (see, for example, Kellam et al., 1975).

Psychological Well-Being in the First Grade

Data on psychological well-being were collected from struc-tured clinical observations, from the mothers, and from children in the third grade. We will discuss only the first grade measures in this chapter. The Mother Symptom Inventory (MSI), completed by the mothers in the home interview in 1966–1967, was a 38-item inventory adapted from previous investigations of the epidemiology of symptoms among children (Kellam et al., 1975). The mothers were asked to rate their children on each symptom on a four-point scale, from "not at all" to "very much." These 38 items as used here are combined into a single total morbidity score reflecting psycho-logical distress. While unaware of the teacher's actual ratings, moth-ers may have been aware of the teacher's views of her child's social adaptation.

We also obtained measures of psychological well-being from Direct Clinical Observation (DCO). At both the beginning and the end of the first grade, pairs of clinicians (a male and a female) observed groups of 10 children, five girls and five boys, randomly drawn from each classroom and, in standardized group play situ-ations, rated each child on six symptoms (Kellam et al., 1975). For this analysis, we have grouped all children who were rated as other than "not sick" by either clinician as having "signs of symptom-atology," and contrasted them with the majority of children who had no such signs. This strategy was based on the relatively few children at age six or seven who rated more than mildly symptomatic on any symptom.

Teenage Substance Use

The information on teenage substance use presented in this chapter was gathered from responses to items in *What's Happening?*, one of two questionnaires administered to the 16- or 17-year-old teenagers who participated in the follow-up sessions. The questions concerned the frequency of use of 12 categories of substances, including alcohol and cigarettes. The teenagers indicated frequency of their use of these substances: 1) during the previous two months, and 2) ever. For the analyses in this chapter, we use only responses to the "ever" question. We discuss four categories of substances: 1) beer or wine, 2) hard liquor, 3) cigarettes, and 4) marijuana or hashish. The questionnaire also asked about the use of drugs such as psychedelics, "uppers," "downers," tranquilizers, cocaine, inhalants, heroin, and codeine, but the respondents used these drugs too infrequently for us to report on their antecedents here.

For all categories except cigarettes, rate of use was broken into three categories: 1) never used, 2) used one to 19 times, and 3) used 20 times or more. Cigarette use was broken into: 1) never used, 2) used once or twice, or occasionally, and 3) used regularly.

Both questionnaires were administered by two black college students to adolescents in groups of five to eight persons. The college students rotated partners and the leadership role. The assessment questions were presented visually on slides and orally on audiotape to control for reading ability differences, and to standardize the pace and the general administration of the questions (Petersen and Kellam, 1977). The group process in which the data were gathered focused on the trust issue, allowing the adolescents to express their fears and questions. During the administration, the assessors stopped the slides and tape whenever a teenager had questions about either the purpose or the meaning of the items. Confidentiality of responses was emphasized.

Drug use in the Woodlawn teenagers was heavily centered on beer or wine, hard liquor, marijuana, and cigarettes (Kellam et al., 1980). Males used significantly more beer or wine, hard liquor, and marijuana than did females. There were no significant sex differences in cigarette use and illicit drug use other than marijuana.

Teenage Psychiatric Symptoms

The psychiatric symptom constructs used in this paper are based on factor analyses of the items chosen to represent six a priori constructs in the *How I Feel* questionnaire, the second questionnaire administered in the same session as the questionnaire entitled *What's Happening?* Each of these 42 items were measured on a six-point scale. Psychometric examination of these original constructs is presented in Petersen and Kellam (1977).

Recently, Bohrnstedt and colleagues, in an unpublished manuscript, used exploratory maximum likelihood factor analysis to check whether the data confirmed the existence of these constructs. They examined seven-factor through 10-factor solutions for the original set of 49 items for males and females separately. These analyses suggested that there were six factors, but we subsequently deleted the Anger Outward factor, because the items we found best representing it were entirely self-reports of actual aggressive behavior, which we believed made it more of a social adaptational status measure.

Items included in one of the remaining five constructs had to have a loading of 0.35 or greater in the (non-orthogonal) promax-rotation factor solutions. Next, those items loading on more than one factor were deleted. Finally, to remain on the list, an item had to be more highly correlated on the average with the items on its own factor list than with the items in the other factor lists.

The lists of items, together with the names we adopted for the factors, appear in Table 2. They resemble closely the original a priori symptom constructs.

We next examined differences between males and females in the structure of the five remaining factor-based psychopathology constructs, and concluded that the same set of items could be used in each construct for males and females.

Besides these measures of specific symptoms, we also constructed a measure of overall distress using Rasch's psychometric model (Wright, 1977). The Rasch model provides a method for obtaining scale values for persons and items on an underlying, unidimensional trait, in this case that of overall psychological distress. The Rasch model yields tests of fit of items to the unidimensional model. On the basis of these tests, we eliminated 14 items from the original 49; the remaining 35 fit the model well and yielded interval Rasch scores of overall distress.

Table 2. Item List for the Five Factor-Based Symptom Constructs

I. Anxiety
1. I feel nervous
2. I feel under pressure
3. I feel tense
4. New situations make me tense

II. Depression
1. I feel sad
2. I cry and don't know why
3. I feel hopeless
4. I feel ashamed of myself
5. I feel guilty
6. People would be better off without me

III. Bizarreness
1. I sometimes hear strange things when I am alone
2. I sometimes think the world is ending
3. I sometimes hear voices or sounds others don't
4. Weird, odd, and strange things happen to me

IV. Paranoia
1. People hide from me what they really feel
2. People have turned against me
3. People talk behind my back

V. Obsessive–Compulsive
1. When things are not neat and orderly, I feel upset
2. If things are not just a certain way, I feel upset

All analyses of the teenage symptom constructs used dichotomies based on summed scores of the items for each construct or on the Rasch score. A high score for a symptom construct or overall distress is defined as any score more than one-half standard deviation above the mean for the entire sample of 705 teenagers. A low symptom score is any score below that value.

In this chapter we examine the long-term outcomes of psychiatric symptoms and substance use predicted by the two social adaptational status measures, teacher observations and test scores, and those predicted by two measures of psychological well-being, direct clinical observation, and mothers' reports of their childrens' symptoms.

The following results are from log-linear analyses, in which data were introduced in a sequence of models testing for 2-, 3-, 4-, and 5-way effects. While the discussion focuses on each of these measures singly, our analyses, which included multiple antecedent measures, have examined the separateness or overlap among the main effects. Only a few important high order associations were found, and these are described here.

Results

First, we describe the relationship between first grade social adaptational status measures and teenage outcomes for both males and females. Next, we present early psychological well-being antecedents.

Shyness

Teacher ratings of shyness among males in first grade are related to an elevated risk of anxiety and to the frequency of substance use. In Figure 1, we see that 37 percent of the males who were rated moderately or severely shy in the first grade reported high levels of anxious feelings as teenagers, as compared to 20 percent of the non-shy males.

Among males, shyness without aggressiveness inhibits the later use of marijuana, hard liquor, and cigarettes (Kellam et al., 1980; Kellam et al., 1983a; Ensminger et al., 1982). Figure 2 shows the outcomes for substance use. For all four substance categories, those males rated shy but not aggressive reported the least substance use as teenagers. However, those males who were rated both shy and aggressive by their teachers in the first grade reported the heaviest use of substances.

Among females, shyness is a much less significant predictor of later outcomes than it is for males. No relationship was found between early shyness and teenage psychiatric symptoms; nor was there any relationship to lifetime frequency of substance use. The only significant relationship we have found is that early shyness in females inhibits the initiation of use of hard liquor in adolescence (Fleming et al., 1982).

Aggressiveness

For males, aggressiveness as rated by first grade teachers leads to increased levels of use of beer or wine, marijuana, hard liquor,

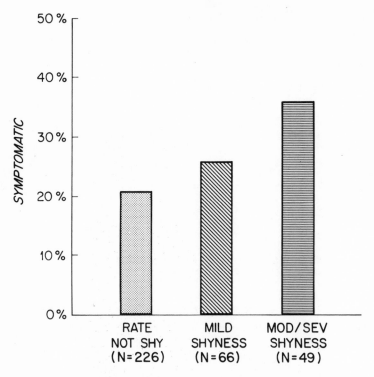

Figure 1. First grade shyness in males, and teenage anxiety

and cigarettes, as well as a higher level of antisocial behavior 10 years later (Kellam et al., 1983a; Ensminger et al., 1983). Those first grade males who are moderately or severely aggressive and shy tend to have even higher levels of substance use 10 years later (see Figure 2). Aggressiveness in males in the first grade (when other variables were controlled) did not lead to later psychiatric symptoms.

While teachers reported aggressiveness as a common maladaptation in males, far fewer females were rated as aggressive. For females, the outcomes of aggressiveness and shy-aggressiveness are quite different. Aggressiveness in females in the first grade does not lead to heavier substance use and higher delinquency in adolescence, as it does in males. However, aggressiveness in females is related to paranoid symptoms, possibly a form of unexpressed aggressiveness (see Figure 3).

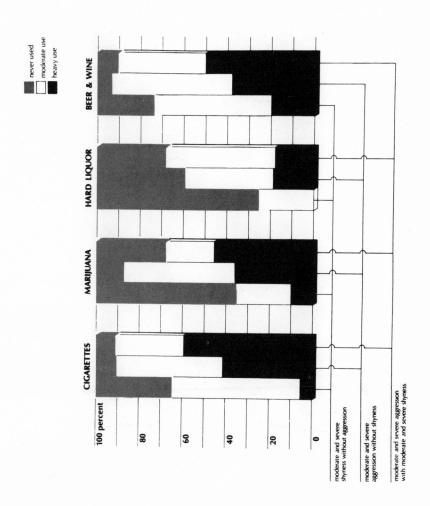

Figure 2. Shyness and aggressiveness in first grade, and teenage substance use by males

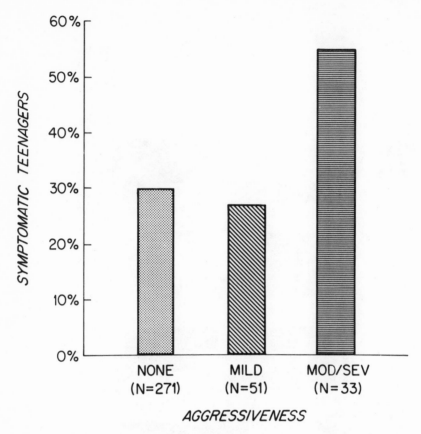

Figure 3.   Aggressiveness in first grade, and paranoia in teenage females

Underachievement

Teacher ratings of this common form of maladaptation in first grade males frequently leads to high levels of depressive symptoms 10 years later. Figure 4 shows that progressively higher levels of first grade underachievement lead to progressively higher proportions of the sample reporting a high level of depressed feelings 10 years later. Almost 50 percent of the males rated as moderately or severely underachieving in first grade reported a high level of depressed symptoms 10 years later. This relationship appears to be specific; underachievement ratings are not related to other symptom constructs or to substance use or to delinquency. Among females, underachievement is related to neither symptoms nor substance

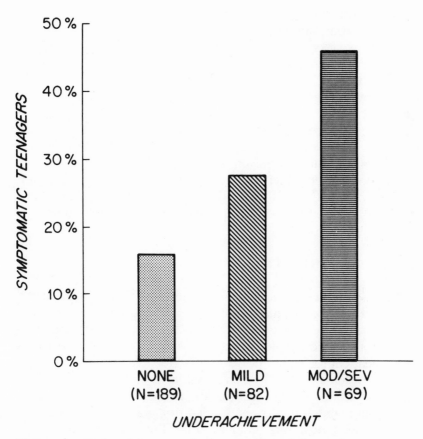

Figure 4. Underachievement in first grade, and depressive symptoms in teenage males

use. This strong association for males—and its total absence for females—appears to be an important difference between the sexes in the meaning of failure to master first grade learning tasks.

Concentration Problems

This teacher rating is of particular interest because it resembles in some respects the central criterion for attention deficit disorder. As noted by Kellam and colleagues in an unpublished manuscript, it is closely related to ratings of aggressiveness (τ–b = .6). In general, concentration problems seem to have outcomes similar to aggressiveness. They are associated, as is aggressiveness, with later substance use and antisocial behavior among males, and with paranoid symptoms among females. When one controls for the effect of aggressiveness, the effect of concentration problems generally disappears or is reduced considerably.

Our conclusion about these relationships is that teachers do not distinguish aggressiveness and concentration problems reliably, especially at the severe end of the scales. The scales appear to substitute for each other in predicting later outcomes. This is most clear for delinquency (Ensminger et al., 1983). Either concentration problems without aggressiveness, or aggressiveness without concentration problems, increase the risk of delinquency 10 years later; but the combination of the two does not raise the risk of antisocial behavior further. In general, aggressiveness has a larger effect than concentration problems.

Readiness for School and IQ

Both IQ and readiness-for-school test scores in first grade had strong relations to psychiatric symptoms 10 years later; lower scores on the first grade tests generally were associated with higher self-reports of specific symptoms at age 16 or 17. This result also seems more clear-cut for males, however, than for females (see Figures 5 and 6). For females, overall distress—that is, the measure based on the Rasch score—does reveal that the intensity of teenage distress was highest among the lowest scoring first graders, and decreased from the least ready first graders to the low normal and average group (see Figure 5). The above average group showed considerably greater risk for overall distress than the average. Obsessive–compulsive symptoms among teenage females showed a simpler relation to first grade readiness, with higher scoring first graders more likely to feel better 10 years later. The other teenage symptoms show no evidence of the relationship between obsessive–compulsiveness and first grade readiness for females, in contrast to the males, where the connection is greater.

Among males, depression was higher among teenagers who had not been as ready as others for first grade 10 years earlier. Anxiety showed much the same relationship, though levels were higher among the above-average than among the average groups (see Figure 6). It appears that better performance on first grade readiness and IQ tests leads to less intense symptoms 10 years later,

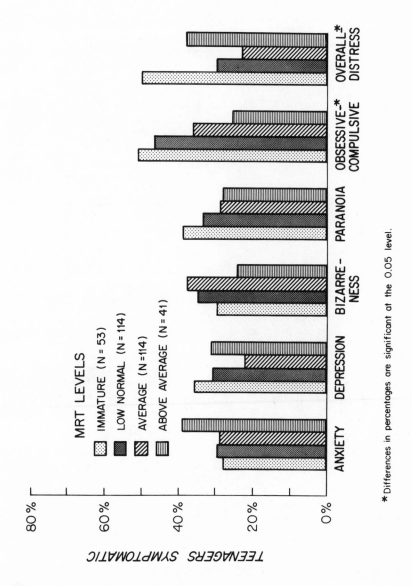

Figure 5. First grade metropolitan readiness test (MRT), and teenage psychiatric symptoms: females

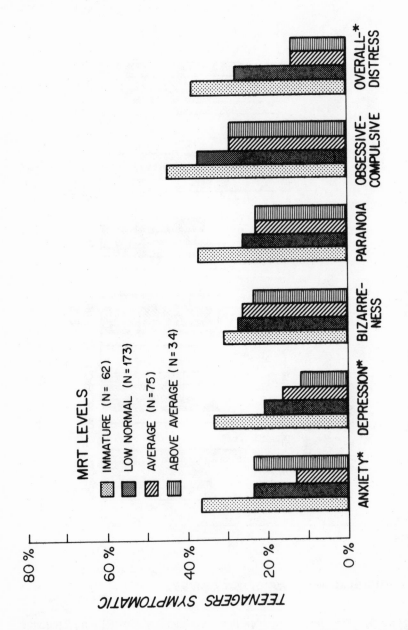

Figure 6. First grade metropolitan readiness test (MRT), and teenage psychiatric symptoms: males

later outcomes. Next, we examine whether the antecedents belonging to the two dimensions of mental health interact with each other in predicting later substance use or symptoms. For instance, we have found that first grade aggressiveness in males predicts substance use 10 years later. One might ask whether this relationship is the same for all males, or whether it operates differently for those exhibiting early psychiatric symptoms. Similarly, while we found very different antecedents of substance use and psychiatric symptoms, one might ask to what extent the substance using population and the symptomatic population overlap. Are the paths and their different outcomes interdependent, or are they empirically, as well as conceptually, distinct?

A multitude of log-linear and other analyses showed that the predictive powers of early social adaptational status and psychological well-being are independent of each other. Early psychological well-being has the same effect among socially adapting and maladapting first graders; early social adaptational status has the same effect among symptomatic and non-symptomatic first graders. The only exception is in the prediction of teenage substance use among females. In the presence of moderate or severe first grade learning problems, but not otherwise, symptoms as measured by MSI appear to inhibit the later use of beer or wine, hard liquor, and marijuana. Log-linear analyses of the effects of first grade social adaptational status measures and MSI confirm that MSI has a different effect at different levels of learning problems. Otherwise, however, specific measures of early social adaptational status and psychological well-being predict specific adolescent outcomes, and these effects are independent of each other.

Furthermore, the two areas of outcome are quite distinct. Table 3 for males and Table 4 for females show that correlations within an outcome area are relatively high (from .23 to .68), while those between the two areas are close to zero or even negative (from − .14 to .15). The adolescent population that uses substances is thus quite different from the population that develops psychiatric symptoms. Note also that this independence is equally true of males and females.

Discussion

These findings show that as early as the first grade, there are clearly identifiable social adaptational and psychological antecedents lead-

Table 3. Correlations Among Categories of Substance Use and Psychiatric Symptoms for Male Adolescents ($N = 338$)

	Beer or Wine	Hard Liquor	Marijuana	Cigarettes	Anxiety	Depression	Bizarreness	Paranoia	Obsessive/ Compulsive	Overall Distress	Average Absolute Value of Correlations
SUBSTANCE USE											
Beer or Wine	1.00										Among Substance Use .48
Hard Liquor	.63	1.00									Among Symptoms .45
Marijuana	.61	.52	1.00								
Cigarettes	.38	.32	.39	1.00							Between Substance Use and Symptoms .07
PSYCHIATRIC SYMPTOMS											
Anxiety	-.11	-.08	-.08	.03	1.00						
Depression	-.11	-.09	-.14	.01	.63	1.00					
Bizarreness	-.02	.09	.04	.08	.43	.41	1.00				
Paranoia	-.05	.07	.06	-.01	.36	.41	.44	1.00			
Obsessive/ Compulsive	-.12	-.01	-.01	.10	.30	.31	.28	.26	1.00		
Overall Distress	-.11	-.01	-.01	.11	.58	.63	.66	.61	.41	1.00	
	SUBSTANCE USE				PSYCHIATRIC SYMPTOMS						

Table 4. Correlations among Categories of Substance Use and Psychiatric Symptoms for Female Adolescents ($N = 357$)

		Beer or Wine	Hard Liquor	Marijuana	Cigarettes	Anxiety	Depression	Bizarreness	Paranoia	Obsessive/Compulsive	Overall Distress	Average Absolute Value of Correlations
SUBSTANCE USE	Beer or Wine	1.00										Among Substance Use .50
	Hard Liquor	.68	1.00									Among Symptoms .41
	Marijuana	.60	.52	1.00								Between Substance Use and Symptoms .07
	Cigarettes	.43	.32	.43	1.00							
PSYCHIATRIC SYMPTOMS	Anxiety	.11	.08	.05	.04	1.00						
	Depression	.11	.14	.03	.08	.68	1.00					
	Bizarreness	.12	.10	.12	.15	.27	.30	1.00				
	Paranoia	.06	.06	.07	.06	.37	.42	.27	1.00			
	Obsessive/Compulsive	.01	.04	.07	.03	.23	.23	.28	.32	1.00		
	Overall Distress	.08	.10	.08	.14	.57	.62	.57	.58	.43	1.00	

SUBSTANCE USE   PSYCHIATRIC SYMPTOMS

ing to specific outcomes at least as far as 10 years into the future. Briefly, the findings are:

1. First grade underachievement as rated by teachers is a strong and specific predictor of teenage depressive symptoms among males; it does not predict substance use.
2. The strongest first grade antecedents of teenage symptom levels in females are in the psychological well-being domain. Both mothers' and clinicians' symptom ratings of first grade females were predictive of high risk of depressed feelings, and mothers' ratings also predicted high anxiety in their daughters 10 years later.
3. Among both females and males, higher scores on first grade readiness and IQ tests in general lead to fewer psychiatric symptoms, but more substance use, 10 years later. However, some teenage symptoms showed a curvilinear relationship, with the highest scoring first grade students reporting moderate levels of distress.
4. Shyness among first grade males, but not females, clearly inhibits substance use at age 16 or 17. For males, early shyness also predicts higher levels of teenage anxiety.
5. First grade aggressiveness without shyness is a strong predictor of increased teenage substance use by males (not by females), but it is not associated with later psychopathology.
6. The combination of shyness and aggressiveness in first grade males is associated with even more frequent use of substances (especially of cigarettes) than aggressiveness alone.
7. With one seemingly minor exception, the social adaptational status and psychological well-being predictors do not interact in their effects on later substance use and psychiatric symptoms.
8. The two outcome areas of psychiatric symptoms and substance use are empirically as well as conceptually distinct. They are barely correlated among male and female adolescents, and the developmental paths leading to them are very different.
9. There are strong differences between males and females in the developmental paths leading to adolescent outcomes. Early school SAS has stronger predictive power for both later social adaptational status and psychological well-being among males (points 1, 4, 5, and 6), while early psychological well-being shows clear continuity with later psychological well-being, but only for females (point 2). The measures of cognitive performance in the first grade have similar effects for both sexes (point 3).

These results show that specific maladaptive behavioral responses to first grade tasks and early psychological measures of distress have specific and important relationships to outcomes 10 years later. From the viewpoint of theory of psychopathology, these data strongly suggest the importance of the distinction between social adaptational status and psychological well-being. It was only by distinguishing these two and studying their interrelationships that the developmental differences between the sexes became apparent. The paths we have found thus far leading to psychopathology in males involve early social maladaptive behavioral responses. For females, the path to psychiatric symptoms in adolescence involves early symptom levels more than classroom maladaptation. The origins of these early symptoms in females are important to study, but the symptoms are even now an important target for prevention research, as are the maladaptive responses.

The social adaptational status predictors are behavioral responses to specific classroom task demands the teacher sets for the children. We have shown in an unpublished paper that the maladaptive behavioral responses in first grade operate mainly separately, not as clusters or syndromes. The single exception is the combination of shyness and aggressiveness, which exaggerates the effects of aggressiveness in predicting substance use and delinquency 10 years later among males.

Theoretically, the results suggest that, at least for males, teenage outcomes evolve along developmental paths passing through the specific social task demands and behavioral responses in the first grade classroom. How children react behaviorally to these demands appears to have long-lasting predictive importance in spite of the great span of time, events, and conditions that intervene between the first grade and mid-adolescence. While these antecedents of later symptoms and substance use are clearly discernible by the end of the first grade, no such predictive power was found in analyses using identical early and middle first grade measures (Kellam et al., 1980). This suggests that specific developmental paths begin to form out of successful or unsuccessful adaptational responses to school. Prevention programs designed to modify social maladaptational status in young elementary school children might have positive outcomes for child, teenage, and adult psychopathology, as well as for other outcomes.

One task of prevention research in the light of these results is to identify periods in the life span in which preventive programs would be most effective, both in terms of reaching a high proportion of people with identified risk factors, as well as affecting outcomes for those identified. The first grade classroom provides both a context and the populations. Again, the fact that these social adaptational status predictors worked only at the end of the year suggests the importance of the first grade demand/response process.

The stressful task demands of the first grade classroom and the level of stress they generate are both measurable and can be manipulated by experimentation, both in the natural context as well as in the behavioral laboratory.

The wide experimental knowledge from behavioral laboratories and clinical settings can be used to design prevention trials that inhibit or enhance certain identified behaviors in the first grade. Our current knowledge about early predictors of psychopathology and substance use lead us to suggest several prevention trials aimed at reducing these outcomes. Aggressive responses, in grades one through four, may be reducible by behavior analysis and modification techniques (O'Leary and O'Leary, 1977). One hypothesis is that such a treatment should reduce teenage substance use, particularly in males. It may also affect other outcomes for nonaggressive children as well, by providing a less disruptive atmosphere in which to learn. A second trial intervention can be aimed at increasing each child's learning. The hypothesis is that increased learning competence would reduce the stress of impending failure, and lower aggressive or shy behaviors in children. This treatment may also affect long-term outcomes. A third strategy is to identify and provide early treatment for children with psychiatric symptoms. Because of the continuity between early and teenage psychological well-being for females, we can hypothesize improved teenage psychological well-being from such a treatment.

Other prevention targets include shoring up the social structural articulations between mother and teacher. Aspects of family structure and teenage motherhood also lend themselves to preventive research interventions (Kellam et al., 1977; Kellam et al., 1982a; Brown et al., 1981). Given the close relationships between daughters' and mothers' psychological well-being (Kellam et al., 1983) family strategies may be important preventive measures for females.

Developmental research in epidemiologically definable populations is an integral part of prevention research strategy, and the last few years have seen considerable progress in the empirical data available for such an intensive next stage in this area of research. Definitions of the family itself have been one product of this method in Woodlawn (Kellam et al., 1977). Family investigators have just begun the study of specific kinds and evolution of family structure in research on children and families.

Early predictors have their origins in the interaction between persons with their biological capacities for adaptation, and the environment and its demands. We need to study the origins of specific antecedents genetically, metabolically, social-structurally, social-adaptationally, and psychologically, with models that combine these perspectives. Such research could be more productive than studies of the causes of adult psychopathology, which omit the early antecedents from the analytic models. Studies of antecedents must be an important part of any effort to design specific preventive intervention trials. Such trials will help to illuminate the function of the early predictors, as well as provide for more effective prevention and socialization.

References

Agrawal KC, Kellam SG, Klein ZE, et al: The Woodlawn mental health studies: tracking children and families for long-term follow-up. Am J Public Health 68:139–142, 1978

Borland BL, Heckman HK: Hyperactive boys and their brothers: a 25–year follow-up study. Arch Gen Psychiatry 33:669–75, 1976

Brown CH, Adams RG, Kellam SG: A longitudinal study of teenage motherhood and symptoms of distress: the Woodlawn community epidemiological project. Research in Community and Mental Health: A Research Annual 2:183–213, 1981

Ensminger ME, Brown CH, Kellam SG: Sex differences in antecedents of substance use among adolescents. Journal of Social Issues 38:25–42, 1982

Ensminger ME, Kellam SG, Rubin BR: School and family origins of delinquency: comparisons by sex, in Prospective Studies of Crime and Delinquency. Edited by Van Dusen K, Mednick S. Boston, Kluwer-Nijhoff, 1983

Erikson EH: Identity and the life cycle: selected papers, part 1, in Psychological Issues. Edited by Klein GS. New York, International Universities Press, 1959

Erikson EH: Childhood and Society, second edition. New York, W.W. Norton, 1963

Fleming JP, Kellam SG, Brown CH: Early predictors of age at first use of alcohol, marijuana, and cigarettes. Drug and Alcohol Dependence 9:285–303, 1982

Graham P, Rutter M, George S: Temperamental characteristics as predictors of behavior disorders in children. Am J Orthopsychiatry 43:328–39, 1973

Havinghurst RJ: Developmental Tasks and Education, second edition. New York, David McKay, 1952

Hechtman L, Weiss G, Perlman T, et al: Hyperactives as young adults: prospective ten-year follow-up, in Psychosocial Aspects of Drug Treatment for Hyperactivity. Edited by Gadow KD, Loney J. Boulder, CO, Westview Press, 1981

Jessor R, Jessor SL: Theory testing in longitudinal research on marijuana use, in Longitudinal Research on Drug Use: Empirical Findings and Methodological Issues. Edited by Kandel D. Washington DC, Hemisphere-Wiley, 1978

Johnston L: Drugs and American Youth. Ann Arbor, MI, Institute for Social Research, 1973

Johnston LD, O'Malley PM, Eveland LK: Drugs and delinquency: a search for causal connections, in Longitudinal Research on Drug Use: Empirical Findings and Methodological Issues. Edited by Kandel D. Washington DC, Hemisphere-Wiley, 1978

Kandel DB, Kessler RC, Margulies RZ: Antecedents of adolescent initiation into stages of drug use: a developmental analysis, in Longitudinal Research on Drug Use: Empirical Findings and Methodological Issues. Edited by Kandel D. Washington DC, Hemisphere-Wiley, 1978

Kaplan HB: Increase in self-rejection as an antecedent of deviant responses. Journal of Youth and Adolescence 4:281–292, 1975

Kellam SG, Branch JD: An approach to community mental health: analysis of basic problems. Seminars in Psychiatry 3:207–225, 1971

Kellam SG, Ensminger ME: Theory and method in child psychiatric epidemiology, in Studying Children Epidemiologically. Edited by Earls F. New York, Neale Watson Academic Publishers, 1980

Kellam SG, Branch JD, Agrawal KC, et al: Woodlawn mental health center: an evolving strategy for planning in community mental health, in Handbook of Community Mental Health. Edited by Golann SE, Eisdorfer C. New York, Appleton-Century-Crofts, 1972

Kellam SG, Branch JD, Agrawal KC, et al: Mental Health and Going to School: The Woodlawn Program of Assessment, Early Intervention, and Evaluation. Chicago, University of Chicago Press, 1975

Kellam SG, Ensminger ME, Turner RJ: Family structure and the mental health of children: concurrent and longitudinal community-wide studies. Arch Gen Psychiatry 34:1012–1022, 1977

Kellam SG, Ensminger ME, Simon MB: Mental health in first grade and teenage drug, alcohol, and cigarette use. Drug and Alcohol Dependence 5:273–304, 1980

Kellam SG, Branch JD, Brown CH, et al: Why teenagers come for treatment: a ten-year prospective epidemiological study in Woodlawn. J Am Acad Child Psychiatry 20:477–495, 1981

Kellam SG, Adams RG, Brown CH, et al: The long-term evolution of the family structure of teenage and older mothers. Journal of Marriage and the Family 44:539–554, 1982a

Kellam SG, Brown CH, Fleming JP: The prevention of teenage substance use: longitudinal research and strategy, in Promoting Adolescent Health: A Dialogue on Research and Practice. Edited by Coates TJ, Petersen AC, Perry C. New York, Academic Press, 1982b

Kellam SG, Brown CH, Rubin BR, et al: Paths leading to teenage psychiatric symptoms and substance use: developmental epidemiological studies in Woodlawn, in Childhood Psychopathology and Development. Edited by Guze SB, Earls F, Barrett JE. New York, Raven Press, 1983a

Kellam SG, Simon MB, Ensminger ME: Antecedents in first grade of teenage drug use and psychological well-being: a ten-year community-wide prospective study, in Origins of Psychopathology. Edited by Ricks D, Dohrenwend B. New York, Cambridge University Press, 1983b

Kellam SG, Brown CH, Fleming JP: Longitudinal community epidemiological studies of drug use: early aggressiveness, shyness, and learning problems, in Studying Drug Use and Abuse. Edited by Robins LN. New Jersey, Rutgers University Press, 1985a

Kellam SG, Ensminger ME, Branch JD, et al: The Woodlawn mental health longitudinal community epidemiological project, in Longitudinal Research in the United States. Edited by Mednick SA, Harway M. Hingham, MA, Nijhoff Publishing, 1985b

Kohn ML: Looking back—A 25-year review and appraisal of social problems research. Social Problems 24:94–112, 1976

Mellinger GD, Somers RH, Bazell S, et al: Drug use, academic performance, and career indecision: longitudinal data in search of a model, in Longitudinal Research on Drug Use: Empirical Findings and Methodological Issues. Edited by Kandel D. Washington DC, Hemisphere-Wiley, 1978

Milich R, Loney J: The role of hyperactive and aggressive symptomatology in predicting adolescent outcome among hyperactive children. J Pediatr Psychol 4:93–112, 1979

Neugarten BL: Time, age, and the life cycle. Am J Psychiatry 136:887–894, 1979

O'Leary KD, O'Leary SG: Classroom Management: The Successful Use of Behavior Modification. New York, Pergamon Press, 1977

Parsons T: Social Structure and Personality. New York, The Free Press of Glencoe, 1964

Paton S, Kessler R, Kandel D: Depressive mood and adolescent illicit drug use: a longitudinal analysis. J Genet Psychol 131:267–289, 1977

Petersen AC, Kellam SG: Measurement of the psychological well-being of adolescents: the psychometric properties and assessment procedures of the "How I Feel." Journal of Youth and Adolescence 6:229–247, 1977

Pritchard M, Graham P: An investigation of a group of patients who have attended both the child and adult departments of the same psychiatric hospital. Br J Psychiatry 112:603–12, 1966

Robins LN: Deviant Children Grow Up: A Sociological and Psychiatric Study of Sociopathic Personality. Baltimore, Williams & Wilkins, 1966

Robins LN: A Follow-Up of Vietnam Drug Users. Special Action Office Monograph, Series A, No. 1. Washington DC, Special Action Office for Drug Abuse Protection, 1973

Robins LN: Sturdy childhood predictors of adult outcomes: replications from longitudinal studies. Paper presented at the Paul Hoch Award Lecture, American Psychopathological Association Meeting, Boston, 1978

Robins LN, Murphy GE: Drug use in a normal population of young Negro men. Am J Public Health 57:1580–1596, 1967

Robins LN, Davis DH, Wish E: Detecting predictors of rare events: demographic, family, and personal deviance as predictors of stages in the progression toward narcotic addiction, in The Origins and Course of Psychopathology: Methods of Longitudinal Research. Edited by Strauss JS, Babigian H, Roff M. New York, Plenum, 1977

Rutter ML: Relationships between child and adult psychiatric disorders: some research considerations. Acta Psychiatr Scand 48:3–21, 1972a

Rutter ML: Review of Childhood Behavior and Mental Health. Child Psychol Psychiatry 13:219–222, 1972b

Rutter ML, Tizard J, Whitmore K: Education, Health and Behavior: Psychological and Medical Study of Childhood Development. New York, Wiley, 1970

Sadava SW: Initiation to cannabis use: a longitudinal social psychological study of college freshmen. Canadian Journal of Behavioral Science 5:371–384, 1973

Shaffer D, Stokman C, O'Connor PA, et al: Early soft neurological signs and later psychopathological development. Paper presented at the Annual Meeting of the Society for Life History Research in Psychopathology, and Society for the Study of Social Biology, New York, November 1979

Smith GM, Fogg CP: Psychological predictors of early use, late use and nonuse of marijuana among teenage students, in Longitudinal Research on Drug Use: Empirical Findings and Methodological Issues. Edited by Kandel D. Washington DC, Hemisphere-Wiley, 1978

Stewart MA, Gath A: Psychological Disorders of Children: A Handbook for Primary Care Physicians. Baltimore, Williams and Wilkins, 1978

Stewart MA, Mendelson WB, Johnson NE: Hyperactive children as adolescents: how they describe themselves. Child Psychiatry Hum Dev 4:3–11, 1973

Warren W: A study of adolescent psychiatric in-patients and the outcome six or more years later, II: the follow-up study. J Child Psychol Psychiatry 6:141–60, 1965

Watt NF: Childhood and adolescent routes to schizophrenia, in Life History Research in Psychopathology, vol 3. Edited by Ricks DF, Thomas A, Roff M. Minneapolis, University of Minnesota Press, 1974

Watt NF: Patterns of childhood social development in adult schizophrenics. Arch Gen Psychiatry 35:160–65, 1978

Wright BD: Solving measurement problems with the Rasch model. Journal of Educational Measurement 14:97–116, 1977

Chapter 8

ADOLESCENT LONELINESS: LINKING EPIDEMIOLOGY AND THEORY TO PREVENTION

Tim Brennan, Ph.D.

Chapter 8

ADOLESCENT LONELINESS: LINKING EPIDEMIOLOGY AND THEORY TO PREVENTION

Few adolescents escape the pain of loneliness. For most, the duration and intensity of feelings of loneliness, and their ways of coping and responding to these feelings, may not be damaging. However, for some, loneliness can be a persistent and ultimately damaging aspect of their lives.

The normal adolescent is engulfed in a developmental process in which social and intimate relationships are rapidly changing. These transitions inevitably involve faltering beginnings, disappointments, and endings. The exciting possibility of heterosexual relationships also brings a new reality—strong desires, as well as the possibility of failure, rejection, frustration, and consequent feelings of loneliness and loss.

The very process of becoming a person, of assuming an individual identity and a separate sense of self, leads to the experience of isolation and loneliness. This process of individuation—which every normal adolescent must navigate—includes separation from parents, as well as the assumption of increased autonomy and individual decision making. Personal autonomy is demonstrated by taking greater responsibility for one's thoughts, values, decisions, and behavior. Ostrov and Offer (1980) have noted that the assertion of this autonomy necessitates moving away from others; separation and loneliness are bound together in the unfolding process of the

The research for this chapter was supported by a grant from the National Institute of Mental Health, No. 7 ROI MH3596-02.

development of an individual identity. Confronting separation and assuming responsibility are major sources of growth, change, and development in adolescence. The inability to deal with separation and its associated loneliness is implicated in certain aspects of developmental failure in adolescence.

The Importance of Loneliness in the Study of Affective Disorders and Suicide Among Adolescents

There are a number of reasons for focusing on loneliness within the context of affective disorders and suicide in the adolescent population. First, loneliness has been linked to a number of serious mental health and behavioral problems that beset adolescents. These include: drug abuse and alcoholism (Holzner and Ding, 1973; Pittel, 1971; Konopka, 1966); suicide (Horton, 1973; Tanner, 1973; Ford and Zorn, 1975); delinquency and prostitution (Konopka, 1966; Brennan and Auslander, 1979); exhibitionism (Basquin and Trystram, 1966; Klapp, 1969); and academic failure (Christiaans, 1965; Cutrona, 1982; Brennan and Auslander, 1979). This list could be expanded to include various psychopathologies such as schizoid disorders and depression. Sullivan (1953), for example, asserted that loneliness was a core component of all psychopathology, and that the struggle to find relief from loneliness was a central motivating factor in much of human behavior. Similarly, Fromm-Reichmann (1959) believed understanding loneliness would lead to a better understanding of the etiology of most mental illnesses.

Second, although the connection between adolescent loneliness and the many behavioral and psychological problems has been well established empirically, there is, as yet, no clear understanding of the role of loneliness in the etiology of such pathologies. The study of loneliness itself has, until relatively recently, been neglected. Peplau and Perlman (1982) provide a useful review of the growth of research on loneliness during the 1960s, and the more rapid escalation of interest following the 1973 publication of Weiss's book, *Loneliness: The Experience of Emotional and Social Isolation.* Only a handful of empirical studies have examined loneliness during the adolescent years (see reviews by Ostrov and Offer, 1978; Brennan, 1982).

Third, it appears that loneliness has a particularly widespread prevalence and intensity during the adolescent years. The available epidemiological evidence (Shaver and Rubenstein, 1979; Ostrov and Offer, 1978; Brennan and Auslander, 1979; Lowenthal et al., 1975) suggests that chronic and intense loneliness is experienced by 10 or 20 percent of the adolescent population, and that a majority of adolescents report the experience of intense feelings of loneliness. These studies also suggest that the experience of loneliness is more widespread among the adolescent population than in any other age group.

A final reason for viewing loneliness within the context of affective disorders and suicide is the pain and debilitating effects of loneliness. The experience of loneliness is extremely aversive. The various symptoms and manifestations of loneliness, described below, are almost uniformly painful; so painful that people will do almost anything to avoid loneliness (Peplau and Perlman, 1982; Yalom, 1980). Weiss (1973) describes the hypervigilant behavior of lonely people and their intense desires to find new attachments. They search, often frantically, to find persons who will relieve their loneliness, spending tremendous energy exploring social settings where such persons are likely to be found. Weiss also describes a pattern of apathy, regret, helplessness, and despair that may result from chronic loneliness when these persons give up seeking and become immobilized.

Within the context of this volume, however, the most critical reason for examining loneliness is a need to clarify the damaging effects of loneliness on adolescent growth and development. The association of loneliness with a large range of emotional and behavioral problems suggests the possibility that loneliness may be implicated in the etiology of these problems. Many additional adolescent problem behaviors such as drug abuse, cult-joining, and suicide may be linked by the common motive of avoiding the pain of loneliness. Strategies for preventing such problems may be enhanced if we can clarify the manner in which loneliness and isolation are implicated in impairing the healthy psychological development of adolescents.

Forms of Loneliness

"How many forms of loneliness are there?" is a question that has not yet been answered. Recent empirical research has confronted the issues of operational approaches to measuring and defining loneliness. A number of factor analytic studies have been conducted on item domains focusing on deficits in social and emotional relationships, and the results have helped define some of the main dimensions of loneliness. One recent review provided 12 different definitions of loneliness (Peplau and Perlman, 1982). However, ambiguities persist (Weiss, 1982).

There is, nevertheless, a growing consensus on three basic issues. First, loneliness emerges from deficits in social relationships. Second, the experience of loneliness is subjective and is not synonymous with objective social isolation. Third, the experience of loneliness is extremely aversive. The following are some of the major forms of loneliness identified in the literature.

Emotional Isolation

This is seen as emerging from deficits in intimate relations. Weiss (1973) sees emotional isolation primarily as stemming from loss of attachment figures. This loss can occur, for example, through romantic separations, divorce, bereavement, or when romantic aspirations are frustrated. The individual does not have a close intimate attachment with another, yet desires such an attachment. Emotional isolation can be remedied only by developing a new intimate attachment or recovering the one that had been lost. Adolescents often speak of being "lonely in a crowd," indicating that easing emotional isolation requires attachment to a particular person rather than a more general affiliation with a group.

Adolescents are particularly vulnerable to emotional isolation. Weiss (1973) noted that because adolescents are separating from their parents as primary attachment figures, they are entering a phase of life in which they are without an attachment figure for the first time. Thus, they may go through a period of pining or yearning for the kind of relationship that would provide intimacy. In addition to feeling the loss of parents as primary attachments, the adolescent is experiencing new needs and capacities for intimacy as a natural result of developmental and psychological changes.

Social Isolation

This stems from deficiencies in social connectedness or social integration into a peer network or community. Needs for a sense of belonging or integration are frustrated. The dominant symptoms of social isolation are feelings of boredom, aimlessness, marginality, and rejection.

The need for integration with peers and friends is critically important for adolescents as they move beyond the orbit of their families. Coleman (1974) commented upon the intense need for close relations among adolescent peers, arguing that family kinship groups are increasingly unable to meet the relationship needs of youth. Social and peer relationships beyond the family provide many important provisions to the adolescent (see reviews by Bell, 1981; Konopka, 1976; Rubin, 1982). In some instances, adolescents enlist the support and encouragement of a peer network to help in the often difficult task of separating from parents. Thus, the rewards and payoffs stemming from tight affiliation with peers are potentially many. The isolation and friendlessness reported by many adolescents may constitute a serious handicap as they confront the developmental challenges of this life stage, a theme explored more fully below.

Spiritual Loneliness

This term is used by a number of writers (Fromm, 1955; Buhler, 1969; Gaev, 1976) to indicate a form of loneliness resulting from perceived deficits in the meaning or significance of a person's life. Spiritual loneliness is described as emerging when the need for significant activities or commitments is frustrated. Frankl (1978), Fabry (1968), and others have argued that humans have a deep need or "will" to seek meanings, purposes, and higher values which extend beyond egocentric goals. Fromm (1955) uses the term "moral loneliness" to indicate a lack of relatedness to such values and meanings. Feelings of boredom, aimlessness, emptiness, and despair are used to describe this form of loneliness (Fabry, 1968; May, 1953).

Adolescents are highly vulnerable to spiritual loneliness. The adolescent is overflowing with new capacities, talents, and energies and is confronted with the exploratory task of discovering meaningful goals to provide a focus for these talents. Experimentation with drugs, joining communes, the popularity of a variety of religious and nonreligious cults (from "Jesus freaks" and Hari Krishnas to the LSD cults), the adulation of heroes, celebrities, and assorted gurus, as well as the search for meaningful educational and work commitments, may all be seen as reflections of the active search for morality and value. An enormous gulf exists between this "will to meaning" of the adolescent population and the range of tasks provided by our society. Marcia (1980) used the term "adolescent moratorium" to describe the stage of identity development in which the adolescent is exploring and searching for meaningful commitments. It can be assumed that while the adolescent is in this stage, he or she has not yet found such commitments.

A massive literature describes the loss of challenge and meaninglessness of contemporary adolescent life in America (Gordon, 1976). The adolescent may experience spiritual loneliness in two basic ways. First, as noted above, adolescents may not be able to discover any meaningful commitments or challenges that evoke their energies, and may remain in an uncommitted state. Second, they may be co-opted into commitments that are basically not of their own choosing. They may not have the strength to resist the commands of their parents, or other significant agents, and they may enter into commitments or take on challenges imposed upon them by others. Marcia (1980) refers to this as the "foreclosed" identity status. Almost by definition, the identity stage of foreclosure is characterized by spiritual loneliness.

Existential Loneliness

This term is used to describe a form of loneliness that is seen as stemming from an awareness of the basic human condition of separateness, a consciousness of mortality, death, and human finiteness, as well as the complete personal responsibility for one's life (Burton, 1961; Loucks, 1974; May, 1953). May (1953) refers to an "inner sanctum" where each person must stand alone. This form of loneliness is seen as emerging from a reflexive self-awareness of individuality and separateness. Confrontation with this form of isolation is fundamentally tied to the process of individuation and to assuming autonomy and independence. The literature describes this form of isolation as evoking feelings of panic, terror, fear, and despair (Yalom, 1980).

The adolescent, in struggling for autonomy, independence, and identity, separate from that of his or her parents, is likely to experience the anxiety of existential isolation for the first time. Mijuskovic (1979) and others have emphasized the cognitive developments leading to a reflexive self-awareness, and an awareness of finitude and death, which are also precursors to experiencing existential loneliness. The adolescent is confronted with a dilemma in which choosing the path of independence, autonomy, and individuation carries the attendant risk of existential loneliness; while the path of security, foreclosure, and avoidance of responsibility is, unfortunately, an option devoid of any real growth. Yalom (1980) provides graphic descriptions of this dilemma and explores the psychological cost of the choice to avoid personal autonomy.

Temporary Versus Chronic Loneliness

This division introduces a time dimension, as well as the difference between chronic characterological causes and situational precipitators of loneliness. It emphasizes the difference between state (situational) and trait (characterological) loneliness. Thus, loneliness can be examined according to the cause as well as the persistence of the experience. In situations such as a family break-up, a relocation, or school change, virtually everyone would be lonely, at least temporarily. On the other hand, the presence of certain personality features, such as shyness, suspiciousness, aggression, fear of taking social risks, low social desirability, and so on, may result in a stable pattern of impaired relations. Much of the current research on loneliness is concerned with identifying the personality features and interpersonal styles of lonely people (Peplau and Perlman, 1982).

What Does the Adolescent Gain From Relationships?

If the lonely adolescent is experiencing a deficit in relationships, it seems appropriate to explore exactly what constitutes this deficit. What is it that relationships provide? The answers to this question may indicate why loneliness is so aversive to most adolescents. It is interesting to note that two separate literatures—the literature on loneliness, and the literature on social support—seem to be converging on this topic (see Weiss, 1974). The following is an outline of some of the main provisions of relationships.

Reassurance of Worth

Affirmation of worth and competence helps the adolescent as he or she takes the first tentative steps into new roles. Young people wish to know whether they are "good enough" and whether or not they have been accepted. The development of social competence and self-esteem partially may hinge upon the provision of such reassurance.

Self-Understanding

Through interaction with others, adolescents attempt to clarify and validate their own feelings, thoughts, opinions, and behaviors. Konopka (1976) provides graphic portraits of this provision in her descriptions of the friendships of adolescent girls. The uncertainty and confusion experienced by adolescents in their rapid state of growth has been noted by many observers. There seems to be a tremendous need to turn to the opinions and evaluations of others—particularly intimate others—who are going through many of the same experiences. Isolation and loneliness would clearly deny the young person such feedback and clarification.

The adolescent is deeply involved in creating a new "self" independent from the family. At the same time, defenses are being erected against any family invasion of this new, autonomous self. Among adolescents, a mutual hostility against family authority may provide an important basis for friendship. The adolescent may also gain support and validation in particular areas that are denied within the family (for example, heterosexual relations, or the questioning of adult authority in areas of morality, dress, behavior, and so on).

Overcoming Separateness

Relationships can alleviate the fear of confronting existential isolation, a form of loneliness that becomes much more likely at adolescence. Intimate relationships, in particular, may alleviate this fear by providing a sense of emotional attachment. Since socially sanctioned intimate heterosexual relationships are remote for most adolescents, particularly very young adolescents, peer relations often assume a highly intimate character during these years.

Social Integration

Social relationships give the adolescent the opportunity for social integration through companionship, participation, and sharing common interests. The management of time and the provision of a structure for the adolescent's life are enhanced by a strong level of social integration. Isolation, on the other hand, is clearly less stimulating and may result in boredom. Adolescents appear to be highly vulnerable to this deficit. It can be noted that boredom seems to exist in large segments of the adolescent population (Brennan and Auslander, 1979; Smith, 1981).

Guidance and Help

Relationships provide a variety of practical and material supports, as well as guidance and information. Adolescents are inexperienced and often insecure. Yet, they are confronted with profound developmental changes and are challenged at the same time with negotiating the difficult tasks surrounding individuation and identity building (Marcia, 1980). Guidance and help are critical provisions of their relationships. Mentors, teachers, and heroes; intimate friends and peers; and parents and other family members, may all become important to the adolescent in different kinds of help needed by the adolescent.

The Importance of Caring for the Other

While the above provisions emerge from being cared for by others, an equally important set of benefits emerge from the discovery and development of caring commitments to others. The adolescent who has discovered appropriate and significant others to care for is provided with an outlet for energies, talents, and enthusiasms, and an organizing principle for his or her life. Such "appropriate others" may consist of vocational and educational goals, values, causes, or particular persons. Meyeroff (1971) explores the many positive results that accrue to the person who has discovered meaningful commitments. The inability to develop such commitments often results in an alienated apathetic condition of aimless drifting, in which the adolescent has no focus for energies and abilities. Fun, entertainment, fads, fashions, and other diversions may become the primary focus of their lives. They remain unchallenged and their abilities remain dormant or misplaced. Aimlessness and meaninglessness have been identified as widespread among American youth (Fabry, 1968; Brennan and Auslander, 1979; Konopka, 1976). This, again, is the condition just referred to as moral or spiritual loneliness. In Marcia's (1980) model of identity development, the successful resolution of the moratorium phase is the discovery and development of appropriate caring relationships. The findings of the incidence studies of the various identity stages (Marcia, 1980) support the suggestion of widespread spiritual loneliness, since these studies also indicate that a substantial proportion of youth do not successfully negotiate the moratorium identity stage, and may remain stuck in the stages of diffusion and foreclosure. Thus, they do not receive the provisions that accrue to the persons who have discovered and developed appropriate and meaningful commitments.

Extent of Loneliness at Adolescence

The available data suggests that adolescence is characterized by higher levels of loneliness than are other stages of the life cycle (Shaver and Rubenstein, 1980; Lowenthal et al., 1975). Brennan and Auslander (1979), in studying more than 9,000 adolescents aged 10 through 18, estimated that 10 to 15 percent were seriously and recurrently lonely; 54 percent agreed that they often felt lonely. Studies by Collier and Lawrence (1951), Ostrov and Offer (1978), and Wood and Hannell (1977) also confirm that large segments of the adolescent population suffer from loneliness of some kind.

Some preliminary findings from an ongoing national study (Brennan and Camilli, 1983) regarding loneliness at adolescence can be noted. Girls report more loneliness than boys, particularly in the family context. Loneliness generally increases across the adolescent years for both sexes in all three contexts of family, school, and peer relationships. There is a rapid escalation of self-reported loneliness in the early teenage years. The age of onset seems to be between 12 and 14 for both sexes. Available evidence suggests that self-reports of loneliness reach a maximum by age 16 and may flatten out after this age. Social class differences have been found. Lower-class youth report higher levels of loneliness in both family and school contexts.

Adolescents are clearly vulnerable to situational changes that disrupt their relationships and precipitate loneliness. For example, youth whose parents have separated or divorced in the last year report more loneliness in the family context. Similarly, youth who have changed schools in the last year report more loneliness.

This NIMH-funded study of adolescent loneliness involves a

national probability sample of youth followed for a five-year period. This study incorporates both self-report as well as scaled measures of loneliness in the social contexts of school, peer, and family relations. The numerous findings will be presented more fully in a separate report.

Theories of Loneliness

Work on loneliness remains primarily at the descriptive phase. In the last few years, however, a large body of descriptive data has emerged regarding the characteristics of persons who are lonely. Peplau and Perlman (1982) have presented a general framework for organizing this knowledge. This framework identifies the major antecedents of loneliness. At least three classes of antecedents can be seen in Figures 1 and 2: 1) personal predisposition (shyness, introversion, and the like); 2) sociocultural processes that disrupt or weaken relationships; and 3) disruptive changes (either developmental or situational) that may be seen as pushing, or precipitating, the person into isolation or loneliness. For the adolescent, developmental changes are particularly important. This framework emphasizes precipitators and predispositions that disrupt either the initiation or the quality of relationships. Another feature of this framework is that cognitive attributions regarding the causes, duration, and control over loneliness have a moderating influence on the experience of loneliness, and may strongly influence coping strategies. Major components of this model are now discussed from the perspective of adolescent loneliness.

Developmental Changes and Adolescent Loneliness

Changes of almost any kind can disrupt or impair one's relationships. The adolescent years are a time of profound change. Relational deficits may arise as a result of new needs or desires for specific kinds and qualities of relationships. New capacities for intimacy may increase the experience of loneliness if there is no corresponding development in actual relationships. Sullivan (1953) suggested that loneliness first becomes possible during the preadolescent stage when a "need for intimacy" emerges. Deficits in relationships can also arise from the loss or transformation of existing relationships. We now examine some of the more important

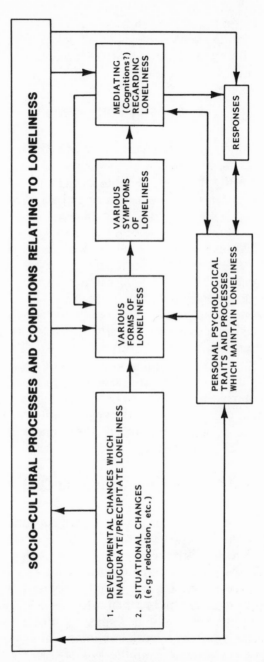

Figure 1. A generalized model of the main interacting domains of variables in the study of adolescent loneliness

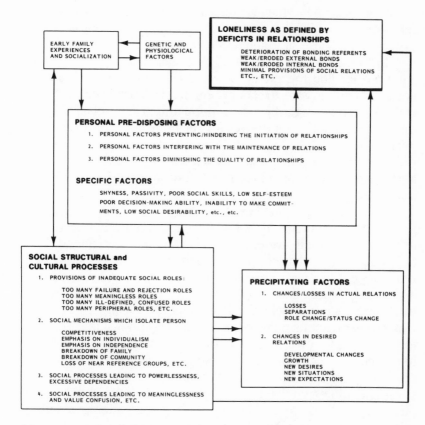

Figure 2. Organization of some main antecedents of adolescent loneliness

changes that may influence the levels of loneliness experienced by adolescents.

A first major disruption or loss stems from the transformation of the attachment bond to parents. Relinquishing or weakening this bond has been posited as a critical antecedent of increased loneliness at adolescence (Weiss, 1973; Ostrov and Offer, 1978). Weiss suggests that emotional isolation will emerge as a result of this change in the attachment system.

A second profound change is the loss of childhood identity. Ostrov and Offer (1978) have argued that the loss of the childhood identity and of its psychological and social reference points leaves the adolescent in a state of extreme uncertainty and confusion. This intensifies the adolescent's needs for reassurance, guidance, and self-understanding, which in turn lead to increased demands for relationships. Until such needs are met the adolescent is likely to experience a sense of loneliness.

In the same period, both physiological and emotional maturation are leading to new desires and capacities for intimate relationships. Furthermore, the adolescent may face strong cultural norms and expectations regarding social popularity. These social processes can intensify adolescent desires for relationships. Unless the young person develops the confidence and skills necessary to achieve success in peer and heterosexual relationships, he or she may face a protracted period of deficit in which desires for relations remain unfulfilled.

The adolescent is also experiencing an increased awareness of separateness. Cognitive development at adolescence has been linked to a new form of self-awareness and separate identity (Elkind, 1968). Mijuskovic (1979) has recently argued that the development of a reflexive self-consciousness is a necessary basic condition for the experience of loneliness to be possible. The adolescent struggles to assume cognitive, behavioral, and emotional autonomy together with greater responsibility for personal decision-making. This drive for autonomy involves both a separation from parents as well as an increased sense of isolation. The adolescent tries to build a sense of identity that is often defined in contradistinction to parental desires. The adolescent attempts to separate from the childhood dependency on the parents. In many cases, parents attempt to subvert this process of separation. This may result in estrangement between parent and adolescent, with an increased likelihood of the adolescent feeling lonely and misunderstood. Thus, the process of individuation and the struggle for autonomy may lead to greater awareness of the self as "separate" and, at the same time, to various forms of loneliness.

Such changes inevitably disrupt both the actual relationships and the needs for relationships of the adolescent. Loneliness arises as a concomitant of either the losses and changes of existing relationships, or the increased desires for new relationships.

Personal Predispositions Toward Loneliness

Empirical research has entered the phase of establishing the personal characteristics of adolescents who report high levels of loneliness. This research may clarify characterological predispositions toward loneliness. In this section, a brief review is given of the psychological characteristics of adolescents distinguished by atypically high levels of loneliness.

Low self-esteem is generally associated with high loneliness. The tendency of people to blame themselves for their loneliness and to underestimate situational causes has recently been noted (Weiss, 1982). The suggestion is that people tend to overestimate the relative importance of their own characters and actions. All of the research findings to date have confirmed that among the adolescent population, loneliness is strongly correlated with low self-esteem (Brennan and Auslander, 1979; Wood, 1978). The lonely adolescent may feel worthless, unattractive, unpopular, and stupid. The causal direction of this association remains in dispute (Peplau et al., 1982). One view is that persons of low self-esteem may have difficulty in initiating as well as maintaining social relationships. They may adopt self-defeating interpretations of their social experiences. Ambiguous social interactions may be interpreted negatively. They may adopt self-blaming positions regarding any perceived social failure, or they may be overly sensitive to criticism and unable to accept compliments (Peplau et al., 1982).

A second view is that chronic loneliness may erode self-esteem. The lack of friends within the gregarious and often socially competitive culture of the high school is often interpreted as social failure. Thus the perception of social deficit is transmuted into social failure, which may erode feelings of personal worth. The cognitive attributions adopted by the adolescent are, however, seen as critical mediating variables. Attributions to internal features, such as personality or ability, may foster feelings of incompetence and inadequacy. Over time this process may lead to a generalized pessimism about social relations as well as low self-esteem (Shaver and Rubenstein, 1980). Research findings with adolescents as well as college students (Loucks, 1974; Brennan and Auslander, 1979) have repeatedly confirmed that self-reported "lonely youth" perceive themselves as unpopular, unattractive, and socially stigmatized by others.

A further line of research has established that lonely youth have high scores for external control, powerlessness, and passivity. Studies of boys and girls across the adolescent years have confirmed the generality of this relationship. Separate scales of powerlessness in the family and peer contexts have demonstrated that feelings of powerlessness existed in both of these contexts among the lonely youth (Brennan and Auslander, 1979). Such passivity is also shown regarding time management. The structuring of leisure time can be conducted actively or passively. It has been found that passivity in the structuring of leisure activities correlates with loneliness (Brennan and Auslander, 1979).

Shyness and fear of social risk-taking can hinder the initiation of relationships. Various research studies have confirmed that shyness, self-consciousness, and fear of taking social risks are correlated with loneliness (Konopka, 1976; Brennan and Auslander, 1979). An interesting finding in our own research is that the relationship between shyness and loneliness is substantially higher for boys than for girls. A similar sex difference has been reported for adults (Weiss, 1973). This suggests that difficulty in the initiation of relationships is a more serious factor leading to loneliness for males than for females.

The inability to care for others, or to develop a sense of commitment to the growth and well-being of others, may obviously restrict the initiation, maintenance, and development of social as well as intimate relationships. It is not surprising that loneliness will be experienced when the person cannot discover anything or any person to care about. Selfishness and disinterest in others has been found to characterize lonely adolescents (Brennan and Auslander, 1979). They tend to be more mistrustful and suspicious of others than non-lonely youth (Loucks, 1974). Their interest in gaining social popularity and social affirmation was lower than that of non-lonely youth. Many exhibited a pattern of apathy in regard to peer, parent, and teacher relationships when compared with non-lonely youth.

The task of establishing characteristics that may predispose a young person toward loneliness has received impetus from the development of new test instruments to assess loneliness. Russell (1982) provides a useful review of current progress and problems in conceptualizing and measuring loneliness.

Cultural Factors and Adolescent Loneliness

Many social and cultural factors have been identified that may contribute to loneliness (Gordon, 1976; Peplau and Perlman, 1982). The literature describing these factors are not reviewed here. However, some of the major factors contributing to adolescent loneliness are discussed.

The social roles provided to adolescents are often described as inadequate or marginal. Rappoport (1972) has described the social role of the adolescent as a social "limbo," in which the adolescent enjoys neither the rights nor the psychological supports that are given to adults and children. Role ambiguity, deterioration of role models, absence of identification rituals, confusion regarding rights, duties or privileges, and so on, are often mentioned (Konopka, 1978; Rappoport, 1972). Deficiencies in social role may deprive the adolescent of a clearly defined sense of belongingness or mode of participation. For example, large segments of the adolescent population are cast into rejected failure roles (Konopka, 1966; Stierlin, 1974). Failure in school has been found to have a strong correlation with feelings of rejection and loneliness (Brennan and Auslander, 1979).

Adolescents also have to cope with unrealistically high expectations and social norms. Many become caught up in invidious and damaging comparison against these norms for social popularity, social achievements, dating, and so forth (Gordon, 1976; Peplau and Perlman, 1979). The tendency of young people to compare their social performance against that of others may magnify feelings of social failure and rejection. The mass media as well as the high school culture may encourage and intensify such comparisons.

In dealing with the exploratory, pre-commitment (or moratorium) phase of identity development, adolescents face strong social and family pressures toward foreclosure and conformity (Marcia, 1980). Yet, the moratorium phase of exploration, experimentation, and deferred commitment are critically important for identity development. The struggle for independence, autonomy, and freely chosen commitments by the adolescent is challenging and requires much support. If parents are unsympathetic, peer support may become crucial. Loneliness and isolation might undermine the adolescent in meeting this challenge. Many adolescents are known to give up the struggle and enter a foreclosed identity status (Rappoport, 1972).

Finally, many have argued that contemporary social conditions are such that the challenges and tasks provided to the adolescent are empty and meaningless. Meaningful participation and worthwhile social roles are simply not provided to all adolescents (Konopka, 1966). The more resourceful adolescent may advance in spite of this, and may discover interests or challenges to evoke excitement, creative energy, and commitment. However, many may fail to discover such tasks or interests, and may succumb to a chronic apathy. Boredom and apathy have been found to be widespread among adolescents (Smith, 1981; Brennan and Auslander, 1979). Once again, the suggestion is that a vast segment of the adolescent population is confronted with the problem of spiritual loneliness.

Responding to Loneliness

As noted earlier, people will do almost anything to avoid loneliness. Adolescents are no exception, and an enormous variety of activities can be seen as attempts to escape loneliness. A general dichotomy is whether the coping strategy is functional in dealing with relational deficits, or whether it is dysfunctional—that is, it does nothing to alleviate these problems, and instead leads to new problems (drugs, alcohol, delinquency), deeper levels of despair, or the erosion of the sense of self. The following coping strategies may be useful initially as a framework for discussion.

Many adolescents respond directly to loneliness by attempting to increase their levels of social contact and to develop new friendships. They enter a bewildering range of social activities. A related approach within this strategy is to increase one's social desirability. This may include being more beautiful, skilled, intelligent, strong, wealthier, or more mature. Many will attempt to strengthen their social affiliations by adopting the external signs of belongingness or identification with a particular group (for example, motorcycle gear, punk-rock uniforms, or high fashion). A second direct approach is to make better use of existing networks. This may happen when romantic breakups occur, and the young person energetically explores existing social connections.

An alternative approach frequently used by lonely adolescents is to develop surrogate relationships. Hero worship with celebrities of various kinds has always been rampant in the adolescent population. The absence of a "symmetrical" relationship renders this strategy dysfunctional in certain ways. The adolescent who engages in surrogate relationships will not experience the kind of reassurance, feedback, and validation that is so important in adolescent friendships. Heroes and celebrities may have an important evocative function regarding adolescent goals; however, the one-way nature of this type of relationship would render it only partially effective in a number of critically important provisions of relationships.

Another general response of lonely persons is to reduce their desires for relationships. Adolescents exhibit many strategies falling under this general heading. They may defer romantic attachments until some future "milestone" is reached (such as graduation from high school or college). They may deny the importance of such relationships. A dysfunctional feature of such an adaptation is that the healthy and normal desire for such relationships may be permanently inhibited. A related approach is to engage in relatively nonsocial activities that give alternative satisfactions. For example, some may place strong emphasis upon hobbies, pastimes, school work, sports, and so forth, that can be enjoyed alone and that provide substantial satisfactions.

Others may vigorously deny the existence of personal loneliness. To be lonely in this society is to be a failure; some adolescents may respond by denying or suppressing any acknowledgment of their loneliness. They may dogmatically declare that they have never been lonely. Many adolescents in the Foreclosed Identity Status may be following this strategy (Marcia, 1980). The personal cost of such a denial of loneliness is that its "early warning" promptings remain unheeded, and the young person remains stuck in a web of relationships that is not satisfying or conducive to personal development (Marcia, 1980; Yalom, 1980).

A favorite antidote to loneliness—one especially advocated by the mass media—is to seek alternative "consumer" gratifications rather than attempt to develop better relationships. Gratifications and "fun" such as alcohol, drugs, fast cars, and other consumer diversions and "entertainment," are proposed as cures for loneliness. Gordon (1976) graphically describes the emergence of the "loneliness industry" that exploits the mass loneliness in this society. The allure and selling point of many advertised products is the implicit promise of a cure for loneliness. Fashion magazines tie social and heterosexual success and the avoidance of loneliness to a broad range of advertised consumer products. The lonely and often desperate adolescent is vulnerable to the promises contained in such messages, as well as to other offerings (such as clubs, singles bars, gurus, and cults). Although many of these products and activities are not explicitly aimed at the adolescent market, their apparent message that they banish loneliness clearly reaches most adolescents. This has been a general overview of some common responses to loneliness. Works that examine many of the more specific responses can be found in Cohen and Taylor (1978); Yalom (1980); and Peplau and Perlman (1982).

Linking Loneliness to Suicide

Although not specifically focused on adolescent suicide, some recent typological studies of suicide and parasuicide suggest a strong
association between loneliness and certain kinds of suicide (Henderson et al., 1977; Bagley et al., 1976; Li, 1973). Each of these
typological studies contains subtypes of suicide or parasuicide that
are clearly characterized by loneliness. Bagley and colleagues describe one subgroup of completed suicides with the following defining features: early disruption of family life, and social isolation
and sociopathic traits. Li (1973) describes and presents data on a
subtype "egoistic suicide" characterized by a lack of social integration, and extreme separateness and individuation, coupled with
feelings of suspicion and of being mistreated by others. In the study
by Henderson and colleagues (1977), two of the three classes of
parasuicides were found to have feelings of exclusion, being unwanted, not needed by others, and loneliness. It is also noteworthy
that, although 184 variables were used in creating this latter typology, the indicator of loneliness emerged as one of the most pow-
erfully discriminating variables.

The Effects of Loneliness on
Adolescent Development

It must be stressed that loneliness has some adaptive significance.
If responded to in a positive way, loneliness can motivate an adolescent to seek out relationships that are more satisfying. Temporary
loneliness is experienced by virtually all adolescents, and, if they
heed its warning, it may be useful in keeping their relationship
network well matched to their particular social needs. Chronic
loneliness, on the other hand, may be implicated in a process that
is ultimately damaging to the mental or physical health of the individual. The exact role of loneliness in such damage is not well
understood. What follows is clearly speculative regarding the damaging effects of loneliness.

Fear of Loneliness and the Avoidance of Individuation

One obvious impairment to adolescent development is avoidance of individuation caused by an inability to face the separation

and loneliness that accompany independence and autonomy. As noted earlier, existential isolation is a corollary of independence and personal autonomy. Some adolescents (and adults) may be so fearful of this risky developmental task that they may collude with others to avoid such separation. Yalom (1980) gives a detailed clinical picture of this avoidance of individuation caused by an inability to face existential loneliness. As noted earlier, existential isolation is a corollary of independence and personal autonomy. The costs and symptoms described by Yalom include avoidance of autonomy, avoidance of responsibility, passivity, external control and powerlessness, extreme conformity and other-directedness, fear of rejection, and a needy, anxious, exploitative approach to relationships, as well as an impaired ability to care for others. Many of the symptoms clinically described by Yalom have been found to characterize lonely adolescents.

Failure to Deal Successfully with the Adolescent Moratorium Due to Absence of Supports

Marcia (1980), Yalom (1980), and others have shown that adolescents require substantial psychological resources to successfully tackle the moratorium stage. Such resources include optimism, patience, confidence, ability to be alone, freedom from either internal or external compulsion to end this phase prematurely, and so on. The adolescent who decides to face the moratorium is in a vulnerable position. Even assuming that the adolescent is not colluding with parents or others to avoid this stage, that person may collapse back into a foreclosed identity state if he or she does not receive appropriate support. The isolated or lonely adolescent may be much more vulnerable to the collapse of will, than the adolescent who has secured the encouragement, guidance, and validation of close friends. Thus social and emotional isolation may be implicated in the failure of many adolescents to successfully cope with the moratorium. Daniel Levinson, in Chapter 1 of this volume, points to the existence of "transitional" developmental phases. Persons encountering such phases must successfully deal with autonomy, exploration, and choice, often in the face of unknown outcomes and lack of experience. These "exploratory" tasks clearly imply a phase of detachment from commitments and a willingness to be alone (or uncommitted). The individual who cannot face loneliness will be tempted to curtail this exploratory phase and will be unlikely to make appropriate choices regarding new commitments. The support of friends and the guidance of mentors seems critical for many individuals coping with transitions.

Discussion

Loneliness is a signal that the social relations of the adolescent are deficient in some way that may be important. Temporary loneliness may be beneficial to prompt or motivate the adolescent to take certain coping actions to improve or extend their relationships. Thus, this kind of loneliness should not necessarily be prevented. However, if certain inappropriate responses are adopted, this temporary loneliness may endure and may develop into a more chronic damaging condition. The link between recurrent loneliness and various mental health problems—including suicide—is now documented in an increasing number of empirical studies. This chapter has examined some of the major causes of loneliness among adolescents. The intent is to identify conditions that lead to such chronic loneliness, and to allow the specification of groups of adolescents who may be at risk for the damaging effects of loneliness. We are at the earliest stages in specifying the causal mechanisms linking chronic loneliness to various disorders. The responses to loneliness and the fear of loneliness may be critical in the emergence of causal mechanisms for such damaging problems as drug abuse, denial, narcissism, withdrawal into fantasy, and so forth. The descriptive stage of loneliness research has proceeded fairly rapidly, and some interesting linkages are becoming visible between this research and the more theoretical writings on adolescent development (Marcia, 1980; Yalom, 1980). Such convergence may aid in the development of preventive interventions for the damaging effects of chronic loneliness.

References

Bagley C, Jacobson S, Rehin A: Completed suicide: taxonomic analysis of clinical and social data. Psycho/Med 6:429–438, 1976

Basquin M, Trystram D: Exhibitionism in the adolescent. Annales Medico-Psychologiques 2, 1966

Bell RR: Worlds of Friendship. Beverly Hills, CA, Sage, 1981

Brennan T: Loneliness at adolescence, in Loneliness: A Sourcebook of Current Theory, Research and Therapy. Edited by Peplau LA, Perlman D. New York, John Wiley and Sons, 1982

Brennan T, Auslander N: Adolescent Loneliness: An Exploratory Study of Social and Psychological Predisposition and Theory. Boulder, CO, Behavioral Research Institute, 1979

Brennan T, Camilli G: The epidemiology and dynamics of adolescent loneliness. Boulder, CO, Institute for Research on Social Problems, 1983

Buhler C: Loneliness in maturity. Journal of Humanistic Psychology 9:167–181, 1969

Burton A: On the nature of loneliness. Am J Psychoanal 21:34–39, 1961

Cohen S, Taylor L: Escape Attempts. New York, Penguin Books, 1978

Coleman JS: Youth: Transition to Adulthood. Chicago, University of Chicago Press, 1974

Collier RM, Lawrence HP: The adolescent feeling of psychological isolation. Educational Theory 1:106–115, 1951

Christiaans X: Study of favorable and unfavorable influences on successful study in 200 students in a teacher's college. Tijdschrift Voor Psycho-medisch-Social Werk 12:155–163, 1965

Cutrona CE: Transition to college: loneliness and the process of social adjustment, in Loneliness: A Sourcebook of Current Theory, Research and Therapy. Edited by Peplau LA, Perlman D. New York, John Wiley and Sons, 1982

Elkind D: Cognitive development in adolescence, in Understanding Adolescence. Edited by Adams JF. Boston, Allyn and Bacon, 1968

Fabry JB: The Pursuit of Meaning. Boston, Beacon Press, 1968

Ford EE, Zorn RL: Why be Lonely? Niles, IL, Argus Communications, 1975

Frankl VE: The Unheard Cry for Meaning: Psychotherapy and Humanism. New York, Simon and Schuster, 1978

Fromm E: The Sane Society. New York, Holt, Rinehart and Winston, 1955

Fromm-Reichmann F: Loneliness. Psychiatry 22:1–15, 1959

Gaev DM: The Psychology of Loneliness. Chicago, Adams Press, 1976

Gordon S: Lonely in America. New York, Simon and Schuster, 1976

Henderson AS, Hartigan J, Davidson J, et al: A typology of parasuicide. Br J Psychiatry 131:631–641, 1977

Holzner AS, Ding LK: White dragon pearls in Hong Kong: a study of young women drug addicts. Int J Addict 8:253–263, 1973

Horton PD: The mystical experience as a suicide prevention. Am J Psychiatry 130:294–296, 1973

Klapp OE: Collective Search for Identity. New York, Holt, Rinehart and Winston, 1969

Konopka G: The Adolescent Girl in Conflict. Englewood Cliffs, NJ, Prentice-Hall, 1966

Konopka G: Friends-loneliness, in Young Girls: A Portrait of Adolescence. Englewood Cliffs, NJ, Prentice-Hall, 1976

Li WL: Durkheim's typology of suicide: some observations from Taiwanese data. International Review of Modern Sociology 3:214–223, 1973

Loucks S: The dimensions of loneliness: a psychological study of affect, self-concept, and object-relations. Dissertation Abstracts International 35:3024B, 1974

Lowenthal MF, Thurner M, Chirboga D: Four Stages of Life. San Francisco, Jossey-Bass, 1975

Marcia JE: Identity in adolescence, in Handbook of Adolescent Psychology. Edited by Adelson J. New York, John Wiley and Sons, 1980

May R: Man's Search for Himself. New York, Delta Books, 1953

Meyeroff M: On Caring. New York, Harper & Row, 1971

Mijuskovic BL: Loneliness in Philosophy, Psychology and Literature. Assen, Netherlands, Van Gorcum, 1979

Ostrov E, Offer D: Loneliness and the adolescent, in Adolescent Psychology. Edited by Feinstein S. Chicago, University of Chicago Press, 1978

Ostrov E, Offer D: Loneliness and the adolescent, in The Anatomy of Loneliness. Edited by Hartog J, Andy JR, Cohen YA. New York, International Universities Press, 1980

Peplau LA, Perlman D: Blueprint for a social psychological theory of loneliness, in Love and Attraction. Edited by Cook M, Wilson G. Oxford, Pergamon, 1979

Peplau LA, Perlman D: Perspectives on loneliness, in A Sourcebook of Current Theory, Research and Therapy. Edited by Peplau LA, Perlman D. New York, John Wiley and Sons, 1982

Peplau LA, Miceli M, Morasch B: Loneliness and self-evaluation, in Loneliness: A Sourcebook of Current Theory, Research and Therapy. Edited by Peplau LA, Perlman D. New York, John Wiley and Sons, 1982

Pittel SM: Developmental factors in adolescent drug use: a study of psychedelic drug users. J Am Acad Child Psychiatry 10:640–660, 1971

Rappoport L: Personality Development: The Chronology of Experience. Glenview, IL, Scott, Foresman, 1972

Rubin Z: Children without friends, in Loneliness: A Sourcebook of Current Theory, Research and Therapy. Edited by Peplau LA, Perlman D. New York, John Wiley and Sons, 1982

Russell D: The measurement of loneliness, in Loneliness: A Sourcebook of Current Theory, Research and Therapy. Edited by Peplau LA, Perlman D. New York, John Wiley, 1982

Shaver P, Rubenstein C: Living alone, loneliness, and health. Paper presented at the Annual Meeting of the American Psychological Association, New York City, 1979

Shaver P, Rubenstein C: Childhood attachment experience and adult loneliness, in Review of Personality and Social Psychology, vol. 1. Edited by Wheeler L. Beverly Hills, CA, Sage, 1980

Smith RP: Boredom: a review. Human Factors 23:329–340, 1981

Stierlin H: Separating Parents and Adolescents. New York, Harper and Row, 1974

Sullivan HS: The Interpersonal Theory of Psychiatry. New York, Norton, 1953

Tanner IJ: Loneliness: The Fear of Love. New York, Harper and Row, 1973

Weiss RS: Loneliness: The Experience of Emotional and Social Isolation. Cambridge, MA, MIT Press, 1973

Weiss RS: The provisions of social relationships, in Doing Unto Others. Edited by Rubin Z. Englewood Cliffs, NJ, Prentice-Hall, 1974

Weiss RS: Issues in the study of loneliness, in Loneliness: A Sourcebook of Current Theory, Research and Therapy. Edited by Peplau LA, Perlman D. New York, John Wiley and Sons, 1982

Wood L: Loneliness, social identity and social structure. Essence 2:259–276, 1978

Yalom ID: Existential Psychotherapy. New York, Basic Books, 1980

Chapter 9

Personality, Life Events, and Other Psychosocial Factors in Adolescent Depression and Suicide

Robert M.A. Hirschfeld, M.D.
Susan J. Blumenthal, M.D., M.P.A.

Chapter 9

Personality, Life Events, and Other Psychosocial Factors in Adolescent Depression and Suicide

The phenomena of depression, nonfatal suicidal behavior, and completed suicide are related to one another. Affective disorders and alcoholism have been associated with approximately 70 percent of completed suicides (Dorpat, 1960; Barraclough, 1974). A history of prior suicide attempts is common in those who completed suicide. On the other hand, the majority of people who suffer from depression do not attempt suicide, and very few of those who attempt suicide actually commit suicide. Thus, although these three phenomena overlap, they are not congruent. A pressing public health concern is to identify characteristics that will help to predict which people will make suicide attempts, and which people will complete suicide. Such information may allow early and effective preventive therapeutic intervention.

Research on these phenomena in younger groups has been limited. Whether the characteristics that distinguish among depression, nonfatal suicidal behavior, and completed suicide among adults are the same for younger age groups has received little attention.

Risk factors for these phenomena may exist in several areas, including the sociodemographic, psychosocial, biological, and genetic domains. This chapter focuses on psychosocial risk factors for depression, suicidal behavior, and completed suicide in adolescents and young adults. Two specific questions will be addressed:

The authors wish to express special appreciation to Leora Rosenthal, Ph.D. for the significant contributions she made to this manuscript.

215

1. Are there differences in psychosocial risk factors among depression, suicidal behavior, and completed suicide among adolescents and young adults?

2. How do psychosocial risk factors for these three phenomena in adolescents and young adults compare with psychosocial risk factors for these phenomena in adults?

An answer to the first question will help to identify specific risk factors for each phenomenon in adolescents and young adults. An answer to the second question will help us to understand what distinguishes these phenomena in adolescents and young adults from the same phenomena in adults. Similarities in the risk factors for the two age groups would support the hypothesis that there is a continuum between adolescence and adulthood. Differences in the risk factors in the two age groups would support the notion of a difference in these phenomena between adolescence and adulthood.

After a section on definition of terms, there is in this chapter a brief overview of child and adolescent depression. The next section reviews the research literature on personality, life events, and other psychosocial factors in adolescent and young adult depression. Next, there is a review of these factors in suicide attempts, followed by an examination of these risk factors in completed suicides for adolescents and young adults. In order to provide a basis for comparison, the adult literature on personality and life events is summarized in the same order: depressive syndrome, suicide attempts, and completed suicide. A discussion follows, which focuses on the similarities and differences among these three clinical phenomena and their overlap in adolescent, young adult, and adult populations. An overview of methodological issues in suicide research completes the discussion section.

Definition of Terms

The *clinical depressive syndrome* is defined as a psychiatric disorder in which the major feature of the clinical picture is dysphoric mood or pervasive loss of interest or pleasure, accompanied by a number of the following symptoms: sleep and appetite disturbances, loss of energy, psychomotor retardation or agitation, feelings of self-reproach or excessive or inappropriate guilt, and reduced ability to concentrate. In this chapter we will exclude bipolar disorder—that is, one in which at some time in the past, a manic or hypomanic episode has occurred. A manic or hypomanic episode is characterized by elevated, expansive and/or irritable mood, accompanied by increased activity and talking, flight of ideas, grandiosity, decreased need for sleep, and/or distractability. Depressive episodes also occur in bipolar disorder. Nonbipolar disorder involves only depressive episodes. The reason for the exclusion of bipolar disorder is the lack of studies conducted on psychosocial factors in adolescents and young adults with bipolar disorder.

Adolescence and *young adulthood* will be loosely defined to include the age range from puberty to approximately age 30.

Suicide attempts refer to deliberate, conscious, self-destructive acts that might lead to death, even if the individual does not intend to die. *Completed suicides* refer to such acts that do result in death. *Suicide ideation* has been excluded from the paper in order to simplify the review.

An Overview of Childhood and Adolescent Depression

Until recently, the existence of depression as a syndrome in childhood and adolescence was controversial. In their excellent review of this issue, Kovacs and Beck (1977) quote Toolan as stating that overt manifestations of depression are rare in children and adolescents, but that depressive feelings and equivalents are frequent. This approach led to the concept of "masked depression," in which depression may be expressed as hyperactivity, aggressiveness, school failure, delinquency, or psychosomatic problems. Kovacs and Beck take issue with this approach, and present a number of studies in which all elements of adult depression—including affective changes, cognitive changes, motivational changes, and vegetative and psychomotor disturbances—have been found with reasonable frequency among children. They and others subsequently have recommended abandonment of this term, "masked depression." In recent years, depression in childhood and adolescence has been measured and assessed in a number of studies, and instruments have been developed to standardize this measurement and assessment.

Research Literature on Personality, Life Events, and Other Psychosocial Factors

Depression

Empirical research on personality and other psychosocial factors in depression in adolescence and young adults is limited. Much of it involves normal college student samples in which various measures of the personality, performance, and depressive symptom measures are intercorrelated. The relevance of these studies to the clinical syndrome of depression and to premorbid personality is unclear, as we will discuss. Most of the articles on the syndrome of depression do not deal with personality or other psychosocial factors. Nonetheless, there are a few articles in which clinical interviews are performed, and at least some characteristic interpersonal patterns are considered. A sampling of the recent literature follows (see Table 1).

An example of the college student study occurs in the paper by Peterson (1979), in which scores on the Beck Depression Inventory (BDI) were correlated with measures of locus of control in an attempt to test the paradoxical view that depressives blame themselves for outcomes over which they have no control. The sample includes 80 undergraduates recruited through notices on campus. The mean score on the BDI was 7.0 with a standard deviation of 5.1, indicating that more than two-thirds of the sample were well below even the mildest threshold for depression. Peterson concludes that individuals with mild depressions do have illogical cognitions based on modestly positive intercorrelations among self-blame, helplessness, and depression.

In another study, Johnson and colleagues (1982) investigated hypotheses regarding the pathogenesis of depression, particularly in terms of parent–child expectations in a sample of 48 undergraduates. Subjects were considered to be depressed if their BDI scores were above 12 or more. A comparison group of subjects with BDI scores of 5 or less were used. Parent–child expectations were assessed using a version of the semantic differential, although no attempt was made to contact parents. The authors concluded that depressogenic parents negatively evaluate their children, and that depressed college students show lowered self-evaluations. They were not able to support the hypothesis that depressogenic parents

Table 1. Depressive Symptoms in Adolescents and Young Adults: Psychosocial Factors

Study	Sample	Attribute	Findings
Peterson, 1979	Normal college students: 40 males and 40 females	External locus of control (externality)	Depression associated with externality and undesirable social roles
Johnson et al., 1982	Normal college students: 24 males and 24 females	Self-esteem, parental attitudes	Lower self-esteem and greater negativity about parental perceptions characterize depressed subjects
Kandel and Davies, 1982	214 normal high school students aged 14–18 years, and 5,574 of their parents	Degree of attachment to peers and parents	Reliance on peers rather than parents and isolation from peers or parents correlates with depression
Hammen and Cochran, 1981	400 normal college freshmen aged 17–19 years	Life stress	Depressed subjects had lower emotional tolerance for stressful life events than non-depressed subjects

maintain unrealistically high ideals for their offspring. Unfortunately, this study is methodologically flawed in that the population sample cannot be considered to be representative of depression, and assessments of parental expectations do not include information from the parents.

A study on the epidemiology of depressed mood in adolescence by Kandel and Davies (1982) is more relevant to clinical depression. They assessed depressed mood in an epidemiologic sample of 14- to 18-year-old public secondary school students in New York State, using the depression subscale of SCL–90. Although the study did not directly address personality, several findings relevant to personality emerged. Depressed mood was positively correlated with degree of peer orientation, with distance from both parents, and with minor delinquency. There was some evidence to suggest that minor delinquency, especially in boys, might represent some expression of depression. The levels of the correlations were quite modest, but were the highest among a number of other variables, including parental substance abuse, extracurricular activities, academic performance, medical care utilization, and drug and alcohol abuse. The issue of familiar versus peer orientation appears to be important in adolescent depression and suicide, as we will demonstrate.

Kumchy (1981) examined 32 adolescents who had been referred to a family court because of delinquent behavior. He found that depressive symptomatology correlated with an external locus of control, most notably helplessness, fatalism, and externalization of blame. The more depressed youngsters perceived themselves to be in poor control in both peer and familial relationships.

Hammen and Cochran (1981) used a college students sample, but interviewed students above a cut-off score of 15 on the BDI to confirm a clinical diagnosis of moderate depression. They compared 34 moderately depressed students and 30 nondepressed students with comparably higher levels of personal stress, and 35 nondepressed low stress controls. They were not able to support the Seligman's learned helplessness notion of depressives having internal, stable, and global attributions. They found that the depressives were more likely to get upset at a given level of stress.

One study deserves special mention because its methods and design meet criteria of adult clinical research. Cohen-Sandler et al. (1982a, 1982b)(see Table 2) studied 76 children ranging in age from five to 14, who were consecutively discharged from a psychi-

Table 2. Depressive Syndrome in Adolescents and Young Adults: Psychosocial Factors

Study	Sample	Attribute	Findings
Carlson and Cantwell, 1980	102 psychiatric clinic outpatients aged 7–17	Behavior problems in affective disorders	Behavior problems as reported by parents were more serious in children with secondary affective disorders than primary. Children with primary affective disorders self-report less irritability than those with secondary affective disorders.
Chiles et al., 1980	120 adolescents aged 13–15 admitted to a correctional facility	Behavior problems	23 percent of delinquent adolescents met RDC criteria for major depressive disorder. Acting out behaviors with the exception of abuse of drugs and alcohol did not distinguish depressed subjects from nondepressed subjects.
Cohen-Sandler et al., 1982a, 1982b	76 discharged psychiatric inpatients aged 5–14	Life stress in year prior to admission	Depressed children experienced more rejection by peers one year prior to admission.

atric inpatient unit over a 2½-year period. These children were
assigned to one of three diagnostic groups: suicidal, nonsuicidal
depressed, or psychiatric controls. Diagnoses were made from case
records on the basis of explicit operational criteria. An age-specific
life events inventory was used to record and weight psychological
stress (Coddington, 1972). The suicidal children differed considerably from both the nonsuicidal depressed adolescents and the
psychiatric controls. In the area of life stress, the nonsuicidal depressed children had experienced rejection by their peers prior to
entering junior high school, and this rejection had continued for
the 12 months prior to admission. In contrast, the suicidal children
were more often faced with a major disruption at home, such as
parental death or divorce. In the year prior to admission, the depressed and other psychiatric disorder group had each experienced
stress at the level of death of a sibling or protracted jail sentence
of a parent (Coddington, 1972). The suicidal group had experienced
greater than twice that level of stress, including stress resulting from
broken homes due to parental death, separation, or divorce, witnessing attempted murder of one parent by the other, and other
significant deaths.

It is difficult to summarize the findings from these disparate
studies, as they do not converge. However, there is the suggestion
that depressed children are more oriented toward their peers than
their parents compared to other children, yet perceive themselves
to be rejected by their peers.

Suicide Attempts

Most recent studies of suicide attempts on the part of adolescents and young adults have reported on samples drawn from general and psychiatric hospital emergency rooms and psychiatric units
in various parts of the world. In addition is a nationwide sample of
suicidal behavior, as well as a recent review of the literature in the
area. The extent to which these samples are generalizable is not
clear, although we would expect that most relatively serious suicide
attempts on the part of children or adolescents would find their
way to hospital emergency rooms.

The study by Cohen-Sandler and colleagues (1982a, 1982b)(see
Table 3) separated into three groups: suicidal, nonsuicidal depressed, and psychiatric controls, based on explicit operational criteria for all three groups. Using Coddington's Social Readjustment

Scale for Children and a Life Stress Inventory, they found that the suicidal group was distinguished by substantially increased stress scores beginning in early childhood and persisting into later childhood, compared with the other two groups. This difference was two or three times that of the other two groups in later childhood, and especially characterized the year prior to the suicide attempt. In contrast to the other groups who also had substantial stress in the year prior to admission, the suicidal group had severe disruptions at home, such as substantial separation and/or divorce of parents, witnessing a death of a grandparent or friend, observing the attempted murder of one parent by the other parent, and having a parent hospitalized. The suicidal group was much less withdrawn than either of the other two groups and scored substantially higher in the area of threatening behavior, suggesting increased general aggressiveness. Home conditions were not extensively examined, although the authors did report that parental alcohol and drug abuse was substantially greater in the suicide group. They conclude that suicidal children experienced a "disproportionate number of losses of all kinds" compared with other groups prior to their admission.

Garfinkel and colleagues (1982) reviewed hospital charts of all children and adolescents who presented to a large children's hospital emergency room in Canada, who had attempted suicide over a seven-year period. They identified 505 cases. The sample had three times as many girls as boys, with a mean age of approximately 15. A control group matched for sex and age who had been admitted to the emergency room at nearly the same time for reasons other than suicide was selected. Life events were not included in the study. The familial background of the suicidal children was more distinguished by broken homes, and nearly one-quarter had both parents absent from the home. There was a much higher frequency of previous contact with psychosocial services. The overall frequency of familial history of suicidal behavior was eight times higher in the suicidal group, and a history of mental illness was also much higher. The suicidal group also reported a much higher rate of substance abuse (37 versus six percent). Although the variables selected in this study were, by and large, not relevant to this review, the findings do support a picture of suicidal adolescents as coming from broken and disturbed homes.

Tishler and colleagues (1981) reported similar findings in a study of 108 adolescent suicide attempters evaluated over a two-year period at a children's hospital emergency room in Columbus,

Table 3. Attempted Suicide in Adolescents and Young Adults: Psychosocial Factors

Study	Sample	Attribute	Findings
Goldney 1981(a)(b)(c), 1982	110 female suicide attempters aged 18–30 years, admitted to hospital; 25 age- and sex-matched controls from a women's health center	Obsessoid versus hysterical personality traits	Increasing depression correlated with increasing obsessoid personality. Suicide attempters scored higher on the obsessoid scale than on the hysteria scale.
		Personality, substance abuse, sociodemographic variables	Suicide attempters with greatest lethality lacked a significant other, had less history of violence and a greater number of schizoid personality traits than did controls. Lethality of attempt associated with decreased death anxiety.
		Parental loss or deprivation	Suicide attempters had greater incidence of childhood broken homes due to parental loss, separation or divorce, parental quarrelling, disagreements with parents, poor physical health, and a negative perception of their parents' character, than did controls.
		Locus of control	Suicide attempters had higher externality scores than controls. Lethality associated with internality.

Study	Sample	Category	Findings
Inamadar et al., 1982	Adolescents (aged 12–17 years) hospitalized for the first time (n = 30 females and 21 males)	Psychosis	80% of psychotic adolescents had a history of violent and/or suicidal behavior; 40% a history of violent acts; 16% had a history of suicidal acts; 25% had a history of both. Suicide attempters M:F was 1.5:1.
Hawton et al., 1982 (a) (b) (c)	Adolescents (12–18 years old) admitted to hospital after self-poisoning (n = 45 females and 5 males)	Life stress	28% reported problems with parents, opposite sex, or schoolwork in the 48 hours prior to the suicide attempt. 18% had a recent hospitalization for medical/surgical problems. 1/3 were physically ill, and 20% had psychiatric difficulties at time of the suicide attempt (80% of these adolescents were worse or unchanged at 1-year follow-up).
		Motivation and personality characteristics	Suicide attempters show increased anger, isolation, and impulsivity. 1/3 wanted to die at the time of the attempt. Suicide attempters report little feeling of sorrow, shame, or failure compared with adults.
		Sociodemographic	Suicide attempters had more familial disruption and problems than published norms.

Table 3. Attempted Suicide in Adolescents and Young Adults: Psychosocial Factors (continued)

Study	Sample	Attribute	Findings
Tishler et al., 1981	108 adolescent suicide attempters followed over a 2-year period from an emergency room. The sample is primarily white and female	Life stress	Suicide attempters had increased family disruption. 50% had divorced parents; 60% said their parents' marriage was bad; 18% had alcoholic parents; 22% had parents who had exhibited suicidal behavior. Most common precipitating events: 52%—parental problems; 30%—school problems; 16%—sibling problems; 15%—peer problems; 5%—psychotic symptoms; 20%—some recent death.
Cohen-Sandler et al., 1982	75 5- to 14-year-olds consecutively discharged from the inpatient psychiatric unit. Cases assigned to 3 groups: (1) suicidal; (2) depressed, nonsuicidal; and (3) psychiatric control	Life stress	Suicidal children experienced an increased amount of life stress as they matured, especially over the one year prior to admission (similar to Paykel's study of adults and life events). Suicide completers had more temporary/permanent loss of parent or grandparent and psychiatrically traumatic experiences.

Garfinkel et al., 1982	505 children and adolescent suicide attempters from a pediatric hospital emergency room studied over a 7-year period. Matched with controls (physical or psychiatric illness) for age, sex, and time of admission.	Life stress, sociodemographic variables	Ratio of M:F suicide attempters was 3:1. Suicide attempters had more drastic living situations, increased substance abuse, current psychiatric illness, prior psychotherapy, and current medical illness. Their families had greater psychiatric incidence of psychiatric illness, alcohol abuse, suicide history, paternal unemployment, and parental absences than controls.
Marks et al., 1977	Emotionally disturbed adolescents selected for: (a) suicide attempters ($n = 31$ boys and 67 girls); (b) suicide attempters as well as suicidal thoughts and threats ($n = 7$ boys and 22 girls); (c) suicidal thoughts and threats only ($n = 13$ boys and 12 girls)	Personality, social supports	Few differences were found between attempters and ideators. Suicidal boys, as compared with other emotionally disturbed male adolescents, were more worried, impulsive, suspicious, perfectionist, had mothers who abused alcohol, were not close to their fathers during childhood, and lacked close relationships with male peers. Suicidal girls, as compared with other emotionally disturbed female adolescents, were more tearful, hopeless, despondent, had more sex difficulties, and were less resilient. They are more socially isolated and estranged from their parents.

Ohio. There was a predominance of females at the time of admission, including 14 percent living in institutions. Drinking problems, separations, and general marital discord were prevalent in the families of these adolescents, although no control group was included. The most common precipitating event was a problem with parents, followed by problems with members of the opposite sex and school problems. More than one-fifth of the adolescents had experienced recent suicidal behavior in their families. Thus, this study is very consistent with the findings reported by Garfinkel and colleagues.

Hawton and colleagues described a report on a study of adolescent suicide attemptors in three recent articles in the *British Journal of Psychiatry* (1982a, 1982b, 1982c). The sample included 50 adolescents between the ages of 13 and 19 who were referred to a general hospital psychiatric service in England over a six-month period following a suicide attempt. Most of the attempts were relatively mild. One-third of the adolescents reportedly wanted to die, and less than one-sixth of these attempts were considered this serious by a clinical evaluator. In terms of family background, 48 percent did not live with both parents, compared with 16 percent in the general population. Unfortunately, no specific control group was included. The families were characterized by considerable discord and disturbance. A relatively high percentage of the families had had contact with professional social services groups.

The Hawton findings were similar to the previous studies regarding life events and stress. Nearly three-quarters had had significant problems with their parents, and more than one-half had serious scholastic and peer problems. Three-quarters of the precipitating events included problems with members of the opposite sex or with parents. Nearly one-third had a chronic physical disorder such as asthma or juvenile arthritis. This study did not look at personality variables directly, although a picture of angry and lonely children emerges, many having a history of impulsiveness. The motivation for the suicide attempt in this group was overwhelmingly an attempt to communicate unhappiness or anger rather than escaping from a difficult situation. Less than 10 percent of the sample had considered the attempt for more than 24 hours, and one-half had thought seriously about the fact for less than 15 minutes.

Goldney reported in a serious of four articles (1981a, 1981b, 1981c, 1982) on a study of 110 young women between the ages of 18 and 30 who had attempted suicide by drug overdose and who had been admitted to a large city general hospital in Australia. The average age of the women was about 23. He divided the sample into three groups based on the degree of lethality. The highest lethality group was marked by decreased current or past use of alcohol. Approximately five percent of the group had experienced parental death during childhood, and 10 percent had experienced parental separation or divorce. Compared with a control group of 25 women attending a community mental health center with no history of suicidal behavior, Goldney reported a significant difference in parental separation and divorce during childhood, but not death. In reviewing seven studies of attempted suicide and parental separation, Goldney describes a consensus of broken homes and parental divorce and separation.

Goldney assessed several aspects of personality, including locus of control and the hysteroid-obsessoid dimension. The suicidal group scored higher on externality and obsessoid features than the controls. Unfortunately, the assessments were made during the hospitalization, and therefore may be affected by the clinical state. These findings relative to obsessionality are nearly all consistent with nine previous studies reviewed in this paper. Some increased hysteroid features have been found in low lethality attempters.

Marks and Haller (1977) reported on a nationwide study of 830 emotionally disturbed adolescents aged 12 to 18, who were divided on the basis of whether or not there had been suicidal behavior. Minnesota Multiphasic Personality Inventories (MMPIs) and Personal Data Questionnaires were completed by the patients, and a Q sort, an adjective checklist, and case data questionnaire were completed by the psychotherapist. The suicide group included 67 girls and 37 boys. Findings for the boys and girls differed. The boys tended to be more depressed and were considered to be impulsive, isolated, and perfectionistic. They tended to have an exaggerated need for affection and to react to frustration intropunitively. The girls also tended to be sad and very isolated, but more resentful. Hysteroid features were very low in both groups. The girls also tended to react to frustration intropunitively. Marks and Haller concluded that the suicidal boys "in contrast to other emotionally disturbed male adolescents, are referred because they are impulsive and run away, are worried, suspicious, perfectionistic, and sometimes physically handicapped." They were not seen as resentful. Suicidal girls, "in contrast to other emotionally disturbed adolescent females, are referred for treatment because of tearfulness and sex difficulties." They were viewed as despondent, resentful, weak, and unstable.

Although the data base is limited, there is remarkable convergence of findings in this area. Adolescents who make suicide attempts are characterized by considerable increased life stress, and have had many losses and significant changes within the nuclear family as compared with other psychiatrically disturbed youngsters, depressed adolescents, and the general population. They have had both physical and psychiatric illnesses. Precipitating events are almost invariably interpersonal problems between the adolescent and his parents or peers. The social and familial background of those adolescents is marked by parental death, divorce, and separation. The general relationship with parents is often troubled and there is considerable marital discord. Less information on personality exists than on other factors, but the picture of the suicide attempters tends to include isolation and impulsiveness in people who perhaps have limited coping skills as compared with other people, although this last aspect is speculative. The suicide attempt is more often an attempt to communicate anger or frustration than necessarily an attempt to die, although this varied considerably. Thus, adolescents who attempt suicide have a greater number of negative life events, have fewer social supports, and have fewer personal resources, than adolescents who do not.

Completed Suicide

To our knowledge, only one study of completed suicide in adolescents has been performed, although several studies of adult suicides included a significant number of people in their early thirties. Shaffer (1974)(see Table 4) studied all of the suicides reported among children under the age of 15 occurring in England and Wales during a seven-year period, obtained by a coroner's records. The sample of 31 children included 21 boys and nine girls. There were no suicides below age 12, and only two occurred at age 12, which .s consistent with other reports of the rarity of suicide in prepubertal children (Shaffer and Fisher, 1981).

With regard to life events, approximately one-third of children in this study were involved in a "disciplinary crisis" involving truancy, or other related school problems. Another one-third of the sample had interpersonal problems with peers, parents, or close friends of

Table 4. Completed Suicide in Adolescents and Young Adults: Psychosocial Factors

Study	Sample	Attribute	Findings
Shaffer, 1974	31 cases of completed suicides of children aged 12–15 years	Precipitating events, personality traits	The most common precipitating events were: (1) disciplinary crises (36%); (2) fights with peers (13%); (3) fights with opposite sex friend (19%); (4) had no precipitating event. All had above-average IQs. One-half had hostile affect—mostly outwardly directed. Personality descriptions included: (1) paranoid, suspicious, critical; (2) explosive; (3) quiet, uncommunicative; (4) perfectionist; (5) miscellaneous. 17%—antisocial symptoms; 13%—affective symptoms; 57%—antisocial and affective symptoms

the opposite sex. In 10 percent of the sample, no precipitant was apparent. Nearly one-half had previously threatened or attempted suicide, and two of the 30 were suffering from a chronic illness. The children in this study had normal or slightly superior intelligence. Approximately 70 percent had antisocial features including fighting, stealing, truancy, and other delinquency.

The home environment of these children contrasted with that reported in the Cohen-Sandler study. More than 90 percent of the children were living at home with one or both of their natural parents, with approximately 20 percent coming from broken homes. However, the home environment was far from ideal, with over one-half of the parents or siblings having a recorded psychiatric disorder, and approximately 13 percent having attempted suicide.

Shaffer concluded that there are two types of children who commit suicide. The first lead a solitary, isolated existence and are often of superior intelligence and have mentally ill mothers. Prior to their deaths, depression and antisocial behavior increased. The second group is more impulsive, impetuous, prone to aggressive or violent outbursts, and sensitive to criticism. Obviously, this group displayed considerable antisocial behavior and had school problems.

In an extensive review on psychosocial and cognitive aspects of adolescent suicide, Petzel and Riddle (1981) concluded that adolescent completers are even more isolated, less visible, and more disturbed than suicide attempters. They described a host of familial, social, school, and emotional problems, as well as physical illness as interacting to increase the suicide risk. Petzel and Riddle concluded that a disrupted nuclear family is the most common distinguishing feature of suicidal adolescents. Social isolation and impulsiveness were reported in a number of studies. Suicidal behavior within the family was associated with increased adolescent suicide attempts. Petzel and Riddle concluded with a recommendation for an approach using an interrelationship of multiple factors.

Research Literature on Personality, Life Events, and Other Psychosocial Factors in Depression and Suicide in Adults

In order to provide a basis for comparison of personality, life events, and other psychosocial factors for depression and suicide in adolescents and young adults, a summary of the adult research literature in this area will be presented.

Personality and other psychosocial risk factors in adults have recently been reviewed by Hirschfeld and Cross (1982). They distinguished three major diagnostic categories: depressive symptoms, nonbipolar depressive syndrome, and bipolar depressive syndrome. Because bipolar depressive syndrome and depressive symptoms are not reviewed in the adolescent literature, they will be excluded from discussion in this chapter.

Depressive Symptoms

As is evident from Table 5, no systematic studies of personality characteristics have been undertaken that are relevant to depressive symptoms. In the area of life events, there is support for a positive relationship between level of depressive symptoms and number of life events experienced in the months prior to the interview. Ilfeld (1977) found that marital stress, along with parental stressors for women and job stressors for men, accounted for nearly 25 percent of the variance in the level of depressive symptoms while demographic characteristics accounted for less than eight percent.

As regards personal resources, including social and other supports, the quality of the marital relationship or that of a confiding relationship has been shown to be the most important resource, the lack of which is associated with depression. Contrary to some sociopolitical arguments, higher rates of depression have been found among the unmarried, not the married, for both women and men.

Depressive Syndrome

There have been a number of studies relating depressive syndrome and psychosocial variables (see Table 6). Nonbipolar patients with major depression whose personality has been *assessed during nondepressed states* have been found to be introverted, and interpersonally dependent. Only those depressives with premorbid maladaptive characters have been found to exhibit neurotic characteristics. With regard to life events, most investigators have generally found that depressed patients experienced a greater number of life events in the six months prior to onset than do normals or patients with nondepressed psychiatric disorders. Life events such as exits from the social field, or undesirable events, are especially likely to have

Table 5. Depressive Syndrome in Adults: Psychosocial Factors

Attribute	Findings
Sociodemographic characteristics, personality, life events, social supports.	Rate of depressive syndrome in M:F was 2:1. Rates of depressive syndrome were inversely related to social class and age. No racial differences in prevalence were reported. Rates of depressive syndrome were somewhat lower in persons with a significant intimate relationship.
	Depressive syndrome associated with such personality characteristics as introversion, interpersonal dependency, low self-esteem, and general neuroticism.
	Onset of depressive syndrome correlated with an increased number of life events (particularly undesirable and exit events) particularly one month prior to onset.
	An increased risk of depressive syndrome associated with lack of confiding relationship with spouse/partner, unemployment, three or more children under the age of 14 in the home, and loss of parent before age 17.

Based on findings reviewed in Hirschfeld and Cross (1982; 1983)

Table 6. Attempted Suicide in Adults: Psychosocial Factors

Study	Sample	Attribute	Findings
Henderson et al., 1977	350 patients admitted to hospital as a result of a suicide attempt in Tasmania and in Australia from 1974–1975	Life stress, suicidal intent	3 personality types for suicide attempters emerged from cluster analysis: (1) patients not characterized by high scores on any of the variables who remain a puzzle; (2) depressed, alienated, with a higher suicide intent and greater amount of marital discord; (3) angry, alienated, with a lower suicide intent, but a greater intent to be punitive and a higher degree of marital stress.
Luscomb et al., 1980	47 male psychiatric patients admitted to a VA hospital following a suicide attempt. A control group of non-suicide attempting male psychiatric patients admitted to the VA hospital ($n = 51$)	Life stress, locus of control	Suicide attempters were significantly younger and more likely to have a diagnosis of depression than controls. In the young and middle-age groups, no significant differences in amount of life stress was found between suicide attempters and controls. Older suicide attempters and those who scored as high trust, high externals had significantly more life events than controls.

Table 6. Attempted Suicide in Adults: Psychosocial Factors (continued)

Study	Sample	Attribute	Findings
Bancroft et al., 1977	143 suicide attempters in the Oxford area between June–December 1972. Three groups were defined: (1) those admitted as inpatients; (2) those treated as outpatients; and (3) those referred by general practitioners	Life stress, precipitating events	Most common precipitating life event was a quarrel with a key person (48%) in the 7 days prior to the suicide attempt (more common among women than men). Significantly more male than female suicide attempters had extramarital affairs during the preceding year. The lack of a confidant was similar for men and women. One-third of the sample were receiving nonpsychiatric medical treatment. At the time of the suicide attempt, 1/4 were receiving psychiatric treatment, and 1/2 had received psychiatric treatment at some time.
Rygnestad, 1982	257 self-poisoned patients (155 females, aged 13–79); (102 males, ages 14–88) living in Trendheim	Sociodemographic variables	An increased incidence of divorce, separation, and unemployment was found in suicide attempters. More than 50% had seen a physician one month prior to the suicide attempt. Poor social and economic conditions, alcoholism, and an increased incidence of psychiatric disturbance was found in the sample.

Adams et al., 1982	98 patients admitted consecutively to hospital following a suicide attempt. 102 matched controls (age and sex) from general practice population with no history of suicide behavior	Parental loss, family stability	Suicide attempters experienced more parental loss (mainly due to separation/divorce rather than death) than controls. Death of a father was higher for suicide atempters. Significantly more female suicide attempters had experienced loss due to death before age 25. Suicide attempters had more chaotic unstable family environments than controls. In those cases when parental loss had occurred, more suicide attempters than controls had chaotic or unstable family environments prior to the loss, as well as in the long-term period following the loss.
Slater and Depue, 1981	Hospitalized suicidal patients aged 18–65 who met RDC for primary depressive disorder, with serious suicide intent ($n = 14$). Nonsuicidal depressed controls matched for age, sex, race, and social class ($n = 14$)	Life stress, social supports	Suicide attempters experienced significantly more independent life events (especially exit events) than nonattempters, both before and after onset of depression. 75% of the suicide attempters lacked a confidant or social support as compared with 25% of the controls.

occurred. Interestingly, these rates do not change with endogenous symptomatology—that is, endogeneity is *not* associated with lack of precipitating stress. Lack of a confiding relationship increases the likelihood of depression.

Suicide Attempts

Studies on suicide attempts in adult populations vary widely in sample and methodology (see Table 7). They range from random epidemiologic subsamples of suicide attempts in a community, to consecutive admissions to a general hospital emergency room, to admissions to Veterans Administration Hospitals. Some of the studies involve no controls, while others use controls drawn from non-suicidal general psychiatric patients; still other studies use general populations matched for age and sex. Despite this considerable variability in sample and in approach, remarkable convergence of findings emerges. The proportion of women in the samples varies from 60 to 70 percent, except of course in the VA sample, and suicide attempts seem more prevalent in the younger age groups.

The most striking finding is a significant increase in life events compared with any control group, particularly exit events. For example, in their classic 1975 study, Paykel and colleagues compared 53 suicide attempters admitted to a general hospital emergency service with matched nonsuicidal depressed patients and subjects in the general population. They found that the suicide attempters have four times as many life events in the six months prior to the attempt as compared with the general population, and 1½ times as many as the depressed patients. Entrance and exit events were equal in number. These results may be limited in their generalizability as Slater and Depue (1981) pointed out: 1) the diagnostic compositions of the three groups is not specified; and 2) the suicidal group is predominantly young and female, with low intent of lethality. Therefore, the suicide group is probably not representative of the more severe primary depressive group, which is at highest risk for completed suicide.

Slater and Depue (1981) addressed these issues in their study of high lethal intent suicidal patients compared with nonsuicidal controls, all meeting Research Diagnostic Criteria (RDC) for primary major depressive disorder. They reported that the suicidal group had a greater number of independent events both prior to—and after the onset—the depression, and that they had nearly three times

Table 7. Attempted Suicide in Adults: Psychosocial Factors

Study	Sample	Attribute	Findings
Patsiokas et al., 1978	Male psychiatric patients aged 19–59 admitted to a VA hospital for a suicide attempt. (n = 49). The control group was male psychiatric patients with no history of a suicide attempt (n = 48)	Cognitive rigidity, impulsivity and field dependence	Suicide attempters had greater cognitive rigidity, were younger and more depressed than controls. The control group had more psychotics than the suicide attempter group.
Paykel et al., 1975	53 suicide attempters admitted to general hospital emergency service, and matched depressive and general population control.	Life stress	Suicide attempters reported 4 times as many life events 6 months prior to the attempt than general population controls, and 1½ times as many as reported by depressed patients. Suicide attempters were preceded by entrance and exit life events equally.

the number of exits prior to the onset of depression. This distinction of continued negative life events *after* the onset of depression may be critical to the precipitation of the suicide attempt.

Bancroft and colleagues (1977) investigated approximately 50 percent of all self-poisoning or self-injuries in three samples drawn from general health practices in England. They reported that nearly one-half of the suicide attempters had had a quarrel with a key person within the past seven days, most within the past two days. Nearly one-half of the patients had been medical or psychiatric patients within the last year. Teenagers, especially, had a higher percentage of separation from a key person in the days preceding the suicide attempt. Unfortunately, Bancroft included no control group, so that base rates of these events cannot be determined.

A study of 257 patients with self-poisoning referred from medical services to a psychiatric service in Norway (Rygnestad, 1982), found alcohol abuse in nearly 60 percent of males and 24 percent of females. Eighty percent of the patients had a psychiatric disorder, and approximately 60 percent had visited a health professional in the month prior to the suicide attempt. A follow-up of these patients revealed a mortality rate of 168 times the expected value in the year after discharge!

Somewhat different findings were reported by Luscomb and colleagues (1980) in their study of male suicide attempters in a Veterans Administration Hospital compared with nonsuicidal psychiatric patients. They reported that suicide attempters were younger but had similar levels of stress to the controls. Only in the older patients were exit events more prevalent.

Therefore, with the exception of the Luscomb findings in a specialized population, suicide attempters experienced greater stress, especially due to exit events, than did various controls in the period preceding the suicide attempt. Especially prevalent are quarrels and other interpersonal problems. Those with exits and independent events that occur *after* the onset of depression may be at especially high risk.

The findings are similar with regard to early life experience and family background. Adams and colleagues (1982) compared 93 suicide attempters with matched controls in a study of life experience in a sample of consecutive admissions to the accident and emergency department of a hospital in New Zealand. They report a significantly higher prevalence of parental loss among the suicide attempter group, especially due to parental divorce or separation.

Nearly one-half of the group of suicide attempters had lost one or both of their parents early in their lives, as compared with less than one-quarter of the control group. Nearly all of the attempted suicide group came from a family environment rated as unstable or chaotic, as compared with less than one-half of the control subjects.

With regard to current social supports, Slater and Depue (1981) reported that only 40 percent of the serious suicide attempters had confidant support, compared to more than 85 percent of the depressed controls. The overwhelming majority of the nonsuicidal controls who suffered an exit event had a confidant, while the suicide attempter group contained a large number of people who had recently lost their confidant. Thus, the presence of a confidant may play a crucial role in mediating against a suicide attempt.

Rygnestad (1982) reported that fewer than one-half of the suicidal females and only one-quarter of the suicidal males were married. Significantly higher rates of divorce, separation, and widowhood were reported among both men and women than expected from general population figures.

The literature regarding personality of adult suicide attempters is limited. Luscomb and colleagues (1980) reported no differences in locus of control between attempters and controls. Patsiokas (1978) did find personality differences in essentially the same sample in cognitive rigidity, but not impulsivity. However, these findings are of very limited generalizability due to the narrowness of the sample and many methodologic problems in the study.

Completed Suicide

Completed suicide in an adult population has been studied from several vantages (see Table 8), including long-term prospective epidemiologic studies, prospective studies of psychiatric patients, and retrospective investigations of patients who have committed suicide. In general, these studies of completed suicides show a preponderance of men, an increased prevalence among people living alone, those having a physical illness, the unemployed, and those with a previous psychiatric history (particularly affective disorders and alcoholism). Patients who commit suicide are likely to have made prior attempts compared with nonsuicidal populations. Whether alcoholism or physical disorder is a risk factor is controversial (Roy, 1982), as is the importance of parental loss during childhood (Tennant, 1980).

Table 8. Completed Suicide in Adults: Psychosocial Factors

Study	Sample	Attribute	Findings
Evenson et al., 1982	207 white suicides in Missouri during 1972–1974.	Sociodemographic variables and psychiatric history	Males had a higher suicide rate than females. A history of psychiatric treatment increased the suicide risk for women. Age-adjusted rates within each sex is highest for those with a diagnosis of major affective disorder.
Borg and Stahl, 1982	2 inpatients and 184 outpatients treated at a psychiatric hospital in Linkoping, Sweden in 1976.	Life stress, sociodemographic variables	Suicides had a higher incidence of being widowed, abusing drugs and alcohol, and having neurotic or depressive symptoms than controls. Previous suicide attempters and loss of key persons by death occurred more frequently among the suicides but was not statistically significant.
Dorpat and Ripley, 1960	114 consecutive suicides in Seattle between 7/1/57–7/1/58 obtained from county coroner. Data obtained from public agencies.	Life events, psychiatric and medical history	Suicide was often a deliberate act, and intent was usually communicated. One-third had made prior attempts. M:F suicide completers was 2:1. Loss of a significant relationship with a prolonged grief reaction was found in many cases. 51% had a serious medical illness that contributed to the suicide. Most common psychiatric diagnosis: depressive illness—28%; alcoholism—26%; schizophrenia—11%; personality disorders—9%. 22% had seen a psychiatrist, and 87% had seen a physician in the previous year.

Barraclough et al., 1974	Retrospective study of 100 suicides obtained from coroner's records. Data obtained from interviews with surviving relatives.	Life events, psychiatric and medical history	93% were diagnosed as having a psychiatric disorder; 70%—depressive illness; 15%—alcoholism. 80% were seeing a doctor and were given psychotropic drugs. 25% were seeing a psychiatrist. 50% had previous psychiatric histories. Between 50–60% made a previous suicide attempt. Over 50% had expressed suicidal intent. Social stresses (especially interpersonal) increased risk of suicide for depressed and alcoholic subjects.
Robins et al., 1959	134 consecutive suicides during 1956–1957 in St. Louis, based on coroner reports. Data obtained from interviews with family, physicians, friends and others after the suicide.	History of psychiatric and physical illness; sociodemographic variables.	98% of sample were clinically ill. 94% had a psychiatric disorder. 47% had an affective disorder, depressed phase; 25% suffered from alcoholism, 73% had seen physicians/ psychiatrists in the last year of life. Over 70% of depressives and alcoholics communicated their suicidal intent. Factors other than diagnosis that increased risk for successful suicide: increasing age, being male, being white, and having a physical illness.

However, three studies of completed suicides with more than 100 cases conducted over a 10-year period (Dorpat, 1960; Barraclough, 1974) clearly demonstrated that depressive illness and alcoholism were the predominant diagnoses in approximately 70 percent of the cases associated with completed suicide, and that a significant percentage of the sample had a physical illness at the time of death. Dorpat (1960), in a retrospective study of 114 consecutive suicides in Seattle over a one-year period from 1957 to 1958, analyzed data obtained from public agencies and the county coroner's office. A questionnaire was completed by the interviewers on each case eliciting information about social background, drinking history, medical and psychiatric history, and questions on the circumstances of the suicidal act. Sixty-six percent of the suicides were committed by men. The mean age of the men was 52.4 years, and the mean age of the women was 48.9 years. There was a high percentage of unmarried individuals who had committed suicide in the sample. Eighty-three percent of the subjects in this study indicated their suicidal intent in some manner. Approximately 33 percent had made previous suicide attempts, and all patients in this study were found to have a psychiatric illness. The most common psychiatric diagnoses were depressive illness in 28 percent of the cases, alcoholism in 26 percent of the cases, schizophrenia in 11 percent of the cases, and personality disorders in nine percent of the cases. Twenty-seven percent of those who had completed suicides had experienced the recent loss of a loved person (by death, separation, or divorce) in the year prior to their suicide. A significant number had one or more serious physical diseases at the time, or one year prior to the suicide. Eleven percent of the cases had had major surgery in the year preceding their death. In 51 percent of the group (the group suffering a physical illness), it was felt that their medical or surgical illness contributed in some way to their suicide. Like other studies, this investigation showed that a majority of the subjects who commit suicide have been under the care of a physician. Twenty-two percent had seen a psychiatrist, and 87 percent had seen a nonpsychiatric physician in the year prior to their suicide.

Barraclough (1974) investigated retrospectively 100 cases of suicide by interviewing surviving relatives. A questionnaire was used by the interviewers. To insure uniformity of coding, the three interviewers reviewed jointly each case record, item by item, when it was completed. The study design involved achieving high interrater reliability as well as high interpsychiatrist agreement in psychiatric diagnosis.

A high number of the suicides in this study were men in the older age groups and women over 65. The sociodemographic characteristics of the sample resembled the national suicide statistics in England. Therefore, the authors believed the cases were representative of suicides in their country. Ninety-three percent of the sample were diagnosed as having a psychiatric disorder. Seventy percent had a depressive illness, and 15 percent suffered from alcoholism. Social stresses (especially interpersonal) increased the risk of suicide for depressed and alcoholic subjects. A history of attempted suicide was eight times more frequent than in a sample of living depressives. More than 50 percent of the subjects had expressed suicidal intent, and nearly 60 percent had made a previous suicide attempt. Eighty percent of the cases were seeing a doctor and had been given psychotropic drugs prior to the suicide. Twenty-five percent of the sample were seeing a psychiatrist, and one-half had seen the psychiatrist one week before the suicide.

The study by Robins and colleagues (1959) examined consecutive suicides in St. Louis over a one-year period from 1956 through 1957 using coroner reports and data obtained from interviews with family, physicians, and friends after the suicide. Diagnoses were made by two psychiatrists who reviewed the records independently. Ninety-eight percent of the sample were clinically ill, with 94 percent having psychiatric disorders. Of these, 47 percent had an affective disorder, and 25 percent suffered from alcoholism. Sixty-two percent of those with affective disorder and alcoholism had medical and psychiatric care for their illness within one year of their suicide. More than 70 percent of this group had communicated their suicidal intent in some way.

Hagnell and colleagues (1980) investigated 28 persons who committed suicide during a 25-year prospective study of over 3,500 persons in Sweden. The suicide group was compared with two groups drawn from the same population: age- and sex-matched normal groups, and a sex-matched group of individuals who died of nonviolent causes at the same age as the corresponding suicide victims. The suicide group, which was overwhelmingly male (23/5), had in the week prior to the suicide experienced humiliating situations, object loss situations, and acute psychiatric illness. The humiliating situations included having been discovered at illegal activity, being fired from work for drinking, and being turned down

for training. Object loss included marital or interpersonal separations and loss of a family firm. An acute change in behavior occurred
in nearly one-half of the subjects, especially among those who had
had a history of mental illness. The suicide group was also characterized by presence of long-term social and occupational stresses
leading to a general personal deterioration. Previous suicide attempts were common in the suicide group. The one finding that
may be relevant to personality is that nearly one-quarter of those
who committed suicide had a history of aggressive behavior, including actual or threatened assaults, as compared with less than
two percent of the normal group.

In another prospective study of 2,000 Swedish psychiatric inpatients and outpatients, Borg and Stahl (1982) identified 34 patients
who had committed suicide in a one- to two-year period. This rate
was four to five times higher than expected in a general population,
and included a predominance of males. A control group of psychiatric patients was selected, matched for age, sex, diagnosis, and
in/outpatient status. The suicide group had a significantly higher
prevalence of being unmarried, living alone, and history of substance abuse or neurotic character. In terms of life events, they
found a significantly higher proportion of loss of key persons by
death (not by divorce or other causes) in the suicide group, although
the time period was not specified. It is difficult to interpret the
significance of these life event findings because of the lack of a
specified time period. There were no differences in employment
or social isolation between the two groups.

Roy (1982) identified 90 patients who had committed suicide
in a one-year period who had been psychiatric patients at the Clark
Institute in Toronto. He matched them with the next consecutive
patient meeting age and sex criteria at the hospital. His findings
were similar, but not identical to, those of Borg and colleagues. He
found a prevalence of men whose mean age was nearly a decade
younger than the women. Eighty-five percent were unmarried, and
more than one-half lived alone. A difference in unemployment was
significant only for the male suicide completers. In terms of background variables there was a modest increase (42 versus 31 percent)
in the prevalence of parental loss prior to age 17 in the suicide
group as compared with the controls. The suicide group had a
higher history of psychiatric illness, especially affective illness. Interestingly, drug and alcohol abuse did not differ between the groups.
Nearly one-half of the suicide group had made a prior suicide

attempt. Roy concluded that risk factors for completed suicide in adults include "depression, past suicide attempts, chronic psychiatric disorder, recent admission, living alone, being unemployed, unmarried, and vulnerable to depression."

In summary, these studies demonstrate that the psychosocial risk factors for completed suicide in adult populations are a history of psychiatric illness (particularly affective disorder and alcoholism), the presence of physical illness at the time of death or one year prior to the suicide, a history of previous suicide attempts, an increased number of negative life events or object loss, and poor social supports (including living alone and lacking an intimate social confidant). Limited data on personality exist, although there is a suggestion that aggressive behavior, including threatened or actual assault, is associated with increased risk of completed suicide.

Discussion

This chapter has examined ways in which personality, life events, and other psychosocial factors are associated with—and whether they differentially predict—adolescent depressive syndrome, suicide attempts, and completed suicides. Similar comparisons with adults have been made in order to ascertain whether there were distinctive adolescent phenomena. It has become apparent that this goal cannot be fully achieved for several reasons.

First, has been the paucity of studies of depression and suicide in adolescents that examined personality and other psychosocial factors. Most of the literature has dealt with the existence of depression in younger age groups. A large part of the reason for this has been that the syndrome itself has been controversial until quite recently. Other nosological problems in the literature include multiple definitions of suicide, the combining in samples of suicide ideators, attempters, and completers, and the lack of a standardized typology of suicides.

The second issue is that the samples of adolescents and adults are not comparable. Adult samples tend to be drawn from epidemiological population surveys, or from inpatient or outpatient clinical psychiatric facilities. Many of the studies of adolescents and young adults utilize normal college students in psychology classes, or recruited subjects in other ways. College students are hardly representative of the population at large, and their life experience is quite unique. Furthermore, in most of these samples, the threshold for depression is significantly below that which would be considered depressed, often even mildly depressed, in other studies. There is no standardization of age boundaries in the literature. Problematically, many studies combine samples with children, adolescents, and young adults. We know that these groups are quite distinct, and therefore the conclusions reached about risk factors for depression and suicide may differ among them. Therefore, comparability across studies in the literature is limited.

A further problem is that studies with college students include intercorrelations among various self-reports, personality measures, performance tests, and self-report depression measures. Therefore, any associations discovered are with the *depressive state*. It has been shown (Hirschfeld et al., 1982) that assessments of personality performed on an individual who is depressed are significantly influenced by the depressive state. This is hardly surprising, since it has been demonstrated that significant cognitive distortions occur during depression. It cannot be assumed that these disturbances are characteristic of the individual when he or she is not in a depressed state.

The retrospective nature of many of the studies on suicide limits interpretation. This is particularly problematic in the area of suicide because of underreporting, the difficulties inherent in reconstructing a person's life, and the reluctance of relatives to discuss the issue due to stigma and guilt surrounding the suicide. Of course, all information about the individuals must be gained second-hand and, therefore, may be distorted.

Another problem in comparing adults and adolescents is lack of comparability in methods, study design, and generalization. With the exception of locus of control, no single measure crosses categories even within the adolescent groups, and much less so in comparisons of adolescents and adults. This is unfortunate because a number of personality inventories widely used in adult research have versions that are suitable for use with children and adolescents. The most frequently used method has been the use of questionnaires, but issues of reliability and validity rarely have been addressed, nor has the same measure been used in other studies.

The problem is compounded because not only do the measures differ, but the concepts measured differ. Formal psychometric measurement techniques have not been vigorously used in many of the studies.

Finally, the nature of control groups is problematic and the issue of what group constitutes the appropriate control is unanswered in the literature. Some studies compare against normal adolescents, while others use psychiatric controls. Often no control group is used at all.

Conclusion

We have examined personality, life events, and other psychosocial factors in three interrelated phenomena: depressive syndrome, nonfatal suicide attempts, and suicide completions in adolescent and young adult populations, and in adult populations. Our first purpose has been to identify differential risk factors for each phenomenon in the younger population. Our second purpose has been to compare these risk factors between the two age groups in order to examine whether the phenomena differ between them.

In the population of adolescents and young adults, the psychosocial risk factors for depression and nonfatal suicidal behavior appear to be similar, and lie on a continuum. They occur much more frequently in girls than in boys. Life events tend to be negative and undermining of the self; home situations are unsupportive and stressful; a family background of illnesses (especially psychiatric) is prevalent; and individual personality qualities include poor ability to cope with stress. These factors are uniformly worse in individuals who attempt suicide than in those with depression only. In contrast, suicide completers are overwhelmingly boys, tend to be more active, aggressive, and impulsive than either the depressives or the suicide attempters. Also, confrontation with authority for some event (such as poor grades, truancy, or antisocial behavior), with possible subsequent public humiliation, is a more prevalent theme than interpersonal loss among adolescent suicide completers.

The findings in the adult literature are strikingly parallel to those for adolescents and young adults. For adults, depression and suicide attempts have similar psychosocial risk factors, with a severity continuum between them. They occur more frequently in women with negative precipitating life events, especially undesirable interpersonal ones. Depression and suicide occur more frequently in women who are lacking in social supports and who often do not have an intimate confidant. A history of psychiatric and other medical illness is frequent. An impoverished childhood is more likely. Personality findings have been restricted to depression, and include introversion and increased interpersonal dependency. In contrast, suicide completers are nearly exclusively men who are often faced with humiliating situations. They often live alone and have few, if any, social resources. A history of psychiatric and other medical illnesses is common.

A review of adolescent and adult literature in personality, life events, and other psychosocial risk factors for depression and suicide supports a continuum between depression and nonfatal suicide attempts in both age groups. Suicide completers seem to be drawn from different populations in both age groups. All three phenomena appear to have similar risk factors in the two age groups, suggesting that the phenomena themselves do not differ with age.

Future research needs to further clarify what is similar and what is different about personality, life events, and other psychosocial factors in adolescent and adult depression and suicide, integrate the many biological factors in adolescence that have distinct impact on this developmental period (that is, endocrine, neurotransmitters, heredity, menstruation, pregnancy, and abortion), and compare them to the biological factors known to be associated with depression and suicidal behavior in adults.

Finally, research in suicide would benefit from a standardized nosology for suicidal ideation, gestures, attempts, completions, and other self-destructive behaviors. Better reporting of suicides, combined with systematic well controlled studies by investigators examining life events, psychosocial variables, personality, sociodemographic factors, and biological vulnerability, will contribute greatly to our understanding of depression and suicide in adolescents and adults.

References

Adams KS, Boukoms A, Streiner D: Parental loss and family stability in attempted suicide. Arch Gen Psychiatry 39:1081–1085, 1982

Bancroft J, Skrimshire A, Casson J, et al: People who deliberately poison or injure themselves: their problems and their contacts with helping agencies. Psychol Med 7:289–303, 1977

Barraclough B, Bunch J, Nelson B, et al: A hundred cases of suicide: clinical aspects. Br J Psychiatry 125:355–73, 1974

Borg SE, Stahl M: A prospective study of suicides and controls among psychiatric patients. Acta Psychiatr Scand 65:221–232, 1982

Carlson GA, Cantwell DP: Unmasking masked depression in children and adolescents. Am J Psychiatry 137:445–449, 1980

Chiles JA, Miller LM, Cox GB: Depression in an adolescent delinquent population. Arch Gen Psychiatry 37:1179–1184, 1980

Coddington RD: The significance of life events as etiologic factors in the diseases of children, I: a survey of professional workers. J Psychosom Res 16:7–18, 1972

Cohen-Sandler R, Berman A, King R: Life stress and symptomatology: determinants of suicidal behavior. J Am Acad Child Psychiatry 21:178–186, 1982a

Cohen-Sandler R, Berman AL, King RA: A follow-up study of hospitalized suicidal children. J Am Acad Child Psychiatry 21:398–403, 1982b

Dorpat TL, Ripley HS: A study of suicide in the Seattle area. Compr Psychiatry 1:349–359, 1960

Evenson RC, Wood JB, Nuttall EA, et al: Suicide rates among public mental health patients. Acta Psychiatr Scand 66:254–264, 1982

Garfinkel B, Froese A, Hood J: Suicide attempts in children and adolescents. Am J Psychiatry 139:1257–1261, 1982

Goldney RD: Attempted suicide in young females: correlates of lethality. Br J Psychiatry 139:382–390, 1981a

Goldney RD: Parental loss and reported childhood stress in young women who attempted suicide. Acta Psychiatr Scand 64:34–59, 1981b

Goldney RD: Are young women who attempt suicide hysterical? Br J Psychiatry 138:141–146, 1981c

Goldney RD: Locus of control in young women who have attempted suicide. J Nerv Ment Dis 170:198, 1982

Hagnell O, Rorsman B: Suicide and endogenous depression with somatic symptoms in the Lundby study. Neuropsychobiology 4:180–187, 1978

Hagnell O, Rorsman B: Suicide in the Lundby study: a controlled prospective investigation of stressful life events. Neuropsychobiology 6:319–332, 1980

Hammen CL, Cochran SD: Cognitive correlates of life stress and depression in college students. J Abnorm Psychol 90:23–27, 1981

Hawton K, Cole D, O'Grady J, et al: Motivational aspects of deliberate self-poisoning. Br J Psychiatry 141:286–291, 1982a

Hawton K, O'Grady J, Osborne M, et al: Adolescents who take overdoses:

their characteristics, problems, and contacts with helping agencies. Br J Psychiatry 140:118–123, 1982b

Hawton K, Osborne M, O'Grady J, et al: Classification of adolescents who take overdoses. Br J Psychiatry 140:124–131, 1982c

Henderson AS, Hartigan J, Davidson J, et al: A typology of suicide. Br J Psychiatry 131:631–641, 1977

Hirschfeld RMA, Cross CK: Epidemiology of affective disorders: psychosocial risk factors. Arch Gen Psychiatry 39:35–46, 1982

Hirschfeld RMA, Cross CK: Personality, life events, and social factors in depression, in Psychiatry Update: The American Psychiatric Association Annual Review, vol. 2. Edited by Grinspoon L. Washington DC, American Psychiatric Press, 1983

Ilfeld FW: Current social stressors and symptoms of depression. Am J Psychiatry 134:161–166, 1977

Inamadar S, Lewis D, Siomopoulos G, et al: Violent and suicidal behavior in psychotic adolescents. Am J Psychiatry 139:932–935, 1982

Johnson JE, Petzel TP, Dupont MP, et al: Phenomenological perceptions of parental evaluation in depressed and non-depressed college students. J Clin Psychol 33:56–62, 1982

Kandel DB, Davies M: Epidemiology of depressive mood in adolescents: an empirical study. Arch Gen Psychiatry 39:1205–1212, 1982

Kovacs M, Beck AT: An empirical approach towards a definition of childhood depression, in Depression in Childhood: Diagnosis, Treatment and Conceptual Models. Edited by Schulterbrandt JC, Raskin A. New York, Raven Press, 1977

Kumchy CIG: The CIP battery: identification of depression in a juvenile delinquent population. J Clin Psychol 37:880–884, 1981

Luscomb RL, Clum GA, Patsiokas AM: Mediating factors in the relationship between life stress and suicide attempting. J Nerv Ment Dis 168:664–650, 1980

Marks PA, Haller DL: Now I lay me down for keeps: a study of adolescent suicide attempts. J Clin Psychol 33:390–400, 1977

Patsiokas AT, Clum GA, Luscomb RL: Cognitive characteristics of suicide attempters. J Consult Clin Psychol 47:478–484, 1979

Paykel ES, Prusoff BA, Myers JK: Suicide attempts and recent life events: a controlled comparison. Arch Gen Psychiatry 32:327–333, 1975

Peterson C: Uncontrollability and self-blame in depression: investigation of the paradox in a college population. J Abnorm Psychol 88:620–624, 1979

Petzel SV, Riddle M: Adolescent suicide: psychosocial and cognitive aspects. Adolescent Psychiatry 9:343–398, 1981

Robins E, Murphy GE, Wilkinson RH, et al: Some clinical considerations in the prevention of suicide based on a study of 134 successful suicides. Am J Public Health 49:888–899, 1959

Roy A: Risk factors for suicide in psychiatric patients. Arch Gen Psychiatry 39:1089–1095, 1982

Rygnestad TK: A prospective study of social and psychiatric aspects in self-poisoned patients. Acta Psychiatr Scand 66:139–153, 1982

Shaffer D: Suicide in childhood and early adolescence. J Child Psychol Psychiatry 15:275–291, 1974

Shaffer D, Fisher P: The epidemiology of suicide in children and adolescents. J Am Acad Child Psychiatry 20:545–565, 1981

Slater J, Depue RA: The contribution of environmental events and social support to serious suicide attempts in primary depressive disorder. J Abnorm Psychol 40:275–285, 1981

Tennant C, Bebbington P, Hurry J: Parental death in childhood and risk of adult depressive disorder: a review. Psychol Med 10:289–299, 1980

Tishler CT, McHenry PC, Morgan KC: Adolescent suicide attempts: some significant factors. Suicide and Life Threatening Behavior 11:86–92, 1981

Toolan JM: Depression and suicide in children: an overview. Am J Psychother 35:311–322, 1981

Chapter 10

WELL-BEING IN ADOLESCENCE: PAST AND PRESENT

Pamela J. Perun, Ph.D.
Sumru Erkut, Ph.D.

Chapter 10

WELL-BEING IN ADOLESCENCE:
PAST AND PRESENT

It has become increasingly clear to developmental researchers in recent years that our ability to comprehend the course of human lives will always be limited. We realized earlier in this century that our understanding of developmental processes in individual lives was necessarily relative; that is, relative in regard to such individual attributes as class, gender, and race. But we have just begun to see that fundamental processes of social organization and historical change impinge upon individual lives. A principle of relativity therefore applies to developmental research, because there is little we can know absolutely about human lives. While there is also much we can learn about human life relative to the time and place in which a life is lived, we must always be careful to recognize the limits of that knowledge. It is with this understanding—that our knowledge of human lives is relative to time and place—that we approach the study of adolescence.

Of all periods of life, adolescence is perhaps the one most subject to the vicissitudes of social and historical change. Its designation as the time of transition between the major life stages of childhood and adulthood makes adolescence particularly vulnerable to redefinition. As cultural ideas change about the nature of either childhood or adulthood or both, the meaning of adolescence in the life course correspondingly changes. It can be argued, then,

Research for this work was supported by Grant HL–0742–7 from the National Heart, Lung, and Blood Institute to Harvard Medical School.

that adolescence is one of the most flexible of developmental periods. The definition of what constitutes psychological well-being
in adolescence is also subject to redefinition. Our thesis is that
understanding the structure and content of well-being, necessary
for the formulation of any preventive strategies for improving adolescent mental health, requires careful examination of the historical and sociocultural context of the adolescent experience.

In this chapter we demonstrate, first, that the period designated
as adolescence in the life course is a social construction whose
significance and duration varies over historical time and across
cultures. Second, we demonstrate that well-being in adolescence is
to be understood in the context of the timing of events in individual
lives, and relative to sociohistorical changes in the social construction of adolescence. Thus, we take issue with contemporary stage
theories of adolescence (such as Erikson's), in which a defined
series and sequence of events is designated as normative. However,
our rejection of contemporary stage theories of adolescence should
not be understood to mean that we see no utility in describing
specific components of development in terms of hierarchical models within well-defined sociohistorical contexts. Rather, we are per-
suaded of the utility of conceptions of the life course that organize
developmental processes by time rather than by stage (Perun and
Bielby, 1979, 1980; Rossi, 1980). In this chapter, we hope to demonstrate the way that this alternative model of development illu-
minates critical aspects of adolescence not otherwise visible in stage
theories.

The Social Construction of Adolescence

The term adolescence is derived from the Latin "adolescere," meaning "to become an adult," and signifies the period of transition
between childhood and adulthood. As conceptions of adulthood
differ cross-culturally and are subject to change over time, the prevailing social definition of adolescence is also subject to change.
Indeed, whether adolescence has always been recognized as a distinct period of human development is questionable. In the United
States, adolescence as a social status and as a developmental period
emerged in recent times as a consequence of economic and societal
change. Demos and Demos (1969) have argued convincingly that
adolescence became recognized in the United States as a stage of

life in the 1800s, as a consequence of urbanization following the Industrial Revolution. Before the 1890s—that is, before G. Stanley Hall's work stimulated scientific interest in the period now known as adolescence—the term "youth" was used to indicate the years from the middle teens to the middle twenties. The normative content of those years, however, remained undefined (Kett, 1971). By 1870, the chronological ages associated with youth had been narrowed to the ages of 14 through 19, and the meaning of youth had acquired psychological as well as social connotations (Kett, 1971).

As the relatively undefined stage of youth became transformed into the scientifically grounded stage of adolescence, unwarranted assumptions about the universality and normative nature of adolescent behavior were made. The primary fallacy was the assumption that puberty and adolescence are mutually inclusive, with the onset of puberty marking the onset of adolescence. While all known cultures recognize puberty as a transitional marker between childhood and adulthood, not all cultures either have or similarly define a stage of life called adolescence. For example, Kett (1971) notes that in mid-19th-century America, puberty and youth were assigned differential meanings relative to gender:

> Girls were not really viewed as having, like boys, a period of youth ... girls were seen as experiencing a wrenching [physical] adolescence between fourteen and sixteen, but not as having a stage of youth; boys went through a relatively painless physical adolescence, but followed it with a critical period of youth. (Kett, p. 296)

Hence, current theorists of human development, still influenced by Hall's emphasis on puberty and Freudian notions of the biological "sturm and drang" of adolescence, have erred in concluding that adolescence, like puberty, is a universal phenomenon.

When adolescence is viewed as a social status as well as a developmental period—as we believe it should be—and puberty is seen merely as its biological concomitant or precursor, the distinction between the two terms becomes clearer. But even this distinction may promise greater conceptual clarity than it can really achieve because the secular trend in the onset of puberty has not always been synchronous with the period socially understood to be adolescence. Tanner (1968) reports that the average age of menarche, which is itself a relatively late event within the sequence of biological changes constituting puberty, has decreased in Western societies over the last century. For example, statistics show the average age of menarche in Norway dropping from about 17 years of age in 1840 to about 13.5 years of age in 1950. In the United States, the average age at menarche was over 14 years of age at the turn of the century, but under 13 years of age by the mid-1950s. Today the average age of menarche in the United States is considered to be 12.8 years (MacMahon, 1973; Garn, 1980). Schonfeld (1969) reports that for 80 percent of American girls, pubertal development (from the onset of pigmented pubic hair through menarche to the formation of "primary" breasts) takes place between the ages of 10 and 16. In boys' pubertal development, the first ejaculation is not as dramatic a change as first menses is for girls. Therefore, its first appearance has not been studied as carefully as menarche. There is some evidence that, like menarche, first ejaculation is occurring at earlier ages (Eskin, 1977).

Today, adolescence is usually associated with the years from ages 12 to 22, indicating that puberty for a substantial proportion of girls precedes rather than initiates adolescence. Whereas students of adolescence are understandably reluctant to provide exact ages for the beginning and end of adolescence, the age range of 12 to 22 appears to be the one most often associated with the period today. An influential collection of essays (Kagan and Coles, 1972), subtitled "Early Adolescence," had *12 to 16* as its main title, anchoring the onset of adolescence at the age of 12. Since there is a general agreement that college students make up the late adolescent group (witness their use as subjects in studies of late adolescence in the leading journals in the field), we conclude that contemporary adolescence is considered to end at approximately age 22. The 12 to 22 age range is, of course, intended to be a descriptive rather than a normative designation. Hence, an element of relativity applies to even the relationship between puberty and adolescence.

Given that puberty and adolescence are distinct phenomena, we must next consider how adolescence should be defined in order to distinguish its relatively invariant components from those more responsive to sociocultural and historical conditions. Our focus, therefore, must shift from the transition from childhood into adolescence, to the transition from adolescence into adulthood. There, the critical issues are not so much the universality of the phenomenon or its definition, but the ways in which the timing and sequencing of life events in adulthood have changed in the last 100 years. While we do not yet have a complete picture of the ways in which social and historical change in the U.S. have altered the structure and content of adult lives, the recent interest in the transition to adulthood in history, demography, and sociology, does provide evidence of some long-term trends whose developmental consequences we will discuss.

If we take as the period of analysis the late 19th century to the present, the time during which our contemporary views on adolescence were formed and transformed, two phenomena are immediately of interest. The first of these is the empirical finding that during this period, the variance in life structures—defined as typical life events—and the timing of their occurrence, has been considerably reduced. That is, the lives of individuals have become more alike over time, although sex differences in life structures have persisted. Uhlenberg (1969) has analyzed data from both state and federal census sources in a study of cohort life cycles in native-born Massachusetts women from 1830 to 1920. He found an increased prevalence over time in the proportion of women experiencing the "typical" life cycle of marriage, children, and survival until the marriage of the last child. Only one in five women in the 1830 birth cohort followed the typical life course, but nearly three times as many women in the 1920 birth cohort followed this typical life course (Uhlenberg, 1969). This finding was later replicated by Uhlenberg (1974) in an analysis of U.S. Census birth cohort data from 1890 to 1935. Among black women, the proportion experiencing the typical family life cycle was far below that of white women, although both groups exhibited the same trend toward greater conformity in life structures. Confirmatory evidence of these changes in both women's and men's lives has been presented by Modell and colleagues (1976) in an analysis of 1880 Philadelphia data, other 19th-century census figures, and 1970 U.S. Census data. They note:

> The early life course today is to an important degree organized differently, with different consequences for youth. Our qualitative evidence expands and defines Kett's argument that the broad latitude of choice that characterized growing up in the nineteenth century has been replaced today by a more prescribed and tightly defined schedule of life-course organization ... (Modell et al., p. 27).

In addition to the increased uniformity in the typical events occurring during this period, there is also evidence of an increased age congruity in the experience of life events. The classic studies of Glick (1955, 1977; Glick and Norton, 1977) and recent Census data (U.S. Bureau of the Census, 1982) demonstrate that since the late 1800s, the median age at marriage has decreased for both men and women. For example, in 1890 the median age at marriage was 22 years for women and 26.1 years for men (Glick, 1955). By 1962, the median age at marriage was 20.3 years for women and 22.7 years for men (U.S. Bureau of Census, 1982). As the age at marriage fell, so generally did the average age of mothers at the birth of the first and the last child (Glick, 1977). Modell and colleagues (1976) characterized these changes as an acceleration in the pace of transitions from adolescence to adulthood. The period of time during which a birth cohort completes such transitions as finishing schooling, entering the labor force, and marrying, has been shortened over time. They report: "For males, the period (elapsed between the time the first quintile left school or entered the work force and the last quintile became head of a household) was reduced by a third, taking 21.7 years in 1880 but only 14.4 years in 1970" (Modell et al., p. 203).

The same trend is apparent in women's lives. Perun and Giele (1979, 1982), in a study of the life histories of the graduates of a Massachusetts women's college, show that the average age at marriage dropped markedly in the classes that graduated between 1911 and 1960. Among women who graduated between 1911 and 1915, the mean age at marriage (ever-married women) was 30; but for the women who graduated between 1951 and 1955, the mean age at marriage was 23 (Perun and Giele, 1982). During an era when the proportion of women marrying in subsequent classes was linearly increasing, the mean age at marriage was similarly decreasing. The trend in postgraduate education for these women replicates in important respects the marital data. Among the earliest classes, a bimodal age distribution was exhibited in regard to graduate training. In the classes that graduated in the 1910s, 33 percent had attended graduate school within five years of the B.A., but another 25 percent attended 20 years later. Similar distributions are found in the classes of the 1920s and 1930s. But beginning with the classes of the 1940s and continuing with the classes of the 1950s, attendance at graduate school became concentrated between the ages of 22 and 27 (Perun and Giele, 1979). The trends apparent in the lives of these women, of course, are confounded by secular trends in the numbers and types of women who attended college. Prior to the 1940s, a college education was largely reserved for the privileged; since then a college education has become available to others by virtue of aptitude rather than by class, race, or gender characteristics. Nevertheless, given the paucity of data on women's lives, these descriptive statistics do indicate changes in the structure of women's lives across many generations that parallel those in men's lives.

Looking back over the period from the late 19th century to the present, then, we have assembled evidence of two important changes that span many generations in the late adolescent period. First, we have shown that over time the lives of individuals have become more alike in regards to the timing and sequencing of the life events that encompass the transition to adulthood. Second, we have shown that until the 1950s, an acceleration in the timing of life events has occurred with the result that many important transitional events in the areas of work, education, and family became normatively associated with the early twenties. Hence, there is documentation that a long-term historical process has been at work whereby both the range of developmental tasks prescribed for individuals in late adolescence, and the time by which they are to accomplish them, have been markedly narrowed.

These changes in individual lives that were largely induced by processes of social and historical change appear to have been uniform in nature. If we had been writing this paper 25 years ago, it would have been appropriate for us to point out how linear, and therefore how irreversible, these changes appear to be. But because we are writing this paper in the 1980s, we have far different observations to make. From the available evidence, which admittedly is only tentative at this point, it appears that the trends we cited earlier came to an abrupt halt with the birth cohort of 1935–1939, which came of age in the late 1950s. Census figures indicate that the end point in the trend of earlier ages at marriage occurred in 1955, when 25 percent of the women (then mostly teenagers) born in the 1935–1939 cohort had been married. Comparison figures show that for women born in the 1950–1954 cohort, only 17 percent had been married in their teenage years (U.S. Bureau of the Census, 1972). Similar trends are evident in regard to the age of women at birth of their first child. In 1975, the 1950–1954 cohort had just completed their teenage years, with the lowest levels of fertility of any cohort of women born after 1930. In contrast, women born between 1935 and 1944 had much higher rates of teenage childbearing (U.S. Bureau of the Census, 1978).

Even this trend of delayed childbearing involves an element of relativity. The trend is associated with greater affluence, education, and employment outside the home, which were on the rise in the period discussed. Poor women with less education and no outside employment, or lower occupational status, continued to have earlier first birth and higher completed fertility (Presser, 1971). Indeed, in this same period there has been a decrease in the average age of women bearing an illegitimate child (U.S. Bureau of the Census, 1978). It has been widely documented that this increase in teenage motherhood is associated with low socioeconomic status and race, which then result in truncated educational and occupational opportunities (McKenry et al., 1979).

In the late 1970s, the reverse in trends present earlier in the century continued. From 1970–1981, the median age at first marriage increased from 23.2 years to 24.8 years for men, and from 20.8 years to 22.3 years for women. In addition, the proportion of never-married men and women was decreasing, with 22 percent never-married women aged 25 to 29 in 1981, as compared with only 11 percent in 1970 (U.S. Bureau of the Census, 1982). All of these trends support our basic contention that adolescence, the period of transition from childhood to adulthood, has not remained constant, but has been both shortened and lengthened—in other words, altered—in response to social and historical process of change.

Adolescence and Psychological Well-Being: The Myth and the Reality

Until recently, the notion that adolescence is a stormy period has dominated our understanding of adolescent psychological well-being. This view was promulgated primarily by researchers working in the psychoanalytic tradition. The internal and external conflicts viewed as normative for adolescents within the psychoanalytic tradition are seen to be derived not from the everyday trials of adolescence, but from the reactivation of childhood conflicts. Adolescence, in general, and early adolescence, in particular, has therefore been viewed primarily as a period of regressive change with the major developmental task defined as the recapitulation of childhood issues, rather than the mastery of new, more mature behaviors. Within this school of thought the road to becoming an adult is viewed as taking a detour into childhood. Hence the expectation that adolescents will throw tantrums, be irrational, and behave in otherwise "child-ish" ways (Blos, 1962; Freud, 1958; Josselyn, 1952; Wittenberg, 1955). The unleashing of sexual drives in puberty was seen to coincide with a resurgence of the oedipal feelings, this time with a mature biological capacity to engage in an incestuous relationship. The adolescent was seen to be preoccupied with repudiating all ego ties to the parents in order to ward off unacceptable oedipal impulses. Josselson (1980), in her discussion of this earlier view of adoles-cence, adds that the adolescent's

... ego, besieged by drives and unable to rely on the now-dangerous parental ego for support, was seen to be in "turmoil," shifting un-predictably from one state to another. Turbulence, maladjustment, even psychoticlike states were described as normal (even necessary) aspects of adolescent development. (Josselson, p. 188)

By virtue of their developmental status, adolescents were sup-posed to be experiencing turmoil that greatly strained relationships with their parents. Hence, the notion of discontinuity with parents, or in popular terms a "generation gap," has often accompanied the storm and stress view of adolescent development, placing the locus of the storm squarely between adolescents and their parents (Cole-man, 1978).

Growing empirical evidence from large sample studies that have utilized nonclinically identified populations contradict the stormy view of adolescence. In particular, the notion that adolescents are preoccupied with repudiating their parents has been discredited (Bandura, 1972; Douvan and Adelson, 1966; Offer and Offer, 1975; Offer et al., 1981). This raises the possibility that the turmoil view of adolescent development may have been inspired more by the-oretical perspectives based on clinical studies of disturbed adoles-cents, than by an examination of adolescent development in the general population. Hence, "normal" adolescent development and well-being have not yet been adequately established, theoretically or empirically.

The emerging view of adolescence from large scale empirical studies is one of much greater continuity and harmony with parents than was previously supposed. The disagreements between parents and adolescents involve not major values or aspirations, but such matters of style as personal appearance, choice and volume of music, leisure activities, and dating (Brittain, 1963, 1966; Coleman et al.,

1977; Douvan and Adelson, 1966). It appears, further, that psycho-pathology is not a "natural" concomitant of adolescent development. The incidence of psychiatric disturbance is only slightly higher in adolescence than in middle childhood (Rutter et al., 1976). More-over, disturbances and symptoms found among adolescents are not necessarily outgrown by the end of that period, but continue into adulthood (Masterson, 1967a, 1967b). This further contradicts the view that adolescent turmoil is a function of being in that social status.

All of this is not to suggest that adolescence is a balmy period, totally devoid of stress. During early adolescence especially, the magnitude of physiological, anatomical, and cognitive change is surpassed only by the rapid growth period in fetal development and the first two years of life following birth (Tanner, 1972). At a time when they are attempting to adjust to their changing bodies, adolescents are initiated into a new set of social roles and their accompanying expectations of behavior. These biological and social status changes inevitably produce stress (Hamburg, 1980). Indeed, in a large scale study of 14-year-olds on the Isle of Wight, Rutter and his colleagues (1976) found that although the incidence of psychiatric disturbance was quite low, as many as 45 percent of the adolescents reported feelings of misery and uncertainty. Curiously, in most cases these feelings had not been recognized by parents or teachers who were also interviewed in this study.

An unpublished smaller scale study conducted in 1983 by Erkut of autobiographical accounts of adolescent development among 30 college students from a women's college in Massachusetts, lends further credence to the view that while adolescence is not a painless period, only rarely does the internal turmoil felt by the adolescent unduly strain relationships with parents or manifest itself in overt maladjustment. Our use of the term maladjustment relies heavily upon Weiner's (1980) sixfold eclectic classification of traditional diagnoses of psychopathology and categories of problem behavior: schizophrenia, depression, suicidal behavior, problems of school attendance, problems of school achievement, and delinquent be-havior. Erkut found that among the 30 women interviewed, 28 re-ported feeling confused, miserable, lacking in self-confidence, or unhappy at least some of the time during their adolescence. Typical were comments such as the following excerpts from three different cases:

My earlier adolescence was characterized by periods of confusion, of stress, and of unhappinesss ... from the time I was in the sixth grade until the end of eighth grade was my conformist stage. During this stage I had no mind of my own. My thoughts and feelings were regulated by my peer group ... I never had enough confidence, or felt secure enough about myself as a person to deviate from the norm created by my peers.

When I became fifteen, I felt my pain had started. ... The nature of my pain was unclear to my young heart, but I just knew it had started. ... Everything had its own place. Yet, as far as I was concerned, I felt as if I was floating around. I could instinctively feel that there was so much possibility and also ambiguity about my future. The world suddenly looked so large and complicated. I felt like I was a helpless baby thrown into the universe. Everything was working in order, and it was my own responsibility to find and secure my place there. I did not know where to start. That was the start of my pain.

... junior high school seemed huge, alien, and full of people who were not like me, and who scared me. The girls were socially and physically much more advanced than I, and because I felt so different I had nothing to say to them. ... I became very quiet, less social, and more studious than I had ever been, because studying was both a sure way to please my parents, and save myself the chance of being rejected. ... There was a rowdy, popular crowd which was still beyond my naive, immature capacity, and yet I was desperate to be a part. The kids who smoked in the bathrooms were tough talking, tough acting kids who terrified me. There were many days when I would not go to the bathroom because I was so afraid that some secret smoker would tackle me—often I would go home with a terrible stomach ache. I would never tell anyone my fears, and although my parents were aware that I was unhappy, I was afraid they would get upset with the school if I explained.

As these cases illustrate, feelings of internal turmoil of varying magnitudes were reported to accompany the vast majority of the young women's adolescent development in the study. However, only five women reported significant psychological disturbances that had come to the attention of parents, schools, and/or psychotherapists. Two of these were cases of substance abuse, two were eating disorders, and one was a suicide attempt following rape. One case of sexual abuse and three eating disorders had been experienced without treatment, and perhaps without having been noticed by others. The case of the young woman who suffered through sexual abuse as a child is an example of trauma experienced well into adolescence, without the victim telling others who could do something about it, and without others noticing it.

> ... I was caught red-handed under the house, which was expressly forbidden. Luckily it was not Mom who caught me or I know I would have the sorest bottom around. Instead it was one of the boys next door. Kevin was a typical 15-year-old teenage hot-shot. Kevin gave me two alternatives, one—tell Mom, or two—follow him into his secret fort. Again, being the naive and innocent girl I was, I chose the latter. Dumb choice! For the next three to four years I was blackmailed, abused, childmolested or raped, whatever you want to call it. I was always too scared to say anything to anybody, even after his younger brother Toby, who was a year or two younger than Kevin, caught us and also took advantage of me after being talked out of telling on Kevin by Kevin. So I started my preadolescence confused, hurt, and very scared, scared to be caught, scared to be in my neighborhood, scared to be in my house, scared to be at friends' houses, because wherever I went I felt as though they knew where I was and if they felt like it I was at their command. ... For many years I never told anybody about it. I kept all my emotions inside me, locked up from those who could find out. Strangely enough it did not affect me with dealing with other kids my age. Actually outside of school, I usually hung around with older kids, but I had always done that before, so on the outside I was your normal "run-of-the-mill" adolescent who showed no resentment against anyone for the past; on the inside I would never forget. ... Today I am as emotionally stable as anyone else my age, if not more. I do not let problems emotionally upset me. I realize these can always work out, at least I like to think so.

The resistance of adolescents to emotional scarring is dramatically illustrated by this last case example. It is also borne out by the study of Rutter and colleagues, already mentioned. The picture that emerges from Rutter's and Erkut's findings is that adolescents have much greater resilience than previously assumed. The misery and pain that may accompany their development rarely leads to overt maladjustment. Thus, psychoanalytic views to the contrary, adolescence is seen here as a period of life with its own legitimate stresses and conflicts, but one with which most individuals are able to cope satisfactorily. Only a minority of adolescents experience the extremes of emotional and behavioral turmoil previously thought to be normative. From this alternative view of adolescent development, then, comes evidence validating the phenomenon of psychological *well*-being during this stage of life.

Well-Being in Contemporary Adolescence

In the previous two sections, we discussed the meaning of adolescence both as a social status and as a development period. In this section, we examine the interaction of these two concepts in order to gain a better understanding of the contemporary adolescence experience. In doing so, we choose to focus on two issues. Because we believe that psychological well-being is an important component of adolescent development, we first suggest the way it evolves in individual lives. Second, we discuss adolescent psychological well-being within the context of recent social and historical changes in the United States.

In light of the many biological and social changes of the adolescent period, it is indeed difficult to trace the course of psychological development. It is important to remember, however, that none of the changes of adolescence appear overnight, or without warning. Whether biological or social in nature, the processes of changes occur over a period of time, and normally with a prescribed sequence of events. In other words, the changes of adolescence, whether biological or sociological in origin, are composed of specific timetables whose duration and sequence are known, although the scheduling of timetables may vary considerably across individuals. Psychological well-being in adolescence, we believe, is a function of the fit of timetables of change in individual lives. While there is no one perfect arrangement of timetables, there are patterns that are more adaptive for psychological development than others. The extent to which an individual achieves an adaptive scheduling of timetables during adolescence in large measure determines his or her psychological well-being over time.

An illustration of the relationship of individual timetables to psychological well-being in adolescence can be found in the work of Coleman (1978). He asks:

> If adolescents have to adjust to so much potentially stressful change, and at the same time pass through this stage of life with relative stability ... how do they do it? The answer ... is that they cope by dealing with one issue at a time. They spread the process of adaptation over a span of years, attempting to resolve first one issue and

then the next. Different problems, different relationship issues, come into focus and are tackled at different stages, so that the stresses resulting from the need to adapt to new modes of behavior are rarely concentrated all at one time. It follows from this hypothesis that those who, for whatever reason, have more than one issue to cope with at a time are most likely to have problems. (Coleman, p. 9)

Coleman's examples of issues that impinge psychological well-being are such concerns as conflict with parents, fears of rejection by peers, and anxiety over heterosexual relationships, which his earlier research (1974) has shown to be experienced at different times by the average adolescent. Coleman's theory of adolescent well-being, in which he attributes maladjustment to an overload of issues occurring simultaneously or in rapid succession, is basically a time-table model for development. That is, he explains adolescent well-being as a consequence of the timing and interaction of psychological issues in individual lives.

As we have posited in the first part of this chapter, however, adolescence defined solely by reference to individual lives fails to capture the multidimensional quality of time. Psychological development at the individual level of analysis (that is, the timing and sequencing of such psychological issues as conflicts with parents, fear of rejection by peers, and the adaptation to new social roles) is, of course, a very important component of the adolescent experience. Yet Coleman's model does not incorporate the equally important but largely overlooked component of *social* timetables, which similarly define and affect psychological well-being in adolescence. For example, we have shown that the period socially defined as adolescence has both expanded and contracted in the last 100 years, and that the social timetable of adolescence has correspondingly changed. As a result, societal expectations of *what it is adolescents are supposed to do and when they are supposed to do it* (for example, going to college; becoming sexually active; getting married) have varied markedly over time. Adolescents' evaluations of their success in meeting those social timetables have similarly varied. There may indeed be eras (or cultures) when social time can be assumed to be constant (that is, unchanging), and where adolescence can therefore be understood solely in relation to individuals' timing and sequencing of psychological issues and social roles. But in the context of contemporary Western societies that exemplify cultures in rapid and continual change, it is clear that the adolescent experience varies markedly for different generations of adolescents. Therefore, adolescent development must be viewed as the product of time-dependent processes of change in individual lives operating within the context of socially imposed deadlines.

An understanding of adolescent development and behavior, which incorporates both individual and social timetables and their interaction, is therefore necessary for predicting which individuals in a given cohort, or which cohorts over time, will experience the greatest levels of stress. Our view is that within a specific cohort, those individuals who are faced with adapting to a multiplicity of issues simultaneously will be the ones to experience the greatest stress. Over time, the cohorts which, by accident of birth, live through important changes in societal expectations of adolescent behavior, will be those most stressed in comparison to other cohorts. In other words, we believe that redefinitions of what it is that adolescents are supposed to do and when they are supposed to do it can account for much of the turmoil traditionally associated with adolescence, both in terms of individual lives and across cohorts.

Our earlier point about the relativity of the adolescent experience to time and place is borne out by recent evidence of significant shifts in adult psychological well-being. Bryant and Veroff (1982), in an analysis of two successive national cross-sectional surveys of subjective mental health in the U.S. (1957 and 1976), present intriguing findings of general stability in the structure of subjective mental health. That is, the same three factors (unhappiness, strain, and personal inadequacy) emerged as major dimensions of subjective evaluation of well-being in both surveys. Confirmatory factor analyses, however, did reveal some important differences in the content of these dimensions over time and between men and women. These analyses suggest that while men 25 years ago defined their well-being primarily in reference to work, and women primarily in reference to family, men and women are becoming more alike in their definitions of well-being. This convergence between the sexes appears to be related to historical changes in sex role definitions between the two survey periods, which have led men to evaluate personal well-being less in terms of their work role and more in terms of their parental role. Women exhibit a parallel trend of smaller magnitude but in the opposite direction.

The generalizability of these reported shifts in the meaning of psychological well-being in adulthood remains untested for adolescents. Nevertheless, they do show that during a period of major social and historical changes, individuals' evaluations of their well-being were altered by shifts in societal expectations. That is, between the two survey periods, the social importance of work and family changed in men's and women's lives as a function of altered sex-role definitions. Similar historical alterations in the construction of psychological well-being in adolescence present themselves as a highly plausible hypothesis.

Conclusion

We have demonstrated in this chapter the relativity of adolescent development and well-being to social and historical change. We have shown that the timing of events in adolescent lives and the normative timing patterns across generations have shifted significantly over historical time. We have also presented evidence of important reformulations of social roles related to recent social change movements, which had important implications for psychological development. All of this suggests that the contemporary adolescent experience is unlike that of earlier generations. In particular, adolescents of the 1980s are faced with a lack of clarity in social boundaries defining both the beginning and the end of the period. They share with many developmental psychologists a sense of confusion over whether the downward secular trend in the onset of puberty also signals an earlier arrival of adolescence in the life course. Similarly, along with historians and demographers, they are uncertain whether the recent upward shifts in the age of marriage and birth of the first child indicates a later departure from adolescence. Moreover, the contemporary adolescent, like his or her elders, is confronted with discrepant prescriptions of behavior which, over the last two decades, have been inspired by the civil rights movements for minorities and women, the nascent men's liberation movement, as well as the renascent conservative movement in reaction to all of the above. Therefore, it is clear that the nature of contemporary adolescence (consequently, the lives of contemporary adolescents) is characterized by multiple standards of behavior, most of which are also in flux and conflict.

The current level of confusion over the nature and timing of adolescence is an important indication that a contemporary definition of adolescence has not yet been achieved by social consensus. The major changes in the expected performance of social roles and social timetables in recent years have invalidated our previous un-derstanding of the adolescent experience. As a society, we are now not at all certain about what it is adolescents are supposed to do and when they are supposed to do it. In the last 25 years, we have been predominantly preoccupied with new definitions of adulthood and old age, and with new formulations of age and sex roles. Not until our social transformation of adulthood has been accomplished, and we have a better understanding of what it is contemporary *adults* are supposed to do and when they are supposed to do it, will there be a new consensus on what constitutes becoming an adult.

Until that time, the adolescent of today is faced with both the presence of conflicting standards of behavior, and the absence of a social consensus of appropriate behavior. Whether or not the current confusion over the boundaries and definitions of adoles-cence is reflected in the internal turmoil so many adolescents report is an empirical question. To date, the epidemiological evidence needed to estimate the prevalence of psychological distress among noninstitutionalized adolescents, or to compare changes in those rates in relation to social and historical change, is lacking. Never-theless, we suggest that, given their magnitude, the social changes of the last 25 years, which have significantly altered the structure of adult lives, will have an enduring impact on the adolescent ex-perience as well. Contemporary adolescents, however, are hardly likely to benefit from the resolution of these changes because, by accident of birth, they are a cohort caught in the middle of social change. Subsequent cohorts, we would hypothesize, will be less stressed once these social changes have been incorporated into a redefinition of adolescent development and well-being. What that redefinition will be is at present a mystery. Its content and meaning will probably be clear to us only in retrospect.

References

Bandura A: The stormy decade: fact or fiction?, in Issues in Adolescent Psychology, second edition. Edited by Rogers D. New York, Appleton-Century-Crofts, 1972

Blos P: On adolescence: A Psychoanalytic Interpretation. New York, Free Press of Glencoe, 1962

Brittain CV: Adolescent choices and parent-peer cross pressures. American Sociological Review 28:385–391, 1963

Brittain CV: Age and sex of siblings and conformity toward parents versus peers in adolescence. Child Dev 37:709–714, 1966

Bryant FB, Veroff J: The structure of psychological well-being: a socio-historical analysis. J Pers Soc Psychol 43:653–673, 1982

Coleman J: Relationships in Adolescence. London, Routledge & Kegan Paul, 1974

Coleman J: Current contradictions in adolescent theory. Journal of Youth and Adolescence 7:1–11, 1978

Coleman J, George R, Holt G: Adolescents and their parents: a study of attitudes. J Genet Psychol 130:239–245, 1977

Demos J, Demos V: Adolescence in historical perspective. Journal of Marriage and the Family 31:632–638, 1969

Douvan E, Adelson J: The Adolescent Experience. New York, Wiley, 1966

Eskin B: When do nocturnal emissions begin in adolescence? Does the date coincide with or resemble first menstruation in girls? Medical Tribune 1977

Freud A: Adolescence. Psychoanal Study Child 13:255–278, 1958

Garn SM: Continuities and change in maturational time, in Constancy and Change in Human Development. Edited by Brim OG Jr, Kagan K. Cambridge, MA, Harvard University Press, 1980

Glick P: The life cycle of the family. Marriage and Family Living 17:3–9, 1955

Glick P: Updating the life cycle of the family. Journal of Marriage and the Family 39:5–13, 1977

Glick P, Norton A: Marrying, divorcing and living together in the U.S. today. Population Bulletin 32:1–39, 1977

Hamburg BA: Early adolescence as a life stress, in Coping and Health. Edited by Levine S, Ursin H. New York, Plenum, 1980

Josselson R: Ego development in adolescence, in Handbook of Adolescent Psychology. Edited by Adelson J. New York, Wiley, 1980

Josselyn IM: The Adolescent and His World. New York, Family Service Association of America, 1952

Kagan J, Coles R: 12 to 16: Early Adolescence. New York, Norton, 1972

Kett JF: Adolescence and youth in nineteenth-century America. Journal of Interdisciplinary History 11:283–298, 1971

MacMahon B: Age at menarche. Vital and Health Statistics, Series II, No.

133. Washington DC, U.S. Government Printing Office, 1973

Masterson JF: The Psychiatric Dilemma of Adolescence. Boston, Little, Brown, 1967a

Masterson JF: The symptomatic adolescent five years later: he didn't grow out of it. Am J Psychiatry 123:1338–1345, 1967b

McKenry PC, Walters LH, Johnson C: Adolescent pregnancy: a review of the literature. Family Coordinator 27:17–28, 1979

Modell J, Furstenberg F, Hershberg T: Social change and transitions to adulthood in historical perspective. Journal of Family History 1:7–32, 1976

Offer D, Offer J: From Teenage to Young Manhood. New York, Basic Books, 1975

Offer D, Ostrov E, Howard KI: The Adolescent: A Psychological Self Portrait. New York, Basic Books, 1981

Perun PD, Bielby DDV: Midlife: a discussion of competing models. Research on Aging 1:275–300, 1979

Perun PJ, Bielby DDV: Structure and dynamics of the individual life course, in Life Course: Integrative Theories and Exemplary Populations. Edited by Back K. Boulder, CO, Westview Press, 1980

Perun PJ, Giele JZ: The changing function of a college education in women's lives: some preliminary results. Paper presented at the Research Conference on Educational Environments and the Undergraduate Woman, Wellesley College, 1979

Perun PJ, Giele JZ: Life after college: historical links between women's education and women's work, in The Undergraduate Woman: Issues in Educational Equity. Edited by Perun PJ. Lexington, MA, Lexington Books, 1982

Presser IB: The timing of the first birth, female roles and black fertility. Milbank Memorial Fund Quarterly 49:329–361, 1971

Rossi A: Life-span theories and women's lives. Signs 6:4–32, 1980

Rutter M, Graham P, Chadwick O, et al: Adolescent turmoil: fact or fiction? Child Psychol Psychiatry 17:35–56, 1976

Schonfeld WA: The body and the body image in adolescence, in Adolescence: Psychosocial Perspectives. Edited by Caplan G, Lebovici S. New York, Basic Books, 1969

Tanner JM: Earlier maturation in man. Scientific American 218:21–27, 1968

Tanner JM: Sequence, tempo, and individual variation in growth and development of boys and girls aged twelve to sixteen, in Early Adolescence. Edited by Kagan J, Coles R. New York, Norton, 1972

Tanner JM: Fetus Into Man: Physical Growth from Conception to Maturity. Cambridge, MA, Harvard University Press, 1978

Uhlenberg P: A Study of cohort life cycles: cohorts of native born Massachusetts women, 1830–1920. Population Studies 23:407–420, 1969

Uhlenberg P: Cohort variations in family life cycle experiences of U.S. females. Journal of Marriage and the Family 36:284–292, 1974

U.S. Bureau of the Census: Marriage, divorce, and remarriage by year of birth: June 1971. Current Population Reports, Series P–20, No. 239, 1972

U.S. Bureau of the Census: Trends in child spacing: June 1975. Current Population Reports, Series P–20, No. 215, 1978

U.S. Bureau of the Census: Marital status and living arrangements: March 1981. Current Population Reports, Series P–20, No. 372, 1982

Weiner IB: Psychopathology in adolescence, in Handbook of Adolescent Psychology. Edited by Adelson J. New York, Wiley, 1980

Wittenberg R: On the superego in adolescence. Psychoanal Rev 42:271–279, 1955

Chapter 11

ADOLESCENT SUICIDAL AND SELF-DESTRUCTIVE BEHAVIOR: AN INTERVENTION STUDY

Eva Y. Deykin, D.P.H.

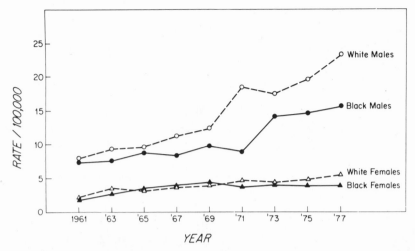

Figure 2. Suicide rate among 15-24-year-old persons by sex and race

at this pivotal stage of human development may have devastating results. The natural emotional liability characteristic of adolescence can produce rapid mood swings and impulsive behavior. The role of impulsive behavior as a determinant of adolescent suicide has not been formally evaluated, but clinical evidence would suggest that it plays an important part. For example, statistics show that almost 70 percent of successful adolescent suicides have employed methods of high and rapid lethality (fire-arms, hangings, or gas poisonings) which substantially diminish the probability of rescue (Shaffer and Fisher, 1981).

Other investigators (Hollinger and Offer, 1982; Hauser, 1981; Easterlin, 1980) have suggested that the rise of suicide in adolescence may be linked to societal or environmental factors that preferentially affect the young. Among such factors are the increase in divorce, the loosening of traditional family bonds, the high rate of geographic mobility, and increased competition for shrinking opportunities such as college and employment (Adam and Bouchoms, 1982; Sabbath, 1966; Cohen-Sandler et al., 1982).

While the factors leading to suicidal behavior may be similar for the young and for the mature adult, the prodromal picture may be quite different in adolescence. During this phase of development, depressive mood is often masked by hyperactivity, boredom, somatic complaints, and listlessness (Toolan, 1978; Weiner and Del Gaudio, 1976). The unfamiliar expression of depressive mood not only fails to alert professionals who are in contact with adolescents, but also may prevent the adolescent from seeking help, as he or she does not experience the subjectively painful feelings of hopelessness, helplessness, and emptiness so common in adult depression (Glaser, 1967).

The Adolescent Suicidal and Self-Destructive Behavior Intervention Study

A study now underway is designed to conduct and evaluate an intervention program geared to reduce the occurrence of suicide, suicide attempts, and self-destructive behavior among adolescents seen in the emergency ward of a large city hospital. The intervention combines a program of direct service to at-risk teenagers with a health education curriculum designed for teachers, probation officers, and community human service workers who have daily contact with adolescents. In addition, a special curriculum is designed for student peer leaders. This intervention is provided at the Boston City Hospital, a municipal hospital open to any Boston resident, but serving largely the inner-city population of Roxbury, South Boston, and Dorchester. The Brockton Hospital, located 40 miles south of Boston, serves as the control site. Assessment of intervention requires a clinical trial with randomization, but ethically this is not possible.

The objectives of the study are as follows:

1. to assess the proportion of suicide attempts and self-destructive behavior among all teenagers who seek medical treatment at the Boston City Hospital and at the Brockton Hospital emergency wards, both prior to and during the intervention program
2. to ascertain whether adolescents who seek help in the emergency ward as a result of a suicide attempt or self-destructive behavior have personal or situational characteristics that differentiate them from other adolescents seen in the emergency ward
3. to evaluate whether the intervention program is effective in:
    a) maintaining and facilitating the follow-up treatment of suicidal or self-destructive adolescents
    b) reducing the recurrence of such behavior
    c) reducing the rate of successful suicide among adolescents

residing in the defined enumerated populations served by the Brockton Hospital

The Setting

The study is conducted jointly at the Boston City Hospital (which is the intervention site) and at the Brockton Hospital (which serves as the control site). The two institutions are comparable in that they both serve largely urban populations with a high percentage of medically indigent individuals. The area served by the Boston City Hospital is an inner-city area with a large black and Hispanic population. The Brockton Hospital serves a population which, while predominantly white, shares many of the problems of unemployment, fragmented services, and high welfare dependency experienced by those residing in the Boston City Hospital catchment area. In both settings, a large proportion of adolescents served come from socially disadvantaged low income families, many of whom are headed by single females. A sizable proportion of adolescents seen at both sites have had problems with education, with the courts, and with alcohol and drug abuse. The occurrence of teenage pregnancy is high in both locations.

The Boston City Hospital and the Brockton Hospital have been selected as the study sites because of the comparability of the disadvantaged populations they serve; because adolescent self-destructive behavior is a problem frequently encountered; and because the two locations are sufficiently distant geographically to preclude the contamination of the control site from the effects of the intervention provided at the Boston City Hospital.

Study Subjects

Study subjects consist of adolescents aged 13 through 17 who are seen in the emergency room of the two study hospitals for injuries resulting from a suicide attempt, a suicidal gesture, or from self-destructive behavior. The major difference between a suicide attempt and a gesture is that in the former, there is a statement of suicidal intent or the presence of a classically suicidal act. In the latter, there is no stated suicidal intent, and the act, while harmful and self-inflicted, has a relatively low lethality. Admissions classified as exhibiting self-destructive behavior are those involving potentially lethal injuries or conditions for which the patient has not indicated a conscious suicidal intent. Self-destructive behavior can be an act of commission, such as driving while intoxicated, or an act of omission, such as a diabetic repeatedly failing to take insulin.

Study Design

The study consists of three facets: a retrospective review of emergency room records at the Boston City Hospital and the Brockton Hospital for a 24-month period preceding the initiation of intervention; a two-year period of intervention with concurrent review of records; and a one-year follow-up to assess the outcome of subjects who did and did not receive the intervention.

The purpose of the retrospective review of the records is to ascertain baseline occurrence of suicidal, self-destructive behavior among emergency room admissions.

For each such admission, a comparison admission matched for date of admission, sex, and age (within one year) is selected from the emergency room records at each of the study sites. The comparison admissions are selected from all emergency room admissions exclusive of those already identified as index subjects. Comparison admissions can result from non-self-inflicted trauma, acute illnesses, or exacerbation of chronic conditions. If no appropriate comparison admission can be found for the date of the index admission, the admissions for the previous and following dates are searched. If more than one comparison admission is available for the date of admission, then the one closest in age to the index admission is selected.

In order to identify any specific personal or situational characteristic that is potentially associated with suicidal or self-destructive behavior, the records of the index subjects are compared to the records of the comparison subjects. Data are collected on prior medical history, circumstances surrounding the present admission, marital status, race, and religion. Where possible, data on family size, living arrangements, and school attendance are also collected.

Statistics on the occurrence of adolescent suicide will be collected for both cities for the two-year period of intervention, and an estimated incidence rate of successful suicide will be calculated based on the number of adolescents in each city, using 1980 U.S. census data to determine the population of adolescents.

Intervention

The intervention consists of two separate but theoretically linked endeavors. One aspect of the intervention involves providing study subjects at the Boston site with the services of a professionally trained outreach health worker; the other facet of the intervention consists of a structured educational program directed at professionals whose work puts them in daily contact with adolescents. In addition, another educational program is designed for student peer leaders who are often in a position to identify an at-risk individual.

Direct Service of a Professional Community Health Worker

The use of a professionally trained outreach health worker is based on clinical and research experience, which indicates that adolescents, and especially those in turmoil, have difficulty in keeping scheduled appointments and in following through on referrals (Petersen and Chamber, 1975; Bogard, 1970). The following interventions are therefore necessary:

- to provide the adolescent with a measure of support, and to serve as a primary resource for his or her emotional, social, or physical needs
- to ensure that the adolescent keep follow-up and referral appointments
- to act as an advocate for the adolescent with his or her family, school, and other community agencies
- to provide a liaison between the subject and the hospital, and between the hospital and the community agencies
- to explore and to document the range of social supports available to the adolescent and, if necessary, to help the adolescent utilize these supports more fully or to develop new social supports

The proposed function of the outreach health worker is not now being filled by any other health provider. Social service, nursing, psychology, and psychiatry are hospital based disciplines, and rarely are equipped to provide aggressive outreach. In some instance, psychotherapy is offered only if the family as well as the adolescent is willing to participate. Given the isolation and alienation of many urban youth, only a few have families sufficiently motivated to begin treatment.

As part of the data collection, the outreach worker keeps detailed records of every contact made with the study subjects, or with third parties on their behalf.

The frequency of contacts between the outreach worker and study subjects is determined by the specific situation presented by the subject and by his or her needs. Usually contacts are quite frequent at the time of study enrollment and diminish as time goes on, unless there is a new crisis. All study subjects are seen by the outreach worker at least four times a year.

Educational Component

The second aspect of intervention is an educational program designed to increase awareness of adolescent depression, to help identify individuals at risk for suicide, and to offer strategies for suicide prevention and intervention. Originally the educational program had been directed at physicians, social workers, nurses, school and court personnel, and other adult providers who had daily contact with adolescents. It became evident, however, that student peer leaders—students who held official or unofficial positions of leadership—were usually the first persons to recognize a deeply troubled schoolmate. Peer leaders often were instrumental in providing support and in facilitating referral to appropriate providers. In addition to the two all-day yearly conferences scheduled for adult providers, we also instituted two all-day conferences for student peer leaders. The content and format of these conferences differed from that of the adult conferences to appropriately address the situations likely to be encountered by the peer leaders. Both sets of conferences informed participants of the range of community resources available to adolescents, and delineated the specific service provided by the community outreach worker at the Boston City Hospital.

Data Collection

Concurrent with the initiation of intervention, we began the review of the emergency room logs and medical records to ascertain the incidence of suicidal, self-destructive injuries among the 13- to 17-year-old youths seen. For every identified subject, we have also identified two control admissions matched for age, sex, and date of admission in order to ascertain whether study-eligible subjects differ from control admissions in terms of sociodemographic characteristics, living arrangements, school enrollment, persons accompanying the patient to the hospital, and type of medical payment. Because initial review of the records revealed that study-eligible subjects had experienced a high occurrence of family violence in their histories, we plan to submit to the Massachusetts Department of Social Services the names and addresses of study admissions and control admissions, to assess whether there had been a differing frequency of child abuse complaints filed for the two groups.

Data Analysis

The efficacy of the intervention program will be assessed by the following measures: the percentage of missed follow-up appointments or incomplete referrals to psychiatry or social service will be calculated and compared for each study site.

Preliminary Results

To date, we have focused our research efforts on identifying children who are study eligible by reviewing the emergency room logs and by abstracting the medical records. We have also identified an age-sex comparison subject for each study-eligible child, but we have not yet collected comparative data on social or background characteristics, or on variables relevant to the admission. The data that have been collected and analyzed to data provide information on the rate of occurrence of emergency ward admissions for suicidal and self-destructive behavior. The data in Table 1 show the overall incidence rate for suicidal, self-destructive admissions of 13- to 17-year-old adolescents at the two study sites. The data are for the 12-month period preceding intervention. Table 2 shows a similar analysis for the first year of intervention.

Data collected both for the 12-month period preceding the study and for the first 12 months of the study indicate that the overall incidence of study-eligible admissions to the emergency room among 13- to 17-year-old youths is somewhat lower at Boston City Hospital than at Brockton Hospital. The difference, while not large, is consistent within the two time periods, and is attributable to the higher

Table 1. Incidence of Suicidal Gestures, Attempts, and Self-Destructive Injuries among 13- 17-year-olds Admitted to the Emergency Rooms During the 12 Months Preceding Study Initiation

	Boston City Hospital	Brockton Hospital
Total ER admissions for 13- 17-year-olds	6485	5292
Number and incidence of eligible subjects	89 13.7/ 1000	91 17.2/ 1000
Total suicidal gestures	28	17
Males	6	6
Females	22	11
Total incidence rate	4.3/ 1000	3.2/ 1000
Total suicidal attempts	27	16
Males	4	3
Females	23	13
Total incidence rate	4.1/ 1000	3.0/ 1000
Total self-destructive injuries	34	58
Males	20	36
Females	14	22
Total incidence rate	5.3/ 1000	11.0/ 1000

occurrence of admissions for self-destructive injuries at Brockton Hospital. The admission rate for suicide attempts and for suicidal gestures is about equal in both institutions. We intend to pursue this finding further by analyzing the occurrence of study-eligible admissions for a period extending back two years prior to study initiation, as well as forward for the duration of the study.

When the three categories of study eligibility are combined, females clearly predominate over males. This trend exists for all subclassifications of study eligibility, with the exception of self-destructive injuries at Brockton Hospital, where males outnumber females 1.4 to 1.

In both institutions, the average age for subjects admitted for self-destructive injuries was slightly older than for subjects admitted for either suicide attempts or for suicidal gestures. This might be due to the involvement of alcohol in many self-destructive injuries.

At both Boston City Hospital and at Brockton Hospital, the month of June had the largest number of study-eligible admissions

Table 2. Incidence of Suicidal Gestures, Attempts, and Self-Destructive Injuries among 13- 17-year-olds Admitted to the Emergency Room During First 12 Months of Study

	Boston City Hospital	Brockton Hospital
Total ER admissions for 13- 17-year-olds	6644	4672
Number and incidence of eligible subjects	76 11.4/ 1000	73 15.6/ 1000
Total suicidal gestures	24	19
Males	7	4
Females	17	15
Total incidence rate	3.0/ 1000	5.7/ 1000
Total suicidal attempts	32	27
Males	6	6
Females	26	21
Total incidence rate	4.8/ 1000	5.7/ 1000
Total self-destructive injuries	20	27
Males	9	15
Females	11	12
Total incidence rate	3.0/ 1000	5.7/ 1000

in the six-month period before study initiation. This was not observed in the 10-month period following study initiation, however, when study-eligible admissions were more evenly distributed throughout the year. Further data collected over a longer span of time will be needed to ascertain whether there is a seasonal gradient in the admission of study-eligible subjects.

The present review of emergency room logs indicates that between one and two percent of all admissions among 13- to 17-year-olds are for some form of suicidal or self-destructive behavior. The excess of females in our sample is consonant with what is known of the epidemiology of suicide attempters. The relative dearth of males should not be interpreted as meaning that males are at lower risk for suicide, but rather that for a variety of reasons they may be less likely to seek treatment for an attempt. The excess of males among completed suicides, and the fact that male suicide attempters tend to select instruments of high and rapid lethality, may effectively remove many males from our sample.

Intervention

Direct work with subjects.   Among the 76 study-eligible subjects identified at the Boston City Hospital, 28 have signed the required consent forms and are receiving the intervention provided by the community outreach worker. This represents an approximately 35 percent yield of study-eligible subjects. A major stumbling block to more complete enrollment has been the difficulty of tracking and contacting youngsters once they leave the emergency room. Many families do not have telephones, and letters are rarely answered. The community outreach worker often establishes contact by making a home visit, and occasionally is successful in involving the discharged youngster in the intervention. It is hoped that, as the study services become better known and understood by the adolescent population, it may be easier to involve a larger proportion of eligible subjects. Recent requests by non-study-eligible adolescents for intervention services suggest that the program is well received and is becoming known. There have been very few outright refusals by study-eligible subjects to the offer of service, and these have been limited to subjects from families who have strong religious convictions against medical involvement.

Community outreach work is personalized to the needs of the individual and differs from case to case. Almost all subjects bear the burden of poverty, fragmented families, violence, and social chaos. School dropout, minor difficulties with the law, and some degree of substance abuse figure prominently in many cases. Chronic illness or physical handicaps are both more common than might be expected in a general adolescent population.

Table 3 shows the distribution of time spent by the community outreach worker. Data for this table come from contact forms completed each time the outreach worker has a contact with a subject or with someone else (school personnel, legal or court official, welfare personnel, or other provider) on the subject's behalf.

Case studies.   The following cases exemplify situations presented by typical subjects, and the service provided by the community outreach worker.

George is a 13-year-old white male admitted to the Boston City Hospital (BCH) pediatric emergency ward for an ingestion of his father's nitroglycerine tablets. Upon admission, George denied any

Table 3. Time Spent by Community Outreach Worker in Various Aspects of Direct Service During First Year of Intervention

	Face to Face Contact with Subjects	Letters to Subjects	Telephone to Subjects	Contacts with Other Persons for Subjects	Total
Total Number of Contacts	141	50	210	72	483
Total Hours	513.5	13	44	98	668.5
Average Hours per Subject	18.3	0.5	1.6	3.5	29.9

suicidal intent and claimed he took the tablets for "a headache." Later, George confided to a nurse that he took the tablets after he and his parents had argued over whether he would be allowed to apply for a part-time job.

George is the eldest of four siblings. A second child, Denise, two years younger, is suffering from end-stage Hodgkins Disease, and is not expected to survive. The two youngest siblings are in good health.

The parents live in subsidized housing, a ramshackle building. Despite a heart condition, George's father continues to work six days a week. George's mother is an obese woman who has devoted much of her time recently attending to her daughter's medical needs. She has a depressed, tired affect and spends her free time smoking and looking out the window. The two youngest children watch television when they return from school.

George is in the eighth grade and gets reasonably good grades, although in the past few months his performance has slipped. George is a strangely overweight child with a very feminized body. Short for his age, he has rounded hips and a perceptible breast formation. He is supposed to receive hormone shots three times a week at the neighborhood health center. Although the shots are necessary for George's sexual development, and will have to be continued through-out his life, George often fails to go to the health center.

George's social interaction is primarily with his sister Denise, whom he fiercely defends against the taunts of neighborhood children. In the home, however, George often resents the added attention Denise gets and frequently becomes angry, or petulant and infantile.

In helping George and his family, the community outreach worker has identified three areas of need:

1. George's need for continued medical care, for increased confidence and self-esteem as a male approaching adolescence
2. the family's impending loss and current difficulty in dealing with the conflicting needs of a terminally ill child and three other children
3. George's and his family's need for pleasurable and self-affirming experiences

The community outreach worker has provided support to George and his family on a weekly basis. She has taken George on special outings, or has spent time with him talking and walking around the neighborhood. On one occasion she has taken George's mother out for an afternoon. The focus of her work has been to encourage (and drive) George to go to the health center for his prescribed injections, and to support him during this difficult time of physical and emotional development combined with a family crisis. She has also helped the family cope with George's angry outbursts and has suggested ways of preventing them.

George has made good use of the direct services. He looks forward to the community outreach worker's visits and is delighted when they go on a special trip. He has become more verbal and expressive and seems to have a higher self-esteem, as evidenced by his attempts to diet. He still has to be encouraged to go to the health center, but his resistance is less. It is hoped that, as the results of the therapy become more evident, he will be motivated to continue his therapy without urging. At the moment, Denise's condition has stabilized, but she still requires a great deal of care. There have been no further ingestions or any self-destructive behavior on George's part. The community outreach worker intends to continue supportive work with this subject and family, cognizant that at the time of Denise's death, George may be at high risk for another suicidal gesture.

> Ann is a 13-year-old black female admitted to the pediatric emergency ward because of a polydrug ingestion of about 20 pills following an argument with an aunt who shares the home with Ann and her mother.
>
> Ann's mother, a 29-year-old woman, is severely diabetic and was receiving inpatient treatment at the time of Ann's ingestion. Ann's family is perpetually shrinking and expanding. Relatives move in, establish relationships, fight over money or possessions, and move out. This pattern is repeated frequently.
>
> Born in Tennessee, Ann was raised partially by her grandmother in Tennessee and partially by her mother in Boston. In the first seven years of her life, she was shuttled between mother and grandmother four times.
>
> The emergency room admission (which identified her as a study subject) was not her first ingestion, or, unfortunately, her last, as she has had a subsequent admission for an ingestion since study enrollment. In each instance, Ann's ingestions have occurred in the context of an argument with a parental figure. Characteristically, Ann's response to family arguments or to discipline imposed by an adult is impulsive self-punishment rather than anger toward others. She has run away from home several times in response to family upheaval.

Most of direct service has been with Ann's mother, since Ann has either been absent from home or has not kept appointments. Ann's school performance has been very low and she is now supposed to repeat the seventh grade. Poor impulse control and her tendency to flee have caused the school to insist on a change of living arrangements for Ann as a prerequisite for school enrollment. The community outreach worker has initiated arrangements for a 766 core evaluation, and has provided the needed comprehensive social evaluation of Ann and her family. (A Chapter 766 core evaluation is mandated by Massachusetts law when a child with any physical, mental, or emotional handicap appears to require a special educational program.)

Work with Ann's mother was focused on the chaotic living arrangements, and on the possibility of providing an alternative living situation for Ann. The mother agrees that Ann needs more control than she can provide, especially since her illness requires frequent hospitalizations. Working with Ann's mother, and coordinating the efforts of school personnel, medical providers, and the Department of Social Services, the community outreach worker is now helping to implement placement for Ann in a residential group setting. A group setting will provide both a measure of control and support unavailable at home. Ann is viewed as a high risk for suicide because her impulsivity and self-imposed isolation make her very difficult to reach. If the residential arrangements can be made, the community outreach worker will concentrate on helping Ann make the transition by providing a great deal of support. The establishment of a meaningful relationship with Ann is crucial if Ann is going to develop a sense of trust in another human being. At the moment, the prognosis for this case is guarded.

Educational component. In the first year of operation, we have held four all-day conference/workshops. Two were targeted for service providers, and two were designed specifically for adolescents who held positions of leadership or who were peer counselors within their schools. The goal of all four conferences was to augment an overall understanding of adolescent depression and suicidal behavior, attending risk factors, and ways of helping at-risk teenagers. Morning sessions were primarily didactic, while the afternoon sessions were devoted to small discussion groups on specific issues.

The conferences that were designed for adolescent leaders stressed the recognition of depressive symptoms in the adolescent, and the types of hidden, ambiguous messages frequently voiced by suicidal youngsters. These conferences utilized innovative educational techniques designed to involve the participants in a dialogue. One such method was the use of the Youth Expression Theater (YET), a semiprofessional group of teenagers skilled in improvisational acting. The YET players improvised six five-minute skits focusing on adolescent depression and suicide. At the end of each skit, the audience was invited to ask questions that the players answered while still in character. It was apparent from the questions that some of the conference participants had encountered similar situations among their classmates. The immediacy of the situations portrayed, and the audience's identification with the actors, sparked a great deal of discussion.

Future Work

We expect that approximately 30 additional at-risk youngsters will receive community outreach intervention services within the next 12 months, bringing the total caseload to about 50. This estimate, based on our experience to date, is conservative, since there is some indication that as knowledge of the intervention spreads, more eligible subjects may be willing to sign participation consent forms. In order to continue to provide optimal direct service to an expanded caseload, we have agreed to serve as a placement facility for a Boston University School of Social Work student. The student will work under the community outreach worker's supervision and carry five to seven selected cases. We believe that this relationship with a school of social work will be mutually beneficial, in that it will provide us with needed assistance, it will offer the student a valuable training experience, and it will establish a mechanism for the continuation of community outreach service to at-risk adolescents beyond the period of study funding. Boston College School of Social Work had also requested that we serve as a student placement facility, but we declined because more than one student would take too much supervisory time at this point. However, it is possible that after the termination of the study, the Division of Social Services at the Boston City Hospital could continue to provide service to suicidal, self-destructive adolescents with the help of several social workers in training.

In the coming year, the educational component of intervention will focus on reaching teachers and counselors in the Boston middle

schools, since many of our subjects are enrolled in grades 7 through
9. We will also be more active in involving police and court personnel who frequently deal with severely self-destructive youths.
The Juvenile Session of the Roxbury District Court has expressed
an interest in having its court personnel attend the conferences,
and we will also contact the Juvenile Sessions of the Dorchester
and Boston courts.

Review of the emergency room logs and medical records will
focus on a comparison of the social, demographic, and admission
process variables of the study subjects and age–sex matched controls. We will continue to monitor all emergency room admissions
to ascertain the occurrence and recurrence rates of suicidal and
self-destructive behavior among study subjects. At the same time,
we will obtain data from the Massachusetts Office for Vital Statistics
on all deaths occurring among 13- to 17-year-olds. Since these data
list the deceased's name, town of residence, age, and primary cause
of death, we will have the opportunity to assess whether any study
subject has died. Death certificates will be located and abstracted.

Finally, we are interested in assessing the possible association
of early child abuse and subsequent suicidal, self-destructive behavior. The medical records of study subjects frequently contain
notation of family violence, child abuse complaints, and removal of
the child from the parental home. However, comparable information is not available for control children, since the reason for their
emergency room admission does not trigger a detailed social or
psychiatric history. To investigate whether receiving abuse as a child
predicts suicidal behavior in adolescence, we have obtained the
collaboration of the Massachusetts Department of Social Services,
which is willing to provide data from its master records within the
legal constraints of confidentiality.

Summary

The Adolescent Suicidal and Self-Destructive Behavior Intervention
Study provides an opportunity to assess the efficacy of an outreach
program involving direct service to at-risk teenagers, and makes
available a specific educational curriculum for service providers. In
addition, this study allows for the estimation of the incidence of
self-inflicted injuries among emergency room admissions, and the
assessment of the possible association of child abuse and subsequent self-destructive tendencies.

References

Adam K, Bouchoms A: Parental loss and family stability in attempted suicide. Arch Gen Psychiatry 39:1081–85, 1982

Bogard HM: Follow-up study of suicidal patients seen in emergency room consultation. Am J Psychiatry 126:1017–1020, 1970

Cohen-Sandler R, Berman R, King RA: Life stress and symptomatology: determinants of suicidal behavior in children. J Am Acad Child Psychiatry 20:178–186, 1982

Easterlin RA: Birth and Fortune. New York, Basic Books, 1980

Glaser K: Masked depression in children and adolescents. Am J Psychother 21:565–574, 1967

Godenne G: The treatment of depressed and suicidal adolescents, in Medical Care of the Adolescent. Edited by Gallagher JR, Heald FP, Garell DC. New York, Appleton-Century-Crofts, 1976

Hauser PM: Our anguished youth: baby boom under stress, in Adolescent Psychiatry, vol. 8. Edited by Feinstein SC, Giovacchini PL. Chicago, University of Chicago Press, 1981

Hollinger PC, Offer D: Prediction of adolescent suicide: a population model. Am J Psychiatry 139:302–306, 1982

Murphy GE, Wetzel RD: Suicide risk by birth cohort in the U.S. Arch Gen Psychiatry 37:519–523, 1980

Peterson DM, Chamber CD: A demographic evaluation of acute drug reactions in a hospital emergency room. Medical Care 13:1061–1069, 1975

Sabbath JC: The suicidal adolescent—the expendable child. J Am Acad Child Psychiatry 5:272–289, 1966

Shaffer D, Fisher P: Suicide in children and young adolescents, in Self-Destructive Behavior in Children and Adolescents. Edited by Wells C, Stuart IR. New York, Van Nostrand Reinhold, 1981

Solomon MI, Hellon CP: Suicide and age in Alberta, Canada, 1951–1977. Arch Gen Psychiatry 37:511–513, 1980

Toolan J: Depression in adolescence, in Modern Perspectives in Adolescent Psychiatry. Edited by Howell J, New York, Brunner/Mazel, 1978

Weiner J, Del Gaudio A: Psychopathology in adolescence: an epidemiologic study. Arch Gen Psychiatry 33:187–193, 1976

Chapter 12

INTERRELATIONS AMONG MEASURES OF DEPRESSIVE SYMPTOMATOLOGY, OTHER MEASURES OF PSYCHOLOGICAL DISTRESS, AND YOUNG ADULT SUBSTANCE USE

Gene M. Smith, Ph.D.

Chapter 12

Interrelations Among Measures of Depressive Symptomatology, Other Measures of Psychological Distress, and Young Adult Substance Use

$\mathbf{A}$s part of a 13-year longitudinal study of substance use, a follow-up questionnaire was completed in 1980 and 1981 by each of 1,521 young adults who had been recruited into the study in 1969. The purpose of the longitudinal study was to identify antecedents, correlates, and sequelae of substance use. Reports already presented have shown that personality and other psychosocial variables, measured prior to onset of substance use, are dependably related to the likelihood and extent of later use of illicit drugs, such as marijuana, cocaine, and LSD (Smith, 1973; Smith, Fogg, 1975, 1979) as well as to precocity of such use (Smith, Fogg, 1978). Self-report and peer rating measures of "socialization" were particularly efficient indicants of later illicit substance use and of escalation in type and amount of substance use. Socialization scores were highest among adolescents who remained nonusers of both licit and illicit substances; somewhat lower for those who became users of cigarettes and/or alcohol but stopped short of illicit use; and lower still for those who became users of illicit substances (Smith et al., 1982).

The follow-up information collected in 1980 and 1981 concerned young adult substance use, but it also measured various aspects of dissatisfaction with life, depressive symptomatology, and other aspects of psychological distress. This chapter describes the use of the follow-up data to develop scales to measure a) dysphoric

This work was supported in part by a grant from the National Institute on Drug Abuse (DA 00065-10), and in part by a grant from the George Harrington Trust.

mood and b) suicidal ideation and suicide attempts in young adults; and it reports the relationship of those two scales to each other, their relationships to other measures of psychological distress, and their relationships to young adult substance use.

Method

During 1980 and 1981, each of 1,923 young adults was sought for follow-up study. Forty-five could not be located (two percent); 18 were deceased (one percent); 339 chose not to participate (18 percent); and 1,521 (79 percent) completed and returned, by mail, the follow-up questionnaire.

Characteristics of the Young Adult Sample

In the group of 1,521 subjects comprising the follow-up sample, 99 percent were between 24 and 28 years of age (median = 26); 53 percent were female; 75 percent had attended school beyond high school; 75 percent were employed full-time, and those full-time workers reported a median income of $13,750; 18 percent were full-time homemakers; six percent were full-time students; four percent were unemployed; 53 percent reported that they were married and were living with their spouse; and 32 percent reported having children.

Forty-nine percent of the respondents reported being current cigarette users and 20 percent reported having quit. Fifty-four percent reported current use of marijuana and 23 percent reported having quit. For other substances, those reporting current use were: alcohol (96 percent), cocaine (23 percent), amphetamines and similar stimulants (19 percent), barbiturates and tranquilizers (nine percent), LSD (four percent), PCP (2 percent), and heroin (two percent).

Measures of Substance Use

For cigarettes, alcohol, and marijuana, an index of young adult use was derived from the subject's 1980-1981 report of number of years of use, number of days of use during the preceding 12 months, and amount of use on a typical occasion of use. For illicit drugs other than marijuana, the index of use was based on years of use, days of use during the preceding 12 months, and the degree of "high" typically achieved.

Measures of Suicidal Ideation, Attempts, and Dysphoric Mood

The items contributing to these two scales vary in format and response options, but they share two characteristics: each is relevant to some aspect of depressive symptomatology, and each can be scored dichotomously to distinguish symptomatic as opposed to nonsysmptomatic responses. Most of the dichotomous cut-points produce a sample split in the vicinity of 12 percent/88 percent; but the splits range from one percent/99 percent to 22 percent/78 percent. The first step in scoring either of the scales is simply to count the number of symptomatic responses given by a subject. For dysphoric mood, a second step involves some compression at the high end of the scale. As seen in Tables 1 and 2, both scales are profoundly skewed. This reflects the fact that our sample is a nonhospitalized group of normal subjects, most of whom report little or no depressive symptomatology.

Measures of Dissatisfaction with Life and Other Aspects of Psychological Distress

Nine measures of life dissatisfactions were derived by factor analysis with an approach similar to that previously used by Andrews and Withey (1976). A weighted average was computed to measure overall dissatisfaction. Other measures of psychological distress were obtained by using selected items from the SCL–90 (Hoffman-La-Roche, 1975); still others were based on the response to the question of whether the subject felt, or had previously felt, that he or she was near to having a nervous breakdown.

Results

Table 1 shows the response distribution and dichotomous scoring for each of the five items used in constructing the suicidal ideation and suicide attempts scale. The subjects who scored positively ranged from a low of one percent (of the total sample) on item 4, to a high of 14 percent on item 1. The distribution of scores for the suicidal

Table 1. Self-Report by Young Adults of Suicidal Ideation and Attempts

Item Number	Question	Response
1)	Have you *ever* thought seriously about taking your own life?	yes = 207 (14%) no = 1,263 blank = 18
2)	If yes, approximately how many times have you had such thoughts during the *past year*?	times 0 1 2 3 4 5 6 7 8 9 or more blank 475 35 31 18 5 7 1 0 0 14 902 111 (7%)
3)	Have you ever actually attempted suicide?	yes = 57 (4%) no = 1,380 blank = 51

4) If yes, approximately how many times have you tried?

(On this item, subjects receive a positive score if they report *more than one* suicide attempt.)

				times		
1	2	3	4	5 or more		blank
39	10	3	1	5		1,430
		{ 19	(1%)	}		

5) Amount bothered or distressed during the *past week* by thoughts of ending your life?

none	some	moderate	lots	extreme	blank
1,417	43	10	6	6	6
	{ 65	(4%)	}		

Five-item scale (bracketed responses are scored positive for suicidal ideation and attempts)

	0	1	2	3	4	5	blank
Number of items scored positive:							
Number of subjects:	1,292	82	70	51	16	8	2
Percent:	(85)	(5)	(5)	(3)	(1)	(1)	(—)

Table 2. Items Used to Measure Dysphoric Mood Among Young Adults

Item Number	Question	Response							
		Satisfaction over the last few weeks							
		delighted			mixed			terrible	blank
		1	2	3	4	5	6	7	
1)	Your general enjoyment of life?	184	654	414	153	40	18	12	13
						223 (15%)			
2)	How happy you are?	201	605	417	154	55	25	14	17
						248 (17%)			
3)	Your prospects for a good life in the future?	192	486	391	316	49	26	15	13
						90 (6%)			
4)	Your success in getting ahead in the world?	104	448	466	284	111	26	16	33
						153 (10%)			

5) Overall life satisfaction *a year ago*

absolute bottom 0	1	2	3	4	neutral 5	6	7	8	9	absolute tops 10	blank
13	20	19	49	81	136	190	351	381	173	52	23

182 (12%)

6) Overall life satisfaction *at present*

0	1	2	3	4	5	6	7	8	9	10	blank
2	11	16	22	45	88	144	313	523	256	62	6

184 (12%)

7) Overall life satisfaction *anticipated for next year*

0	1	2	3	4	5	6	7	8	9	10	blank
2	1	7	6	13	69	79	236	504	402	157	12

177 (12%)

Table 2. Items Used to Measure Dysphoric Mood Among Young Adults (continued)

Item Number	Question	Response					
		true	mostly true	mostly false	false	blank	
8)	I wish I could have more respect for myself.	165 165 (11%)	297	502	513	11	
9)	At times I think I am no good at all.	104 268 (18%)	164	462	752	6	
10)	I certainly feel useless at times.	113 317 (21%)	204	563	597	11	

		Amount Bothered or Distressed in Past Week					
		none	some	moderate	lots	extreme	blank
11)	Feeling blue?	472	709	206	72	22	7
					300 (20%)		
12)	Feeling hopeless about the future?	998	339	77	51	14	9
					142 (10%)		
13)	Feelings of worthlessness?	1150	244	48	17	17	12
				326 (22%)			

13-*item scale* (bracketed responses are scored positive for dysphoria)

	0	1	2	3	4	5	6–7	8–11	12–13	blank
Number of items scored positive:										
Number of subjects:	702	272	166	87	65	61	76	58	32	2
Percent:	(46)	(18)	(11)	(6)	(4)	(4)	(5)	(4)	(2)	(—)

ideation and attempts scale itself is shown at the bottom of Table 1. As seen there, 10 percent of the young adults scored positively on two or more of the five items.

Table 2 shows the response distribution and dichotomous scoring for each of the 13 dysphoric mood items, as well as the distribution of scores for the dysphoric mood scale. As seen at the bottom of Table 2, 11 percent of the young adults scored positively on six or more of the 13 dysphoric mood items.

The 9 × 6 crosstabulation in Table 3 shows a high and positive association between dysphoric mood and suicidal ideation and attempts. The χ^2 is 519.14; the contingency coefficient is 0.50; and the Pearson correlation coefficient is +.46. If the 9 × 6 crosstabulation is collapsed where the heavy lines are drawn in Table 3 (producing a 2 × 2 crosstabulation), approximately 10 percent of the sample is on the depressive side of the demarcation line of each scale. When considered in that manner, subjects in the upper 10 percent on either scale have a 40 to 50 percent chance of being in the upper 10 percent on the other. By any standard chosen, these two measures of depressive symptomatology are highly related.

Table 4 shows the correlation between each of the two depressive symptomatology scales and each of 18 other scales: 10 measures of life dissatisfactions and eight other measures of psychological distress. All 36 correlations are highly significant; and they indicate that among relatively healthy (nonhospitalized) young adults, measures of depressive symptomatology (suicidal ideation/ attempts and dysphoric mood) correlate positively with a wide range of other psychiatric symptoms (anxiety, interpersonal sensitivity, hostility, obsessive-compulsive tendencies, paranoid ideation, and psychoticism) and with a broad spectrum of life dissatisfactions. Note especially the correlation of +.65 between dysphoric mood and the mean of the abbreviated SCL-90 scales, and the correlation of +.67 between dysphoric mood and dissatisfaction regarding cognitive competence and ability to cope.

To explore further the potential usefulness of the information in the dysphoric mood and suicidal ideation/attempts scales, we used the 2 × 2 crosstabulation in Table 3 to define four groups for additional analysis: 96 subjects who scored in the upper 10 percent on dysphoric mood but not suicidal ideation/attempts; 75 who scored in the upper 10 percent on suicidal ideation/attempts but not dysphoric mood; 70 who scored in the upper 10 percent on both; and 1,278 who did not score in the upper 10 percent on

Table 3. Crosstabulation of Dysphoric Mood versus Suicidal Ideation and Attempts

	Dysphoric Mood Score									Row	
	0	1	2	3	4	5	6–7	8–11	12–13	Total	%
Suicidal Ideation and Attempts Score 0	657	241	149	67	52	40	49	30	7	1292	85
1	31	14	9	11	2	5	6	3	1	82	5
2	11	12	7	7	5	5	7	9	7	70	5
3	3	2	1	2	5	8	10	13	7	51	3
4	0	3	0	0	1	1	3	3	5	16	1
5	0	0	0	0	0	2	1	0	5	8	1
Column Total	702	272	166	87	65	61	76	58	32		
Column %	46	18	11	6	4	4	5	4	2		

$\chi^2 = 519.14$; probability $< .0001$
Contingency coefficient $= 0.50$
Pearson correlation coefficient $= 0.46$

Table 4. Suicidal Ideation/Attempts and Dysphoric Mood Correlated With Other Young Adult Measures of Psychiatric Symptomatology and Distress

	Suicide r	Dysphoria r	Number of Items in Scale
Feeling near nervous breakdown	+.47	+.47	1
Life-dissatisfaction scales (adapted from Andrews and Withey, 1976)			
cognitive competence and coping	+.39	+.67	23
work and career	+.23	+.55	11
intimacy/general happiness	+.36	+.59	7
smooth social relations	+.25	+.44	4
current American society	+.13	+.26	4
health	+.31	+.47	3
satisfaction with other people	+.20	+.39	3
financial success	+.18	+.38	3
opportunity for enjoyment	+.28	+.54	4
weighted mean of nine scales	+.38	+.71	62
Scales adapted from SCL–90 (Hoffman-LaRoche, 1975)			
anxiety	+.38	+.57	4
interpersonal sensitivity	+.31	+.55	3
hostility	+.37	+.45	3
obsessive-compulsive	+.26	+.44	2
paranoid ideation	+.30	+.51	2
psychoticism	+.21	+.25	2
weighted mean of six scales	+.42	+.65	16

All correlation coefficients in this Table are highly significant ($p < .0001$).

either. For convenience, we call those four respective groups "Dysphoric," "Suicidal," "Dysphoric *and* Suicidal," and "Healthy."

When compared on responses to the question concerning nervous breakdown, subjects in the "Dysphoric" and in the "Suicidal" groups are equally likely to report having felt in the past that they were near a nervous breakdown. The rates of "positive" response for nervous breakdown in those two groups were 39 percent and 41 percent, respectively. By contrast, only six percent of the "Healthy" subjects responded positively, and 78 percent of the "Dysphoric *and* Suicidal" subjects did so. (Nervous breakdown was scored positively if the subject indicated that he or she had felt near a nervous breakdown in the past and was not completely over it yet.) Thus, the rates of positive response for the "Dysphoric" and for the "Suicidal" groups (although equal to each other) were almost seven times that of the "Healthy" subjects, but were only one-half that of the subjects classified as "Dysphoric *and* Suicidal." The additivity of distress is clearly apparent: a high score on both scales of depressive symptomatology indicates far greater disturbance than a high score on only one.

Although the "Suicidal" and the "Dysphoric" groups are alike on some variables (for example, nervous breakdown, as just cited), they are quite different on others. For example, on the measure of life dissatisfaction that concerns "Competence and Coping," the "Dysphoric" group scores dramatically higher than the "Suicidal" group. Each of those groups scores significantly higher than the "Healthy" group, and scores significantly lower than the "Dysphoric *and* Suicidal" group; but the mean for the "Dysphoric" group is a full standard deviation above the mean for the "Suicidal" group; and the t-value for that difference is 7.47 ($p = .0001$).

Both the suicidal ideation/attempts scale and the dysphoric mood scale tend to correlate positively with measures of young adult substance use, but the correlation coefficients are small. For example, suicidal ideation/attempts correlates +.02, +.09, +.08, and +.10, with amount of young adult use of alcohol, cigarettes, marijuana, and cocaine, respectively; and dysphoric mood correlates +.05, +.13, +.09, and +.04 with those same measures of substance use. For samples of the size used in this analysis, a correlation coefficient of .04 reaches the .05 level of statistical significance; but the practical significance of such a correlation value is inconsequential. A correlation of .13 accounts for less than two percent of the variance.

Comments and Conclusions

The work reported here is still in progress. Our main interest is in examining the longitudinal relationships concerning antecedents and sequelae of teenage and young adult substance use, but the measures in our data base that have most relevance to the subject of suicide and depression among adolescents and young adults are those that deal with dysphoric mood and suicidal ideation/attempts. Analyses of the relationships of those two scales to other measures in our 13-year longitudinal data base are still preliminary, but the work already completed (in evaluating data collected from this non-hospitalized young adult sample) supports the following conclusions:

1. The scales designed to measure dysphoric mood and suicidal ideation/attempts are unmistakably correlated with each other; and both are significantly correlated with concerns about having a nervous breakdown, dissatisfaction with life, and other measures of psychological distress: anxiety, interpersonal sensitivity, hostility, obsessive-compulsive tendencies, paranoid ideation, and psychoticism. Such interrelatedness of symptoms is one reason differential psychiatric diagnosis is difficult—especially when the symptoms are subtle.
2. Despite the high correlation between the two measures of depressive symptomatology, they are by no means conceptually substitutable. They differ in their degree of association with various aspects of psychological distress. Moreover, their diagnostic implications are additive: a high score on both scales indicates far greater disturbance than a high score on only one.
3. Both measures of depressive symptomatology are correlated with extent of use of cigarettes, alcohol, and illicit drugs, but those correlations are quite small and appear to have limited importance—both from a practical and from a theoretical perspective.

References

Andrews FM, Withey S: Social Indicators of Well-Being. New York, Plenum Press, 1976

Hoffman-LaRoche, Inc: Psychiatric Rating Scales, Vol. III: Self-Report Rating Scales, 21–36. Palo Alto, CA, Consulting Psychologists Press, 1975

Smith GM: Antecedents of teenage drug use. Paper presented at the 35th Annual Meeting of the Committee on Problems of Drug Dependence, National Academy of Sciences—National Research Council, 312–317, 1973

Smith GM, Fogg CP: Teenage drug use: a search for causes and consequences, in Predicting Adolescent Drug Abuse: A Review of Issues, Methods, and Correlates. Edited by Lettieri DJ. National Institute on

Drug Abuse Research Issues Series, 11:277–282. Washington DC, DHEW Publication No. (ADM) 76-299, 1975

Smith GM, Fogg CP: Psychological predictors of early use, late use, and nonuse of marijuana among teenage students, in Longitudinal Studies in Drug Use: Substantive and Methodological Issues. Edited by Kandel DB. Washington DC, Hemisphere, 1978

Smith GM, Fogg CP: Psychological antecedents of teenage drug use, in Research in Community and Mental Health: An Annual Compilation of Research, vol. 1. Edited by Simmons RG. Greenwich, CT, JAI Press, 1979

Smith GM, Schwerin FT, Stubblefield FS, et al: Licit and illicit substance use by adolescents: psychosocial predisposition and escalatory outcome. Contemporary Drug Problems 11:75–100, 1982

11

Chapter 13

THE STRATEGY OF PREVENTIVE TRIALS

Ernest M. Gruenberg, M.D., D.P.H.

Chapter 13

THE STRATEGY OF PREVENTIVE TRIALS

Human beings have tried to avoid disease and injury since recorded time began. People have found ways of adapting their patterns of living to widely different ecological niches, with widely different disease hazards. Many protective habits and customs may have evolved as a result of Darwinian "survival of the fittest," without any conscious recognition that a particular disease was being avoided. Did Chinese tea drinking protect against cholera and other waterborne diseases? Did they know it? Did the Arabs have one clean hand and one dirty hand because they wished to avoid all those diseases that result from anal–oral short-circuits, or because they were thinking of propriety or religious observances? No matter. The important thing is to recognize that some life-styles are disease preventing and others (as with cigarette smoking) are disease producing.

Conscious avoidance of disease was, in ancient times, associated with isolation of infected patients, attention to nutrition, avoidance of unhealthy places, and so forth. In ancient Greece, the medical profession regularly gave hygienic advice. Government-sponsored, socially organized disease prevention programs have now become so much a part of our civilization that many people, including those in the medical profession, take them for granted. How many of us lifted our glasses last Thanksgiving and said, "Let us give thanks that in our country no more children will develop brain syndromes from measles or rubella viruses?" (Gruenberg et al., 1986)

319

The progress we have made in disease prevention is due to the socially organized public health movement, which has long worked toward the following goals:

First: To prevent the preventable conditions
Second: To terminate the terminable conditions
Third: To mitigate what can't be prevented or terminated
Fourth: To discover methods of prevention

The first and fourth goals were emphasized in 1978 by Gerald Klerman, M.D., the Administrator of the Alcohol, Drug Abuse and Mental Health Administration (ADAMHA) in the ADAMHA Forward Plan. Prevention should always be the first priority of the public health service. But wise health officers have long known that while prevention is better than cure, it is the cure, rather than the prevention, that is usually emphasized. People do not often appreciate those things that do not happen to them. That is why it is so difficult to make prevention work and to make prevention research a sufficiently high priority.

In the mental health field, there have been some solid victories in lowering the frequency of certain mental disorders: general paresis, pellagra psychoses (Roe, 1973), and equine encephalitis syndromes. We can now add the elimination of the measles and rubella viruses as causes of brain syndromes. These diseases had become general health problems, causes of death and disability; and increased initiative for the elimination of measles and rubella arose from knowledge about mental damage resulting from these diseases. The strategy that added to the plan for 90 percent immunization at school entrance, and the installation of a rigid surveillance system to interrupt each new outbreak among adolescents or preschool children, was motivated by mental health concerns. The knowledge and technology necessary to eradicate measles and rubella came from the Centers for Disease Control (CDC); but the motivation came, in large measure, from mental disorder epidemiology.

To date, we can claim such clear-cut victories for prevention only for brain syndromes. This can be attributed to the research groups that have been established to investigate physical and biological risk factors in a highly developed way. Psychiatric epidemiology is not nearly as advanced as yet. However, it is hoped that the increasing number of qualified investigators and research teams will continue to advance psychiatric epidemiology. Meanwhile, we can learn something useful from the previous successes and failures in efforts to prevent diseases and disorders—any disorders.

Victories for disease prevention have emerged as a result of the practical application of anecdotal observations, clinical observations, and systematic studies. Now and then, new knowledge and techniques are systematically introduced so that the effect of innovative prevention can be measured with precision. The preventive trial design is one such powerful technique, which will be used more often if we are made aware of its potential.

Historical Examples of Preventive Trials

In 1854, John Snow removed the handle from London's Broad Street pump to stop the cholera epidemic. The result was equivocal; perhaps the epidemic would have started to recede that day, anyway (Snow, 1965).

In 1912, Goldberger supplemented diets with brewer's yeast, preventing pellagra from developing. The results were clear, but were not generally accepted (Goldberger et al., 1915).

From 1937 to 1945, Cambridge-Somerville in Massachusetts conducted a trial of delinquency prevention through relationship therapy of high risk youths. The results were clear that relationship therapy had no effect on preventing delinquency (Teuber and Powers, 1953). The treatment group was apparently damaged (McCord, 1982).

From 1945 to 1955, the Newburgh, New York, water supply was fluoridated to prevent dental caries. There, and in Kingston, New York (the control city), children's cavities were monitored. The results were clear, and there was rapid acceptance (Ast et al., 1956).

The Salk polio vaccine trial took place in 1952. The results were clear, and there was rapid acceptance. Polio has been almost eradicated (Francis et al., 1955).

In 1953, Tompkins and Wiehl prenatal diet supplements were tried to prevent congenital birth defects. The results were strongly suggestive, but have not been pursued adequately (Randall et al., 1956).

From 1959 to 1966, Dutchess County, New York, tried to lower the incidence of chronic social breakdown syndrome by providing social support network preservation through rapid, relevant responses to acute manifestations of this syndrome. The results were positive (Gruenberg, 1974; Gruenberg et al., 1969), but they have been misinterpreted (MacMillan, 1958; Gruenberg and Archer, 1979).

In 1964, Fountain House in New York City experimented with prevention of rehospitalization and of unemployment among discharged mental hospital patients through a social rehabilitation program. Results showed two-thirds of careers could not have been affected; the remainder were equivocal (Pitt, 1969).

From 1961 to 1964, Washington Heights, New York tried a chronic social breakdown syndrome prevention program similar to the one tried in Dutchess County, New York. However, the program's execution was faulty.

The Logic of the Preventive Trial

The logic of the preventive trial is simple. It is worthwhile to present it in its skeleton form, because in practice every preventive trial becomes more and more complicated. A clear vision of the analysis that will cap the trial is necessary when deciding how each complication can best be handled, so that any potentially damaging effect will be minimized.

The preventive trial assumes the existence of a population of persons, none of whom have the condition to be prevented. It assumes that the condition is recognizable and ascertainable by a reliable, accurate method, which can be applied to the study population. The trial starts with this study population and divides it into two parts. One part is called the intervention group, the other the control group. This division of the population into two parts is done in such a way that the intervention group and the control group are at equal risk for developing the condition to be prevented.

The simplest way of dividing the study population into two groups that are at equal risk for developing the condition is to randomly assign the individual members of the study population to the two groups. It must always be remembered, however, that random assignment does not guarantee that the two groups end up at equal risk for developing the condition. If the study population is large, then the difference between the two groups after random assignment will be trivial; but if the study population is small, then simply by chance high-risk individuals could disproportionately be assigned to one group, and low-risk individuals to the other.

The study population will, unfortunately, be heterogeneous. Heterogeneity complicates the design. If all the risk factors associated with developing the condition were known, then it would be possible to make the study population homogeneous with respect to those risk factors. It might be possible to match individuals at equal risk and randomly assign members of each pair to the intervention and control group. This increases the power of the subsequent analysis. In practice, random assignment is not always possible.

The Difference Between a Clinical Trial and a Preventive Trial

A clinical trial begins with a group of patients who have the condition to be treated. It divides this population into two groups, each of which is to receive a different treatment for the condition. The outcome being sought is recovery from the condition. This requires a definite condition and a set of criteria for recovery. In practice, many conditions for which clinical trials are done commonly terminate with death. Death then becomes the definition of nonrecovery. This simplifies the execution of clinical trials. Recovery in some conditions (especially cancers) becomes defined as five-year survivorship after treatment. When the initial trial's report emphasizes that treated people died less frequently than the controls, then death is the reported outcome.

In this case, a clinical trial can appear to be like a preventive trial in which the objective is to postpone death. The study population is one at high risk for death because it is made up of patients with a condition that commonly leads to death. The intervention seeks to thwart the fatal outcome. Under these circumstances, the reports of clinical trials take on the appearance of preventive trials. This has become common, as is evidenced by rapid progress in medical technology (Gruenberg, 1977). But even these clinical trials start with a group of persons who are sick, and the investigations are conducted in the course of a relationship between a treating physician or team and a study population of patients.

In contrast, a preventive trial usually has a study population of persons who are not patients, but who represent a sample of the general population, all of whom have a known risk for developing the condition. It is this essential difference of patienthood that dominates the differences in organization, execution, and conceptualization of preventive trials from those of clinical trials.

Trials of Preventive Maintenance Treatment

There is a group of studies—trials of preventive maintenance treatment—that straddles the concepts of preventive trials and clinical trials. One example is the attempt to reduce the complications associated with high blood pressure through prolonged treatment with antihypertensive drugs. In these studies, the study population is identified because of an elevated blood pressure. This condition is frequently asymptomatic, and the study subjects are not seeking help as patients. Under these conditions, the treatment of subjects and controls, and their allocation to different treatment modalities, presents problems similar to those encountered in the preventive trial. The outcomes are undesirable states of health, which are not present in the study subjects at the beginning of the investigation and intervention. The intervention can only be carried out if subjects become patients. This difference makes the intervention more like a clinical trial than like a preventive trial: the intervention itself requires medical supervision, so the study subjects become patients of those administering the continuing intervention. Trials in this category are characterized by the use of long-term treatment for progressive conditions, so that later manifestations of the condition can be either averted or delayed.

The Organization of Preventive Trials

I have emphasized the fact that patienthood among study subjects is the key distinction between a preventive trial and a clinical trial, because I think this determines the main differences in planning organizational and investigative strategies for the two kinds of studies. It is not the logic that distinguishes them; it is the relationship between the investigator and the study subjects that distinguishes them.

The prevention trial must identify a study population to which the planned intervention will be acceptable. The trial must organize the intervention and make it available to the study population without making it available to the control population. The investigator must know that the intervention is harmless, and believe that it may be an effective method of prevention, acceptable to a study population known to be at risk for the disorder. The intervention cannot be so widely available and so acceptable that a majority of people have it.

In the clinical trial, unbiased outcome data is usually obtained through the double blind design, in which neither the patients nor their therapists know which treatment the subjects have been assigned to. It is then possible for the clinical treatment team to monitor the progress of the disorder without bias. But the preventive trial organization partakes of the characteristics of a public health program, and calls upon community organization skills as well as on research skills.

The nature of the interventions varies enormously. This leads to varying degrees of direct contact with study subjects. The Salk vaccine polio trial, for example, only required a few minutes of contact between the intervenors and the study subjects. In those few minutes, all the necessary information had to be gathered to insure later follow-up data in regard to outcome.

The nature of the outcome measurements also determines the amount of direct contact the investigators need to have with the study subjects. When avoidance of death is the outcome, cooperation from the local coroner or the state's Department of Vital Statistics will be enough if sufficient identifying information has been gathered. But when the intervention seeks to lower the frequency of an unreportable disease state or disability, then direct ascertainment becomes necessary, requiring direct contact with the subjects. It is under these conditions that the problem of avoiding bias between the intervention group and the control group becomes difficult, often requiring extremely ingenious arrangements.

There is another factor, the varying nature of which affects the organization of the preventive trial. This factor is the attitude of the intervenor, and whether it plays a role in the preventive trial's effectiveness. Clearly, the Salk vaccine was going to be effective in its generation of antibodies, regardless of the point of view of the person giving the vaccination. But in the Cambridge–Somerville Youth Project (a trial of delinquency prevention through relationship therapy), the attitudes of the intervenors were important. They ranged from psychoanalysts to Boy Scout leaders, with varieties of social workers in between. Each was allowed to do what he or she wished in relation to the youths, but were not permitted to transmit money or arrange for the youths to move away from home.

The organizer and funder of the Cambridge–Somerville study, Dr. Hugh Cabot, firmly believed that the value of these relationships would depend upon the belief system and enthusiasm of the "therapist." That is why the intervenors were not told exactly what to do but were free to do what seemed best for their subjects. In order to insure unbiased follow-up and ascertainment of outcome, the research activities were funded separately from the organization of the intervenors.

When the records were all in, there was no lower frequency of delinquent behavior by the youths who had the relationship therapy. In fact, more of them had performed delinquent acts than had the controls (but the difference was not statistically significant). There was considerable controversy about these findings on the part of many of the professionals who took part in the intervention. However, I think that the paper by Teuber (1953) accurately reports the findings. When McCord followed the same subjects in 1975 she defined "undesireable outcome" as having an FBI-indexed criminal conviction, dying before age 35, or receiving a medical diagnosis of alcoholism, schizophrenia, or manic-depressive disorder (McCord, 1982). The effects of the intervention in the matched pair analysis were adverse ($p < .03$).

This example illustrates the difficulty that can arise when the evaluation of an intervention is in the hands of those who have gone to a great deal of trouble to organize it. It is not always reasonable to expect those who invest a great deal in organizing an intervention to be completely objective. To avoid this problem, a special organizational structure is needed, in which the intervenors are administratively independent of both the data gatherers and the data interpreters regarding outcome. A mutually respectful but independent partnership must be created.

Principles of Organization

There is no standard formula for organizing an intervention. The intervention should be organized by people who are not subservient to the evaluators; and the evaluators should not be administratively subservient to those who organize the intervention. The intervention relies on a delicate balance, and it does not always work. The intervention will not work, for example, if the intervenors are simply looking for research data to support preconceived ideas. The intervention will not work if the evaluators of the research are seeking to denigrate the study. Both sides must have respect for the efforts of their partners as well as respect for the truth. They must not only be able to talk to one another, but they must be able to listen. The intervenors should play an active, and in some matters a decisive, role in specifying the outcome to be prevented. The distinguished British biologist, Sir Peter Medewar, made the perceptive observation that if politics is the art of the possible, science is the art of the soluble (Medewar, 1967). But because a preventive trial is always at least partially a political activity, preventive trials combine the two arts: that of the soluble with that of the possible.

Review committees wanting to know exactly how a study will be executed down to the last detail are sometimes told, "If we knew how it was going to come out, it wouldn't be research, would it?" These trials do not come out entirely as expected. There is an even greater learning process that takes place during the trials than takes place during ordinary research projects. There are always serendipitous findings. Very often it is not until the end of a study that one learns how it should have been conducted properly to begin with. We have not reached a stage in preventive trials in which things are cut, dried, and routine.

For example, in the Fountain House study, we found that one-third of the controls got jobs and were never rehospitalized over the next two years. Therefore, one-third of the treatable group would have had good outcomes without treatment. Another one-third of the treated group were rehospitalized and never got jobs within the next two years. This meant that only one-third of the subjects could show any change according to the agreed-upon outcome and goals of the program. My recommendation was that the data be used to modify intake policy if the intervenors thought that getting jobs and staying out of the hospital was their goal. We could analyze the characteristics of those who would do well without the program and did not need it. We could analyze the characteristics of those who did badly despite the program, and who were not benefitting from help. The managers of Fountain House did not agree to such use of the data.

In the Washington Heights trial, schizophrenics from the neighborhood of the Psychiatric Institute who required hospitalization were randomly admitted to the community psychiatry program instead of being sent to the City Hospital, and from there to state or other facilities. The theory was that these patients would be released quickly from the community service (which was a short distance from their homes) and that patient care would continue on an informal basis, preventing patients from deteriorating. In practice, things did not work out that way, because of the Psychiatric Institute's policy of keeping inpatients until the end of June regardless of the date of admission, so as to start each group of new residents with new patients on July 1. The Psychiatric Institute never did succeed in having a single clinician treat a patient as both an inpatient and an outpatient, so the idea of a unified clinical team never emerged. However, data did provide an opportunity to study the effects of over-hospitalization, since it took more than six months on the average for the intervention patients to be released from the Psychiatric Institute, and approximately three weeks for the controls to be released from the city or state hospitals to which they had been sent. Instead of finding out anything about the prevention of chronic deterioration, we did find out something about the prevention of complete restitution. The findings two years after the index admission were that patients treated at the Psychiatric Institute recovered completely, without clinical or social signs of handicap, only one-half as often as those treated at the city hospital. The report of this study has not been published.

The Funding of Preventive Trials

I have not done a complete investigation of the funding of preventive trials. However, the successful ones that I am acquainted with were never funded on the basis of a government grant. The Fountain House study and the Washington Heights trial were funded by a government grant to a service agency, and the investigator was not free to publish findings independently of the grantee service agency. The pellagra preventive trial by Goldberger, and the Kingston–Newburgh preventive trial of fluoridation of water, were both operated by government agencies, which conducted the studies and organized the cooperation of the service agencies on a partnership basis. The Salk vaccine and the Dutchess County trial of preventing the chronic social breakdown syndrome were financed by foundations that gave separate grants to different aspects of the collaborative work.

There is some question as to whether peer review as currently implemented by initial review groups is capable of funding preventive trials. It would be best for the two groups to present two different proposals as a pair and sent to a single study section, and either be given awards as a pair, or not at all. In this way, it may be possible for the intervention group and the investigator group to remain independent of one another while working in a partnership, and at the same time be mutually dependent, since the two grants would be, in fact, only viable if they were operated in tandem. I do not see how a third entity can act as the organization that keeps the partnership together, except through the proferring of funds to each (each of which is dependent upon continued collaboration in order to receive funds).

Potential Mental Disorder Prevention Trials

Let us look at some of the untested prevention hypotheses currently being advocated for action to see if one can imagine introducing some of them with a preventive trial design.

Maternal Nutrition

The relation of maternal malnutrition (Steichen et al., 1980) to central nervous system development before birth remains cloudy. While there are various programs in existence to raise the nutritional status of marginally nourished young women in this country and elsewhere, none of them is applied with sufficient intensity to get to all of the young women at risk of having a child damaged because of suboptimal nutrition. It certainly would not do such young women any harm if they were systematically educated to feed themselves better and were provided with the nutritional supplements necessary for optimal nutrition.

Such experiments have been tried, but they share one deficiency. From the available evidence, it would be important to start improving nutrition of the treated group of young women long before they became pregnant in order to assure that they had excellent reserves of the essential nutrients at the time they became pregnant. To start supplementation after the first prenatal visit is probably like locking the stable door after most of the horses are already stolen. This would require artful community organization and education programs and not just the erection of a scientific design.

Tyrosine-Rich Diets for the Prevention of Mental Retardation

PKU is a metabolic deficiency sometimes associated with mental retardation. It has been suggested (Bessman, 1972) that if a woman is heterozygous for PKU, she is more likely to have a mentally retarded child if her diet is partially deficient in tyrosine. The complexities of the hypothesis and the reasoning behind it are too detailed to expound here, but they are credible. A woman with a family history of PKU, who had been tested and found to be heterozygous for this gene, could be given an extra supplement of tyrosine during pregnancy. No one thinks that this intervention would do her or her fetus any harm. Passive research does not seem warranted at this stage of our knowledge. The evidence is not strong enough to justify giving every such woman a supplement of tyrosine. Therefore, the next step should be a preventive trial. I do not know how many such women would have to be followed before results could be determined with current methods of appraising central nervous system development in the infants. But I can think of no insoluble ethical, political, or organizational problems in the conduct of such a trial. Yet I know of no agency that is planning one.

Widow-to-Widow Counseling for the Prevention of Depression

The widow-to-widow program, begun at the Laboratory of Community Psychiatry at Harvard in the late 1960s (Silverman, 1970), has been described as a demonstration program in primary prevention. However, the program's effect on the incidence of mental and physical disorders has not yet been demonstrated. The goal of the program is to help recently widowed women under the age of 60 adjust to widowhood through the use of lay counselors who are themselves widows.

The counselors are mostly high-school educated women in their mid-forties, who have been widowed for about three years. Initially, the counselor's role is to share her own experiences concerning financial and emotional problems, and to help the new widow cope with being alone, making decisions, and developing new social relationships. Later, the counselor encourages and supports the new widow's independence.

In many ways, the widow-to-widow program parallels the early programs in community care for the seriously mentally ill. The program is generally thought to provide a humane and socially acceptable intervention; and although its advocates do not specify the condition they hope to prevent, we suspect that this intervention lowers the incidence of clinical depression by preventing undue extension of bereavement in recently widowed middle-aged women. The time is ripe for a preventive trial to either confirm or refute this suspicion.

Because the widow-to-widow program finds its participants by scanning newspaper death notices, and because there are never enough counselors to extend the service to every newly widowed woman, there is no reason why the service should not be offered to a random half of the widows of a given city. The clinical diagnosis of depression can be made accurately enough to measure the reduced incidence of depression. There are, therefore, no major obstacles to initiating such a preventive trial. If the results were positive, we would have learned how to prevent a number of depressions, thereby increasing the number of such programs. If the results were negative, it would not mean that the widow-to-widow program is not good; it would simply mean that it does not prevent depression, and its advocates would have to be more specific about what it does prevent.

Mothers Who Have Negative Perceptions of Their Infants

The results of a carefully organized longitudinal study done by E. Broussard (1976) provide the hypothesis for another preventive trial. It has been shown that a mother's perception of her normal first-born infant during the first month of its life may have a strong influence on the probability of the child later developing an emotional disorder. When a mother thinks her baby is worse than the average child in terms of crying, spitting, sleeping, and a number of other behaviors, the child is at greater risk for developing emotional disorders at age 10 or 11 than children whose mothers perceived them as better than the average child in terms of these behaviors. The mother's perception at one month is somewhat more predictive of later emotional disturbance than is her perception one to two days after birth, but the effect is present when the mother's anticipation of her future child is measured before the child's birth!

Broussard has discovered that the mothers of high risk infants have difficulty anticipating, assessing, and fulfilling their children's needs; they tend to be inflexible and have low self-esteem. She has begun a series of interventions with a small number of these mothers who display negative perceptions of their children during the first month of life. Mother–infant groups meet every two weeks from the time the children are about two months old, and periodic home visits are made by psychiatric professionals, generally on a weekly basis. Broussard has also initiated a program of televised guidance for mothers during their postpartum hospital stay. Early results from these small preventive trials show that the televised instruction does result in a change in maternal attitudes; and that children whose mothers participate in mother–infant groups and receive home guidance are more like low-risk children than high-risk controls whose mothers do not experience any intervention.

Summary

Prevention should have the highest priority in public health work.
     Preventive trials are a powerful design. The design requires not only a recognition that our knowledge and technology are ripe for a crucial scientific test, but also the ability to identify a social and political context in which the test can be carried out (as well as the ability to organize for both the scientific work and the intervention work). Preventive trials have been done and can continue to be done. It is hoped that these trials will be done more often in the future than they have been in the past.

References

Ast D, Schlesinger ER: The conclusion of a 10-year study of water fluoridation. Am J Public Health 46:256–271, 1956

Bessman S: Genetic failure of fetal amino acid "justification": a common basis for many forms of metabolic, nutritional, and "nonspecific" mental retardation. J Pediatr 81:834–42, 1972

Broussard E: Neonatal prediction and outcome at 10 to 11 years. Child Psychiatry and Human Development 7:85–93, 1976

Francis TJ, Korns RF, Voight RB, et al: An evaluation of the 1954 poliomyelitis vaccine trials. Am J Public Health 45:1–63, 1955

Goldberger J, Waring CH, Willetts DC: The prevention of pellagra: a test of diet among institutional inmates. Public Health Rep 30:3117–3131, 1915

Gruenberg EM: The social breakdown syndrome and its prevention, in American Handbook of Psychiatry. Edited by Caplan G. New York, Basic Books, 1974

Gruenberg EM: The Failures of Success. Milbank Memorial Fund Quarterly 55(1):15, 1977

Gruenberg EM, Archer J: Abandonment of the seriously mentally ill. Milbank Memorial Fund Quarterly 57:485–506, 1979

Gruenberg EM, Snow HB, Bennett CL: Preventing the social breakdown syndrome, in Social Psychiatry. Edited by Redlich FC. Baltimore, Williams and Wilkins, 1969

Gruenberg EM, Lewis C, Goldston S: Vaccinating against brain syndromes: the campaign against measles and rubella. New York, Oxford University Press, 1986

MacMillan, D. Hospital–community relationships, in An Approach to the Prevention of Disability from Chronic Psychoses. Milbank Memorial Fund, 1958

McCord J: The Cambridge–Somerville youth study: a sobering lesson on treatment, prevention and evaluation, in Practical Program Evaluation in Youth Treatment. Edited by McSweeny AJ, Fremson UJ, Hawkins RT. Springfield, IL, Charles C Thomas, 1982

Medewar PB: The Art of the Soluble. London, Methuen, 1967

Pitt RB: Experiment to Evaluate the Effectiveness of Rehabilitation for Patients Discharged from Mental Hospitals. Unpublished doctoral dissertation, Columbia University, 1969

Randall A, Randall JP, Kasius RV, et al: Maternal and newborn nutrition studies at Philadelphia Lying-in Hospital, Newborn Studies IV: clinical findings at birth and one month for babies of mothers receiving nutrient supplements. Milbank Memorial Fund Quarterly 34:321–353, 1956

Roe DA: A Plague of Corn: The Social History of Pellagra. Ithaca, Cornell University Press, 1973

Silverman PR: The widow as caregiver in a program of preventive intervention with other widows. Mental Hygiene 54:540–547, 1970

Snow J: Snow on Cholera; Being a Reprint of Two Papers. New York, Hafner Publishing Company, 1965

Steichen JJ, Tsang RC, Gratton TL, et al: Vitamin D Homeostasis in the perinatal period: 1,25–dihydroxyvitamin D in maternal, cord, and neonatal blood. N Engl J Med 302:315–319, 1980

Teuber H-L, Powers E: Evaluating treatment in a delinquency prevention program, in Proceedings of the Association for Research in Nervous and Mental Disorders. Edited by Wortis SB. Baltimore, Williams and Wilkins, 1953

Chapter 14

THE PLACE OF COLLEGE HEALTH SERVICES IN THE PREVENTION OF SUICIDE AND AFFECTIVE DISORDERS

Robert L. Arnstein, M.D.

Chapter 14

THE PLACE OF COLLEGE HEALTH SERVICES IN THE PREVENTION OF SUICIDE AND AFFECTIVE DISORDERS

Suicide and suicide attempts by college and university students have long been a matter of concern (and sometimes consternation) to family, faculty, and other students (Fry and Rostow, 1942; Farnsworth, 1957; Temby, 1961; Rook, 1959). Although a certain incidence of suicidal behavior in the late adolescent–young adult age group has always been recognized (Allison-Tomlinson, 1981; Fawcett, 1982; Holinger, 1978, 1979, 1980; Holinger and Offer, 1982; Inamadar, et al., 1982), the fact of suicidal behavior occurring on campus has always seemed an event of particular poignance (Rook, 1959). This response is probably a result, in part, of the favored position of the college student; and, in part, a result of the view that the college or university is a supportive community. "Why did he do it? He had everything to live for"; and "I could have helped if she had just told me how she felt," are two common reactions. Inevitably, all concerned are interested in prevention of such events, and the university mental health service is an obvious place to turn for help. Understandably, prevention of suicide may involve the alleviation of associated and contributory psychological states, such as affective disorders (Guze and Robins, 1970; Coon, 1961; Minkoff et al., 1973; Weissman et al., 1973), which is also a legitimate goal of a university mental health service. Farnsworth, a preeminent figure in the college mental health field, states: "Almost all the writers in this field thus far have emphasized the importance of depression and suicide in the work of psychiatrists with students" (1957, p. 24).

337

Although university mental health services will do their utmost to contribute to prevention of suicide attempts and suicide in their constituencies (which will include students primarily), there is considerable difference among the resources available to address these problems on any given campus among colleges and universities in the United States (Glasscote and Fishman, 1973). Furthermore, while the mental health component of a student health service will be a major factor in any program that a college develops, there may be equally important mental health professionals operating out of counseling centers, health education units, or other counseling-like endeavors, as well as academic personnel and residence hall supervisors, who frequently provide the first line of aid. Because of my own experience at Yale, I will be referring most often to the mental health division of a university health service; however, many of my comments will apply in general terms to other campus facilities that are concerned with helping students who manifest emotional problems related to affective disorders or potential suicidal behavior.

The Role of the College Health Service in Suicide Prevention

Although it might be more logical to discuss affective disorders first because they presumably precede suicidal behavior, the fact that the latter is more identifiable suggests that a chronologically backward progression may be clearer. A student suicide, if at all widely known on campus, tends to be such a shocking event that it galvanizes much institutional energy into post hoc considerations of how it happened and how future suicides can be prevented. Inevitably, the mental health service will be approached for information and comment, and two questions tend to be addressed to it. If the individual had been seen by a therapist or was in therapy at the time of the suicide, the first question is: "Why was the suicide not prevented?" This, of course, is a legitimate question, although one that may have no satisfactory answer. The second is the more difficult question, and that is: If the suicide victim had no contact with the service, as is usually the case (Fry and Rostow, 1942; Temby, 1961), could not, or should not, the service have had some sort of outreach program that would have increased the possibility that the individual had obtained help prior to the event?

There are, of course, various answers to the first question, some of which have more merit than others. First, the therapist may simply have made a clinical misjudgment. All therapists would like to think that such misjudgments do not occur, but I think few of us would be so certain of our own competence as to deny that possibility. Furthermore, even if one is certain of one's competence, there are a host of variables that may influence the patient after he or she has been seen, and it is very difficult for the therapist to control for all of these. Second, many college services (particularly in recent years as a result of budget pressures) have been cut back or have not enlarged to a reasonable size, so that the demand for service may make it impossible to provide as much support as someone in a suicidal state really needs. Third, partly as a result of the civil liberties movement, many states have tightened up the conditions necessary for involuntary commitment. Although potential danger to self is one that remains, as far as I know, in all states, irrational behavior resulting from a psychotic state is not always a basis for involuntary hospitalization. This may lead to suicidal behavior when no suicide intent is overtly stated (Wilkinson, 1982; Himler and Raphael, 1942; Inamadar et al., 1982). Psychiatrists and physicians will unquestionably vary in their willingness to certify patients when the criteria less clearly meet the relevant statutory requirements, or even when the criteria do (Peszke et al., 1980); but I am quite sure that change in statutes has been a factor in decreasing involuntary hospitalization in Connecticut. Fourth, although some colleges have good insurance coverage, some may not; and, given the hospital bed cost for non-public psychiatric wards or hospitals and the shortage of beds in public psychiatric hospitals, hospitalization, voluntary or involuntary, may not be so easy to achieve. Fifth, and most difficult of all, psychiatric hospitalization for the student may have future consequences that are really impossible to predict, but that are real. Again, it is evident that if one is certain the suicide potential of the individual is high, one would unquestionably hospitalize; but if one is not so certain, one has to balance the immediate risks versus the long-term consequences, and there are times when one may elect to take the immediate risk.

As far as the second question regarding the outreach program is concerned, there are two general approaches. One is some sort of active outreach program, and the other is a more passive approach that involves increasing as far as is possible the access to, and availability of, mental health help. At Yale we tend to take the latter approach, which can be thought of in general terms as increasing everyone's access to the service rather than specifically targeting suicidal individuals. I am, of course, most familiar with the ways we specifically attempt to do this at Yale, and I recognize that what is possible for us is not necessarily possible for colleges with fewer psychiatric resources. However, I do believe that the same principles apply.

First and foremost, we attempt to establish the general acceptability of seeking mental health help. This involves not only public relations work with the student body, but also with faculty and staff who may not necessarily be directly advising a given student but who, by off-hand remarks, may well affect the willingness of a student to seek such help. I believe that the stigma of seeing a mental health professional has decreased over time, but I think it is unrealistic to state that a stigma does not still exist in the minds of some. Thus, informing students that one is not unique if one visits a mental health professional, and taking steps to make such professionals approachable, are both parts of the process.

It is important, if possible, to have someone available 24 hours a day so that the students who feel overwhelmed at any time of day or night can get immediate help, if necessary. We have not established a "hot-line" in the usual sense of that word, but we do publicize the fact that one can call an emergency Health Service number at any time. A mental health professional will respond by telephone, or in person, if indicated.

It is also important to have some sort of relatively rapid assessment for anyone who seeks help. We use an initial evaluation system and a "managed" waiting list if there is no therapy time immediately open. Admittedly this system has its drawbacks, but it does, I believe, allow us to offer service immediately to those individuals in acute distress, of which the suicidal student would certainly be one.

There are certain general policies that influence a student's decision to seek help. One of the most important, we feel, is the reputation of the service for confidentiality. Students are exceedingly concerned that they are being evaluated by faculty and deans, both formally and informally, and they can be totally put off by any suggestion, true or false, that the service will be in touch with deans without their knowledge and permission. A single break in confidentiality can haunt a service for years after it happens.

Continuing education of individuals on campus who may be

in a quasi-counseling role regarding criteria for referral and ways to effect referral is also important. Such individuals will vary, from physicians and nurses in the health service to chaplains, deans, residence hall advisers, coaches, peer counselors, or upperclass individuals who have formalized counseling roles vis-a-vis freshmen. The way in which this is implemented at any given college varies, but at Yale we have a brief orientation program for freshmen counselors; a mental health worker is liaison to each of the residential colleges; we act as backup for two peer counseling services; and we have various interactions with other health care providers in the University Health Services.

The fact that most student suicides occur in individuals who have not been in contact with the mental health service (Fry and Rostow, 1942; Temby, 1961) could be interpreted to mean that an outreach program should be the most significant part of a suicide prevention program. On the other hand, it could also mean that those who are in contact with the service are by that fact somewhat protected. I recognize, of course, that one could say that a person who is in contact with the service never really intended to complete a suicidal act, and, therefore, that the mental health service may be helpful but is not necessarily preventive. I know of no real way to differentiate between these two interpretations of the facts.

Inevitably, the mental health service will see individuals who have taken an action somewhere on the suicidal continuum from gesture to attempt (Blaine and Carmen, 1968; Fry and Rostow, 1942; Hawton et al., 1978b; Raphael et al., 1937). There are some instances in which the action is so minimal that it is uncertain whether it can be even described as suicidal (Birtchnell and Alarcon, 1971); there are other, clear-cut instances, in which an individual has made an attempt that is so serious that its failure is chance. However, there are a series of actions between these two extremes in which the intent is much more difficult to assess (Henderson et al., 1977; Hankoff, 1982; Hawton et al., 1978a). Yet such assessment is a necessary part of clinical evaluation; and the way in which the therapist views it will determine what preventive actions are taken. As I have already implied, these actions may vary from hospitalization in a locked psychiatric unit where full suicide precautions will be taken; to admission to the infirmary, which usually is in no sense suicide-proof, but which may provide a supportive environment; to some other environmental manipulation, with the aim of decreasing stress; to prescription of medication; to the provision of psychotherapeutic support; or some combination of these. These are matters of clinical judgment, each having its advantages and disadvantages. The clinical judgment involves balancing the risks versus the advantages and disadvantages of each therapeutic action. The actions taken are extremely important, however, inasmuch as many studies indicate that anyone who has engaged in suicidal behavior is at risk for repeating the behavior (Hankoff, 1982; Morgan, 1981; Pierce, 1977).

Research on Suicide Among College Students: A Review of the Literature

In regard to specific past research on suicide in college and university students, the literature is rather confusing. In the early days of college mental health, there are frequent mentions of suicidality and the importance of its prevention (Fry and Rostow, 1942); but most of the descriptions are anecdotal, and even an article that purports to apply a statistical approach is rather confusing because it makes no attempt to separate therapists' impressions of a patient's suicidality, reported suicidal ideation, suicide attempts, and completed suicide (Raphael et al., 1937). In the 1950s, there were one or two studies that attempted a more systematic approach (Parrish, 1957; Parnell, 1951), as well as an attempted study initiated at Yale to obtain a broader national sample. It is interesting that the latter was never pursued because the principal investigator, Bryant Wedge, felt that the reports that were returned were either so fragmentary (as a result of inadequate record keeping) or so questionable as to validity (because of the hearsay nature of many of the reported suicides) that they did not permit statistical handling. Wedge believed, however, that two general points emerged:

1. The suicide rate seemed to run in inverse ratio to the drop-out rate, which was interpreted as a possible indication that people drop out before they commit suicide.
2. There was some evidence that the higher the standard of intellectual performance, the higher the rate of suicide, although this could not be proven.

There continued to be sporadic articles describing the experience of one college or another during the 1960s (Temby, 1961; Blaine and Carmen, 1968; Bruyn and Seiden, 1965; Lyman, 1961;

Ross, 1969) and the 1970s (Mishara et al., 1976; Sims and Ball, 1973). In 1970, the American College Health Association began to collect statistics from as many colleges as would participate in an annual survey of mental health services. The number of suicides was one of the questions asked, and rates were derived from such statistics. These varied from four to eight suicides per 100,000, but it is difficult to know how complete the data is. There were also some studies that focused on specific student groups (Pepitone-Arreola-Rockwell et al., 1981; Pitts et al., 1979).

There are many studies to indicate how difficult it is to obtain any kind of accurate statistics on suicide rates (Brugha and Walsh, 1978), partly as a result of the fact that death certificates which report deaths as accidental or suicidal may not reflect the true situation (Holding and Barraclough, 1977, 1978; Holinger, 1979, 1980). The general consensus, however, is that if the sample is large enough, vagaries of death attribution will either cancel out or be consistent, and that in large populations the statistical impact of idiosyncratic death reports will not be substantial. In trying to gather university statistics, however, this is problematic because it is more difficult to gather large statistical samples without running the risk of very great variations in record keeping, completeness, and so forth, as already described. Furthermore, there is no general agreement on when a student is a student. For example, in the Parrish (1957) study, it was decided to define a student suicide as anyone who was enrolled or committed suicide within a year after withdrawal from college. Although this is certainly a possible definition, if the student has withdrawn for psychiatric reasons and then commits suicide months later, it would seem to have a very different implication for a college mental health service concerned about prevention than a suicide that occurs essentially on campus.

It is interesting to note that the public concern over student suicide is a recurring one in which, periodically, an event occurs that spotlights suicidal behavior on campus and leads the media to focus on the subject. This is of some significance because it indicates that there may be a kind of cyclic focusing of attention, and it raises the question of whether reporting of suicide deaths in some way leads to additional acts that are either directly imitative, or indirectly triggered, by the publicity. In a random search of our records I have unearthed newspaper clippings documenting an upsurge of concern in 1927; in 1953 and 1961 in England; and in 1966 in the United States. The content of each clipping is remarkably similar.

Some particular suicide has caught the attention of the reporter, and there follows a crude survey of the situation on various campuses, some discussion of what can be done, and then a decrease in interest until another cycle starts and the pattern recurs.

In regard to the effect of publicity on the incidence of suicide attempts, there have been several studies done, especially in Great Britain, using rather imaginative techniques; but, as far as I could determine, results have been contradictory (Barraclough et al., 1977; Blumenthal and Bergner, 1973). Needless to say, such studies are very difficult to do, but the possibility of "contagion" has been reported (Binns et al., 1966). My own experience is totally impressionistic and is based on one natural sequence of events that occurred several years ago. In May, 1976, just prior to the end of final exams, a senior shot himself. There followed some disagreement among administrators as to how the aftermath should be handled, and the next October the Yale Daily News on four successive days ran a series entitled "Suicide at Yale: Rumors and Facts." In December there were three serious suicide attempts by undergraduates in a short space of time. Although there is no hard evidence linking the publicity and the suicide attempts, it seems highly likely to those of us who have worked in the Mental Hygiene Division for a long time that there was a relationship. This is based partly on a recurring phenomenon involving referrals to the Mental Hygiene Division. A week or two after the Yale Daily News runs an article about the Mental Hygiene Division, there is an unexpected increase in students seeking therapy. In most instances the individual denies any connection between the article and the referral, but over the years it has happened so consistently that it is difficult to ignore the publicity as a causal factor in the decision to seek help, and perhaps as the factor that determined its timing. Although a decision to attempt suicide is very different from a decision to seek help, it seems quite possible that the same general linkage may occur.

Student Suicide: Psychological Development and Predisposing Factors

It is important for the clinician to be aware of the psychological states that may lead to suicide. This has been written about extensively (Allison-Tomlinson, 1981; Blaine and Carmen, 1968; Hankoff, 1982; Hendin, 1975; Ross, 1969; Weissman et al., 1973), and I will not try to summarize. Some years ago, however, the American College Health Association, attempted to develop a position paper on risk-taking among college students. In a sample list of risk-taking actions such as fast driving, drug use, and cigarette smoking, suicide attempts were listed, and I was elected to address the action of suicide attempts. As a result I gave some thought to the motivations and consequences of suicidal behavior, and it may be appropriate to repeat some of my conclusions.

Motivation for Suicide

The use of the term risk-taking brings up the issue of motivation, which cannot be dealt with here in any depth, but which does need to be addressed briefly. When one is talking about suicide in the late adolescent–young adult age group, one must consider it against the background of "normal" development at this stage of life. I believe that any suicidal action is exceedingly complex, and the factors that push an individual from suicidal ideation to suicidal action are, in all probability, multiple rather than single. This is further complicated by the fact that motivation may be both conscious and unconscious. Morgan (1981) states: "A wide range of risk-taking behaviours may be associated with serious damage to the self although not consciously related to a wish for self-destruction. Car driving and chronic alcoholism are two examples" (p. 259). In most, if not all, behaviors, there is a purpose associated with the activity that can be construed as principally positive in the view of the individual concerned. With suicide, however, this seems by definition not to exist, at least on the conscious level (although there may be fantasy elements that appear to be positive to the individual, exemplified by the feeling that "they'll be sorry when I'm dead"). Unconsciously, I suppose it is possible to postulate "positive" results, such as rejoining in death a deceased parent, as some authors have suggested (Hendin, 1975). More precisely, perhaps, a positive result does not exist if the intent of the individual's action is really death. Thus, certain kinds of risk-taking behavior can be "suicidal," but if the primary intent of the action is to take a risk, it becomes a dynamically different act; that is, when it is performed to thrill, to impress, to demonstrate mastery, or to get somewhere in a hurry.

This is not to suggest that a failed suicide attempt may not have positive consequences. Such an action may have considerable positive benefit for an individual because the response of the environment changes his or her view of people's concern, because the action has mediated the expression of certain feelings with a resultant catharsis, or, more abstrusely, because the failure of the attempt suggests that some higher power does not wish the individual to die.

The question then is raised as to whether a suicide attempt in which death is not intended is dynamically different from one in which death is. In this question, if one accepts the existence of the unconscious, an individual may consciously not intend death but unconsciously wish for it, or vice versa. If the former dynamic exists, can the individual calculate accurately the possibility of accidentally achieving the "wrong" outcome? And how does one weigh the factor of knowledge? Most of us would agree that a college student who leaves a suicide note and then swallows eight aspirins does not seriously intend suicide. But if that student swallows eight Seconals, are we as sure? In both instances, the observer is making assumptions about the individual's level of pharmacological knowledge, assumptions that at some point become very speculative. However, when one is postulating an interplay between conscious and unconscious forces, one is dealing with a complex interactive phenomenon. Thus, just as the observer feels that the student who takes eight aspirins is not seriously suicidal, the student may reach the same conclusions; and, if that student's "conscious" intent is suicidal, but the "unconscious" intent is otherwise, the student may find it necessary to take enough to convince the conscious self that the intent is "serious," thereby severely limiting the margin of safety. How able that student is to draw the fine line between satisfying the conscious intent, and fulfilling the unconscious intent of "failing," may depend on a host of factors, some of which may really be unknowable.

Predisposing Developmental Factors

Several psychological developments occur during the college years (late adolescence–young adulthood) that probably make individuals particularly subject to risks that may be life-threatening, or to impulses that may be self-destructive. One such development has already been mentioned—the need to demonstrate mastery. Individuals in this age group are at, or are near, a peak of physical development and power, and some may be tempted to use this power to convince themselves that they have certain highly valued qualities such as courage, competence, and possibly daring. The motivation also may be to impress others, inasmuch as this is an age in which individuals are attempting to develop self-confidence (an element of which is often inferred from the response of a beholder), to make friends, and to find lovers. Thus, climbing a mountain, racing a vehicle, or hang-gliding may be attempted because they are exciting, because they test an individual's skill and bravery, or because they may impress a friend in whom one has a romantic interest. Although there is no conscious suicidal intent, one cannot help but wonder about the dynamic when it is a known fact that a high percentage of racing car drivers, for example, die at a young age from racing accidents.

Another aspect of young adult development relates to drug and alcohol use, which is frequently cited as a factor related to suicidal actions (McGuire et al., 1976; Miles, 1977; Moore et al., 1979). Until recently, experimentation with drugs and alcohol often began at college; and, while use may begin earlier, the development of responsible patterns of use tends to occur during this period. Although drug and alcohol use is by no means restricted to the college period, it is a period when individuals can use drugs with relative impunity. Injury or death that occurs when drugs or alcohol are used once again raises the question of intent.

Several investigators have attempted to delineate suicide from accidental death in statistical studies, and this is not easy to do (Holding and Barraclough, 1978; Holinger, 1980). This may not be a problem in studies that are purely statistical, because "errors" in reporting may be sufficiently consistent so that they do not really affect comparative rate studies (Brugha and Walsh, 1978). When one studies individual cases, however, it may be a different matter. Thus, on the one hand, the suicide attempt or completed suicide may occur because the individual has used drugs or alcohol, and may therefore have impaired judgment, induced a delusional state, or released suicidal impulses that have previously been controlled. On the other hand, the individual may simply have misjudged the effect that a drug or combination of drugs will have. In reporting deaths in which drugs are considered causal, there is a tendency for barbiturate overdoses to be reported as suicide, and opiate overdoses to be reported as accidental death (McGuire et al., 1976). However, if the individual's intent was known, the decision might be different.

A third developmental issue is that of separation from the family, which is considered to be an important psychological task of the late adolescent–young adult period. For those individuals who find the task of separation difficult, there may be violent interactions between the individual and family; some of these may lead to actions that have the potential for injury or death. Furthermore, there is considerable evidence to suggest that the stormiest interactions involve individuals who are quite ambivalent about the separation process, and who may consciously desire to be independent while unconsciously desiring to remain dependent. The suicidal action can, at times, rather neatly reconcile these contradictory feelings. Consciously, the message to parents may be, "The only way I can be free is to kill myself." This is often the individual's response to perceived parental demands to remain dependent. By making a suicide attempt that fails—but that causes injury or hospitalization— the individual may actually elicit more direct care and concern from the parents, and consequently may remain more dependent. In this form, however, the dependency is acceptable.

One aspect of the separation impulse may be the espousal of a cause that very often fulfills idealistic urges as well as separation and identity impulses, if the cause happens to be one that is antithetical to parental values. For example, in the name of a cause or a principle, an individual may either literally or figuratively feel it necessary or desirable to indulge in behavior that is potentially suicidal. "To put one's life or body on the line" is often (and understandably) seen as the ultimate commitment to a belief so that, for purposes of effectiveness or dramatic impact, actions may be taken that are clearly dangerous. Lying down in front of a bulldozer or tank are examples of such actions that have been taken. It can be argued, I suppose, that these actions are taken on the assumption that the driver of the vehicle will not deliberately take human life; but clearly, this assumption is predicated on the belief that the driver holds similar values and has effective control of the situation. This is a questionable assumption on both counts.

Assessment of Risk Factors

One of the most difficult clinical tasks in suicide prevention is the assessment of risk factors when an individual has made a suicide attempt. Various studies have tried to identify risk factors that predict further suicidal behavior (Kirstein et al., 1975; Morgan et al., 1976;

Myers, 1982; Pallis et al., 1982; Paykel and Rassaby, 1978; Pierce, 1977). Other studies have simply described suicide attempters (Wexler et al., 1978; Pallis and Birtchnell, 1977; Blaine and Carmen, 1968; Mishara et al., 1976). Weissman and colleagues (1973) noted the distinguishing characteristic of hostility in comparison with a group of depressed individuals who had not made suicide attempts. Blaine and Carmen (1968) described three major types: the dependent dissatisfied, the satisfied symbolic, and the unaccepting. Hankoff (1982) lists as risk factors suicide in the family and social isolation. Henderson and colleagues (1977) describe three types of parasuicides, of which the depressed alienated were at the highest risk for completed suicide. Many investigators indicate the highest risk factor is the presence of depression (Goldberg, 1981; Guze and Robins, 1970; Hankoff, 1982; Miles, 1977).

In providing an appropriate treatment response to someone who expresses suicidal feelings or who has made a suicide attempt, it is important that the therapist have some awareness of countertransference feelings in such situations. Because the therapist is dedicated to preserving life, the suicidal individual represents a special kind of threat to the therapist's reputation, as well as to the therapist's self-evaluation as a professional. Thus, the therapist's anxiety may rise to a high level, and all sorts of intrusive thoughts and worries may interfere with the primary job of listening to the patient and reacting appropriately. The therapist may be so focused on the question of whether to hospitalize the patient that important messages may be overlooked. Furthermore, the ability of a given therapist to tolerate the anxiety the patient evokes may determine the course of treatment, and not necessarily in the way that is most helpful to the patient.

Affective Disorders

Affective disorders are difficult to discuss because there are various terms used in the literature prior to the publication of the *Diagnostic and Statistical Manual of Mental Disorders, Third Edition (DSM-III)* with no uniform agreement (Kendell, 1976); therefore, comparing studies done over the years is not easy. Furthermore, there have been attempts at subgrouping (Paykel, 1971; Arieti and Bemporad, 1980); a recognition that depression may be masked (Fischer, 1979); and that in adolescence both depression (Inamadar et al., 1979) and mania (Ballenger et al., 1982) may present an "atypical" clinical picture.

The developmental issue of separation may be especially important in vulnerability to a depressive disorder. Depression is often precipitated by a loss or separation; because loss and separation are part of psychological development at this life stage, a late adolescent–young adult may be peculiarly vulnerable to depression. There are several events that are characteristic of this period. First, going to college may be experienced as a separation from parental ties; and, although this is presumably a desirable step in the process of development, not everyone is emotionally ready and some may be overcome by depressed feelings. Second, romantic attachments and detachments are frequent occurrences in this period, and the detachment phase may be especially painful for the late adolescent. Although pain probably always accompanies a loss, the superimposition of the actual loss of a romantic partner on the psychological loss of an attachment to parental figures may multiply the feelings of depression and lead to a state of hopelessness.

The role of the college health service is broad in regard to treating affective disorders if the full range of affective disorders listed in *DSM-III* (Stangler and Printz, 1980) is considered. If the area under consideration is limited to those major affective disorders that might reasonably include a serious suicide potential, the range of affective disorders to be treated by a college service is considerably narrower (Coon, 1961; Himler and Raphael, 1942; Stangler and Printz, 1980; Oliver and Burkham, 1979; Schuckit, 1982). Perhaps it is sufficient to mention briefly the less serious manifestations, and say that a mental health service, in whatever form, will attempt to help students to clarify the problem, to give support, and in some instances to offer brief psychotherapy in an effort to resolve the conflicts that may have led to the depressive symptoms. On occasion, antidepressant medication may be used (Brown BM, 1978), and referral, if feasible, for longer-term therapy may be recommended if the depression seems to be of a chronic, longstanding nature.

The management of an initial episode of major depression or bipolar disorder probably does not vary greatly within the college population from its management elsewhere (Klerman, 1982). If one sees a student with a major depression, one presumably would do as thorough a workup as possible and then choose the appropriate antidepressant medication, admit the patient to the infirmary, possibly attempt to reduce stress by recommending some environmental manipulation such as a lighter academic load, perhaps bring the family into the situation directly, and plan a course of therapy. One's ability to do this is somewhat dependent on the resources available, and the experience of the psychiatrist involved. Some will use cognitive therapy (Rush et al., 1982); some, more traditional psychotherapy (Temby, 1961); and some have suggested new measures such as running (Greist et al., 1979).

If these measures do not alleviate the situation rapidly enough so that the individual can continue with the academic work, it may be necessary for the student to withdraw from college and either be admitted to an inpatient psychiatric program, or return home for outpatient therapy. In a sense, the more problematic epidemiological question centers on the issue of the individual returning to student status if withdrawal has occurred. How does one evaluate: 1) whether the stress of college environment was crucial in precipitating the episode initially; and 2) if so, whether the individual is now ready to cope with essentially the same situation without a recurrence of symptoms?

In the case of bipolar disorders in which the student enters a manic phase while in college, the situation is somewhat similar, but the symptomatology may create different external effects which, in turn, may lead to a different outcome. Because the college is a community, manic behavior that worries others in the environment may create pressure on administrators and mental health professionals to "do something" about the manic individual (Coon, 1961). Unfortunately, the "doing something" is usually not easy, because the manic individual usually does not feel that anything needs to be done. Furthermore, admission to the infirmary, which may be feasible with a depressed student, is unlikely to be feasible with a manic student, because very few infirmaries are staffed or architecturally designed to control manic behavior. Thus, it may be virtually impossible to start a patient on lithium in the infirmary setting; but one is reluctant to try to start lithium on an outpatient basis with such a patient, when one has so little confidence in the patient's judgment or ability to follow directions. Thus, psychiatric hospitalization may be needed sooner with a patient in a manic rather than in a depressed state.

Readmission seems also to be somewhat more problematic for individuals with bipolar disorders. This observation is based on a relatively small sample and is impressionistic, but I do believe that one precipitant of a manic episode can be a feeling of grandiosity that may be triggered by the "success" of being readmitted to college (particularly to selective colleges, admission to which is considered a major achievement).

Future Activities

In terms of future activities, the problem can be divided into three categories: primary prevention, secondary prevention, and research.

Primary Prevention

Various authors have discussed the interaction between the environment and mental health (Freeman, 1978; Greenblatt et al., 1982; Wilkinson and O'Conner, 1982). The role of the mental health professional as a change agent, however, is complex (Arnstein, 1977). It is relatively easy to pick out factors that various investigators and clinicians consider conducive to depression or suicide. These would include, among others, social isolation, family instability, drug and alcohol use, and academic failure. However, the role of the college mental health service in preventing these problems is not clear. Furthermore, there is always the possibility that if an effort is made to alleviate one or another of these problems, it may have a paradoxical effect on a given individual, and lead to further depression or hopelessness.

For example, regarding social isolation: If the individual's feeling of social isolation is related to an inability to engage in some degree of heterosexual socialization, he or she may actually be protected from intense feelings on this point by a single-sex college, where it is possible to blame or explain not having a date on the lack of availability of members of the opposite sex. The same individual in a coeducational college, which presumably should give him or her the opportunity to develop heterosexual socialization skills and thus combat feelings of social isolation and inadequacy, may actually increase these feelings because there is no external excuse possible—the individual must confront his or her own internal difficulties. On the other hand, some colleges have attempted to combat social isolation by establishing social groups (Glasscote and Fishman, 1973), and in some college environments this can work. Other colleges have attempted to create living units within the broader college which, because of their smaller size, may seem less overwhelming.

On a different note, academic pressures and failure may lead to depression and, possibly, to suicidal action. It is reasonable to recommend that a college make every attempt to help the student who is having academic difficulties; but it is not reasonable to suggest that a college should have no academic standards. The existence of such standards, however, always implies the possibility that some students will not be able to meet them and may become depressed as a result (Arnstein, 1972).

Whether one can actually prevent suicide by reducing availability of suicidal methods is an open question. Lester and Murrell (1980), in a provocative study, suggest that strict gun control laws reduce suicide rates for males (who are likely to use guns in suicide attempts) but not for females (who tend to use other methods). Colleges that have regulations against the possession of guns on campus may be taking a preventive measure, although obviously such regulations may be easily circumvented. In a similar vein, the post-World War II campus building boom often led to the construction of high-rise dormitories, which provided greater opportunity for impulsive or premeditated fatal jumps. In an ideal world, mental health consultants may have been able to practice primary prevention by arguing against such buildings, but it is likely that other considerations would take precedence.

Primary prevention may be best attempted by working for the application of such general principles on campus as consistency of rules, some degree of flexibility, and process for orderly change. However, it is difficult to prove that these measures will affect the suicide rate.

Secondary Prevention

As far as secondary prevention measures are concerned, I have already suggested certain measures that I believe in strongly, some of which are more easily implemented than others. First, I believe that colleges should, if at all possible, establish availability and accessibility of helping resources, publicize the existence of such resources, and make every attempt to reduce obstacles standing in the way of the use of these resources by students. Furthermore, I believe that there should be a campus network of individuals prepared to help students in difficulty. This network should include deans, chaplains, residence hall advisors, faculty advisors, career advisors, and peer counselors, as well as general health care providers and mental health professionals. Different groups within this network should work together and not in competition with each other. It is highly desirable to have some resource that is available on a 24-hour basis if emergencies arise in the middle of the night or on weekends. The mental health service should be prepared to offer several modalities of treatment, and, if that is not economically possible, to have established methods of referral to community resources. In this connection it would be advantageous to make some kind of health insurance mandatory, in order to reduce the tendency of students to avoid obtaining help because of financial pressures.

One question related to secondary prevention is, to what extent should assessment procedures for affective disorders and potential suicides be extended beyond a standard clinical interview? This question can be examined from two perspectives: 1) Should some of the newer laboratory tests be used?, and 2) What is the impact of using one or another of the inventory instruments?

In regard to the first perspective, there is an active literature on the use of the dexamethasone suppression test (DST), which suggests that it may be a useful screening test in the treatment planning process (Brown WA, 1981; Carroll, 1982). The few studies that have been done on individuals in the college age group indicate that the test seems to apply to this group as well as to older age groups (Crumley et al., 1982; Gwirtzman et al., 1982); but it still tends to be used primarily with inpatients (Coryell, 1981), and it is not clear whether or how widely it should be applied to a young adult outpatient population (Amsterdam et al., 1982). Furthermore, almost every new issue of the psychiatric journals reports a new laboratory test that is said to add important information (Brown GL et al., 1982; Ostroff et al., 1982; Targum et al., 1982), and procedures have advanced to the point that neuroendocrine profiles are being developed that may have a predictive value in relation to suicidal behavior.

In regard to the second perspective, various scales have been developed (Goldberg, 1981; Goldney, 1981; Moore et al., 1979; Pallis et al., 1982), of which the most widely used is the Beck Depression Inventory (BDI) (Bumberry et al., 1978). The BDI has been used in a variety of research projects (Hammen and Padesky, 1977; Hammen, 1980), often with random samples of students, and seems to provide relatively reliable results; however, its use in a clinic setting must be considered in the context of the total assessment plan. Should it be used routinely with all patients, or only with specific patients if initial clinical evaluation suggests a depressive diagnosis? Finally, it may be helpful to do more traditional psychological testing, which often can evaluate the degree of depression and the suicide potential quite accurately.

One aspect of the suicidal individual's situation that touches on both primary and secondary prevention involves the opportunities available for constructive action. Clinically, the student about whom I worry most is the student who feels "trapped" and who feels suicide is "the only way out." As a therapist, one immediately tries to convince the student that other less destructive actions are possible. These may include withdrawing from college or changing one's environment within the college. If college rules are very rigid about such actions as withdrawal, the student may feel that withdrawal will ruin his life or career anyway, so there is no reason not to commit suicide. The therapist may be helpful in achieving greater flexibility of such rules, and thus provide an alternate course of action that is acceptable to the student. Sometimes, of course, the student's inability to accept withdrawal as a possibility is related not to college rules, but to the expectation of family reaction. In this instance, the therapist may be able to act as intermediary between the student and the family, thereby fostering communication between the two, and giving the student acceptable alternatives to suicide.

Research

I have relatively little to say specifically about research directions. There are many studies that could be done, but given the demand for service it is difficult to find time and support to accomplish them. I believe that college mental health services should continue to attempt, where possible, to evaluate the effectiveness of treatment, as well to study prevalence (Rimmer, 1978). I believe that such services should always attempt to be conversant with the literature on personality development in this age period, and with medical advances in the diagnosis, evaluation, and treatment of affective disorders. It would be useful to have a current survey of suicidal behavior on campus if it could be carried out with enough rigor to be meaningful. Finally, a difficult but important project would be a follow-up study of individuals who were known to have had an affective disorder or to have made a suicide attempt while in college. Hall and colleagues (1982) have published a study on a five-year follow-up of undergraduates with psychiatric illness, and it would be illuminating to have similar studies done on a broader scope.

A further issue that is very difficult to study is the best way to react to a suicide or serious suicide attempt if it occurs within a community. Some feel that it is preferable to discuss openly all that is known about the event, but this has two possible drawbacks: 1) the possible effect of "contagion," and 2) the feelings and wishes of the individual's family, who may not accept the fact that the individual committed suicide or who, if accepting the suicide, may wish to diminish publicity as much as possible. Inasmuch as the family is the most directly affected, it is difficult to proceed against their wishes. Others feel that one should say as little as possible about the event without lying or actively "covering up." This posture also has its drawbacks because rumors inevitably develop, and the rumors may actually exaggerate the facts. A third and perhaps most unfortunate response is one in which officials disagree on the course of action, and the disagreement becomes known to the community at large. This may evoke the kind of troubled response from the community that has been described when there is tension and disagreement among staff members on psychiatric wards.

References

Allison-Tomlinson M: Adolescent suicide. Psychiatric Annals 11:44–52, 1981

Amsterdam JD, Winokur A, Caroff SN, et al: The dexamethasone suppression test in outpatients with primary affective disorder and health control subjects. Am J Psychiatry 139:287–291, 1982

Arieti S, Bemporad JR: The psychological organization of depression. Am J Psychiatry 137:1360–1365, 1980

Arnstein RL: College psychiatry and community psychiatry. J Am Coll Health 20:256–261, 1972

Arnstein RL: The college mental health practitioner as change agent? J Am Coll Health 25:198–200, 1977

Ballenger JC, Reus VI, Post RM: The "atypical" clinical picture of adolescent mania. Am J Psychiatry 139:602–606, 1982

Barraclough B, Shepherd D, Jennings C: Do newspaper reports of coroner's inquests incite people to commit suicide? Br J Psychiatry 131:528–532, 1977

Binns WA, Kerkman D, Schroeder SO: Destructive group dynamics: an account of some peculiar interrelated incidents of suicide and suicidal attempts at a university dormitory. J Am Coll Health 14:250–256, 1966

Birtchnell J, Alarcon J: Depression and attempted suicide: a study of 19 cases seen in a casualty department. Br J Psychiatry 118:289–296, 1971

Blaine GB Jr, Carmen LR: Causal factors in suicidal attempts by male and female college students. Am J Psychiatry 125:834–837, 1968

Blumenthal S, Bergner L: Suicide and newspapers: a replicated study. Am J Psychiatry 130:468–471, 1973

Brown BM: Depressed college students and tricyclic anti-depressant therapy. J Am Coll Health 27:79–83, 1978

Brown GL, Ebert MH, Goyer PF, et al: Aggression, suicide, and serotonin: relationships to CSF amine metabolites. Am J Psychiatry 139:741–746, 1982

Brown WA: The dexamethasone suppression test: a potential tool in the management of depression. Behav Med 8:22–28, 1981

Brugha T, Walsh D: Suicide past and present—temporal constancy of under-reporting. Br J Psychiatry 132:177–179, 1978

Bruyn, HB, Seiden RH: Student suicide: fact or fancy? J Am Coll Health 14:69–77, 1965

Bumberry W, Oliver JM, McClure JN: Validation of the Beck Depression Inventory in a university population using psychiatric estimate as the criterion. J Consult Clin Psychol 46:150–155, 1978

Carroll BJ: The dexamethasone suppression test for melancholia. Br J Psychiatry 140:292–304, 1982

Coon GP: Acute psychosis, depression, and elation, in Emotional Problems of the Student. Edited by Blaine GB Jr, McArthur CC. New York, Appleton-Century-Crofts, 1961

Coryell W, Schlesser MA: Suicide and the dexamethasone suppression test in unipolar depression. Am J Psychiatry 138:1120–1121, 1981

Crumley FE, Clevenger J, Steinfink D, et al: Preliminary report on the dexamethasone suppression test for psychiatrically disturbed adolescents. Am J Psychiatry 139:1062–1064, 1982

Farnsworth DL: Mental Health in College and University. Cambridge, MA, Harvard University Press, 1957

358   SUICIDE AND DEPRESSION AMONG

Fawcett J: The suicide epidemic of youth: how do we understand it and what can we do about it? Current Clinical Briefs 3:3–5, 1982

Fischer HK: Faces and masks of depression: the psychodynamic side. Psychosomatics 20:254–268, 1979

Freeman H: Mental health and the environment. Br J Psychiatry 132:113–124, 1978

Fry CC, Rostow EG: Mental Health in College. New York, Commonwealth Fund, 1942

Glasscote R, Fishman ME: Mental Health on the Campus. Washington DC, Joint Information Service, 1973

Goldberg ED: Depression and suicide ideation in the young adult. Am J Psychiatry 138:35–40, 1981

Goldney RD: Are young women who attempt suicide hysterical? Br J Psychiatry 138:141–146, 1981

Greenblatt M, Becerra RM, Serafetinides EA: Social networks and mental health: an overview. Am J Psychiatry 139:977–984, 1982

Greist JH, Eischens RR, Klein MH, et al: Antidepressant running. Psychiatric Annals 9:23–33, 1979

Guze SB, Robins E: Suicide and primary affective disorders. Br J Psychiatry 117:437–438, 1970

Gwirtzman H, Gerner RH, Sternbach H: The overnight dexamethasone suppression: clinical and theoretical review. J Clin Psychiatry 43:321–327, 1982

Hall ZM, Sheil LP, Waters WE: Psychiatric illness after leaving university: a five-year follow-up of students. Br J Psychiatry 140:374–377, 1982

Hammen CL: Depression in college students: beyond the Beck Depression Inventory. J Consult Clin Psychol 48:126–128, 1980

Hammen CL, Padesky CA: Sex differences in the expression of depressive responses on the Beck Depression Inventory. J Abnorm Psychol 86:609–614, 1977

Hankoff LD: Suicide and attempted suicide, in Handbook of Affective Disorders. Edited by Paykel ES. New York, Guilford Press, 1982

Hawton K, Bancroft J, Simkins S: Attitudes of psychiatric patients to deliberate self-poisoning. Br J Psychiatry 132:31–35, 1978a

Hawton K, Crowle J, Simkin S, et al: Attempted suicide and suicide among Oxford University students. Br J Psychiatry 132:506–509, 1978b

Henderson AS, Hartigan J, Davidson J, et al: A typology of parasuicide. Br J Psychiatry 131:631–641, 1977

Hendin H: Student suicide: death as a life style. J Nerv Ment Dis 160:204–219, 1975

Himler LE, Raphael T: Manic-depressive psychoses among college students. Am J Psychiatry 99:188–193, 1942

Holding TA, Barraclough BM: Psychiatric morbidity in a sample of accidents. Br J Psychiatry 130:244–252, 1977

Holding TA, Barraclough BM: Undetermined deaths—suicide or accident? Br J Psychiatry 133:542–549, 1978

Holinger PC: Adolescent suicide: an epidemiological study of recent trends. Am J Psychiatry 135:754–756, 1978

Holinger PC: Violent deaths among the young: recent trends in suicide, homicide, and accidents. Am J Psychiatry 136:1144–1147, 1979

Holinger PC: Violent deaths as a leading cause of mortality: an epidemiologic study of suicide, homicide, and accidents. Am J Psychiatry 137:472–476, 1980

Holinger PC, Offer D: Prediction of adolescent suicide: a population model. Am J Psychiatry 139:302–306, 1982

Inadamar SC, Siomopoulos G, Osborn M, et al: Phenomenology associated with depressed moods in adolescence. Am J Psychiatry 136:156–159, 1979

Inadamar SC, Lewis DO, Siomopoulos G, et al: Violent and suicidal behavior in psychotic adolescents. Am J Psychiatry 139:932–935, 1982

Kendell RE: The classification of depression: a review of contemporary confusion. Br J Psychiatry 129:15–28, 1976

Kirstein L, Prusoff B, Weissman M, et al: Utilization review of treatment for suicide attempters. Am J Psychiatry 132:22–27, 1975

Klerman GL: Practical issues in the treatment of depression and mania, in Handbook of Affective Disorders. Edited by Paykel ES. New York, Guilford Press, 1982

Lester D, Murrell MA: The influence of gun control laws on suicidal behavior. Am J Psychiatry 137:121–122, 1980

Lyman JL: Student suicide at Oxford University. Student Medicine 10:218–234, 1961

McGuire FL, Birch H, Gottschalk LA, et al: A comparison of suicide and non-suicide deaths involving psychotropic drugs in four major U.S.

cities. Am J Public Health 66:1058–1061, 1976

Miles CP: Conditions predisposing to suicide: a review. J Nerv Ment Dis 164:231–246, 1977

Minkoff K, Bergman E, Beck AT, et al: Hopelessness, depression and attempted suicide. Am J Psychiatry 130:455–459, 1973

Mishara BL, Baker AH, Mishara TT: The frequency of suicide attempts: a retrospective approach applied to college students. Am J Psychiatry 133:841–844, 1976

Moore JT, Judd LL, Zung WWK, et al: Opiate addiction and suicidal behaviors. Am J Psychiatry 136:1187–1189, 1979

Morgan HG: Management of suicidal behavior. Br J Psychiatry 138:259–260, 1981

Morgan HG, Barton J, Pottle S, et al: Deliberate self-harm: a follow-up study of 279 patients. Br J Psychiatry 128:361–368, 1976

Myers ED: Subsequent deliberate self-harm in patients referred to a psychiatrist: a prospective study. Br J Psychiatry 140:132–137, 1982

Oliver JM, Burkham R: Depression in university students: duration, relation to calendar time, prevalence, and demographic correlates. J Abnorm Psychol 88:667–670, 1979

Ostroff R, Giller E, Bonese K, et al: Neuroendocrine risk factors of suicidal behavior. Am J Psychiatry 139:1323–1325, 1982

Pallis DJ, Birtchnell J: Seriousness of suicide attempt in relation to personality. Br J Psychiatry 130:253–259, 1977

Pallis DJ, Barraclough BM, Levey AB, et al: Estimating suicide risk among attempted suicides, I: the development of new clinical scales. Br J Psychiatry 141:37–44, 1982

Parnell RW: Mortality and prolonged illness among Oxford undergraduates. Lancet 1:731–733, 1951

Parrish HM: Epidemiology of suicide among college students. Yale Journal of Biology and Medicine 29:585–595, 1957

Paykel ES: Classification of depressed patients: a cluster analysis derived grouping. Br J Psychiatry 118:275–288, 1971

Paykel ES, Rassaby E: Classification of suicide attempters by cluster analysis. Br J Psychiatry 133:45–52, 1978

Pepitone-Arreola-Rockwell F, Rockwell D, Core N: Fifty-two medical student suicides. Am J Psychiatry 138:198–201, 1981

Peszke MA, Affleck GG, Wintrob RM: Perceived statutory applicability versus clinical desirability of emergency involuntary hospitalization. Am J Psychiatry 137:476–480, 1980

Pierce DW: Suicidal intent in self-injury. Br J Psychiatry 130:377–385, 1977

Pitts FN Jr, Schuller AB, Rich CL, et al: Suicide among U.S. women physicians, 1967–1972. Am J Psychiatry 136:694–696, 1979

Raphael T, Power SH, Berridge WL: The question of suicide as a problem in college mental hygiene. Am J Orthopsychiatry 7:1–14, 1937

Rimmer JD: Systematic study of psychiatric illness in freshman college students: part 1. Compr Psychiatry 19:249–251, 1978

Rook A: Student suicides. Br Med J 1:597–603, 1959

Ross M: Suicide among college students. Am J Psychiatry 126:220–225, 1969

Rush AJ, Beck AT, Kovacs M, et al: Comparison of the effects of cognitive therapy and pharmacotherapy on hopelessness and self-concept. Am J Psychiatry 139:862–866, 1982

Schuckit MA: Prevalence of affective disorder in a sample of young men. Am J Psychiatry 139:1431–1436, 1982

Sims L, Ball MJ: Suicide among university students. J Am Coll Health 21:336–338, 1973

Stangler RS, Printz AM: DSM-III: psychiatric diagnosis in a university population. Am J Psychiatry 137:937–940, 1980

Targum SD, Sullivan AM, Byrnes SM: Neuroendocrine interrelationships in major depressive disorder. Am J Psychiatry 139:282–286, 1982

Temby WD: Suicide, in Emotional Problems of the Student. Edited by Blaine GB Jr, McArthur CC. New York, Appleton-Century-Crofts, 1961

Weissman M, Fox K, Klerman GL: Hostility and depression associated with suicide attempts. Am J Psychiatry 130:450–455, 1973

Wexler L, Weissman MM, Kasl SV: Suicide attempts, 1970–75: updating a United States study and comparisons with international trends. Br J Psychiatry 132:180–185, 1978

Wilkinson CB, O'Conner WA: Human ecology and mental illness. Am J Psychiatry 139:985–990, 1982

Wilkinson DG: The suicide rate in schizophrenia. Br J Psychiatry 140:138–141, 1982

Conclusion

PROSPECTS FOR THE FUTURE

Gerald L. Klerman, M.D.

Conclusion

PROSPECTS FOR THE FUTURE

Since the time of the 1982 Conference on Preventive Aspects of Suicide and Depression among Adolescents and Young Adults (the Conference that forms the basis for this volume), the issue of adolescent suicide and depression has become a matter of public policy and increasing national concern. The epidemiologic evidence is conflicting as to whether or not the rate of suicide is increasing beyond its highpoint in 1979 and 1981. The relationship between depression and suicide so well documented in earlier studies seems to apply to adolescence, although this conclusion remains controversial. Attempts to formulate public policy for possible preventive efforts are underway in Congress and the Executive Branch.

Theoretical and Research Perspectives

A number of different theoretical and research perspectives were represented in these chapters. These included epidemiologic, biological, developmental, social history, demographic, and cultural perspectives.

Epidemiologic Perspectives

Much of this volume follows a public health/epidemiologic model, in which the premise is that in the phenomenon of suicide among young adults, various risk factors can be identified, such as loneliness, low self-esteem, drug and alcohol addiction, and factors in family history (both biological and social). Once risk factors, incidence, and prevalence are established, we can develop the knowledge to develop and undertake strategies for prevention.

An especially illuminating chapter in regard to prevention was written by Ernest Gruenberg. In his chapter, he elucidated the concept of a "preventive trial." In contrast to a clinical trial, which starts with a group of patients who have a condition to be treated, a preventive trial begins with a group of people who do not have the condition to be prevented. This group is divided into a control group and an intervention group. This division is effected in such a way that both groups have an equal likelihood of developing the condition to be prevented. Goldberger's supplementing diets with brewer's yeast, thereby preventing pellagra, as well as Salk's polio vaccine, are two examples of preventive trials. Other experiments, such as Tompkins' and Wiehl's prenatal diet supplements to prevent birth defects, and the Cambridge–Somerville attempts at delinquency prevention, met with less clear-cut success. All in all, however, preventive trials offer a powerful design, integrating scientific, social, and political knowledge, to produce the possibility of widespread results.

A number of risk factors have been identified for depression among adolescents and young adults including youth, family history, recent life events, social class, minority status, female gender, loneliness, and alienation (see also Wells et al., 1985). Many of the psychosocial risk factors for depression are similar for suicide. As described in detail in the chapter by Hirschfeld and Blumenthal, there are some significant differences in risk factors for death by suicide and for suicide attempt. Of particular interest is the chapter by Brennan on the prevalence of adolescent loneliness and alienation as precursors for risk for suicide attempt.

Biological Perspectives

A number of chapters, particularly those by Weissman and by Reich, highlighted biological factors and discussed possible genetic influences.

Family aggregation studies have demonstrated a higher risk among relatives for depressive illness in families where one or more members have been depressed. Family aggregation by itself does not demonstrate genetic transmission. Other studies using twins and adoption studies are more definitive. The Danish adoption studies conducted by Kety et al. (1968), using adoption records in Copenhagen, indicate that the risk for suicide is greatly increased among relatives of depressed patients, even those reared apart after adoption.

In addition to genetic factors, attention has also been given to various endocrine factors, particularly those related to premenstrual tension and postpartum depression (Weissman and Klerman, 1977).

Developmental Perspectives

The extension of the developmental approach to young adulthood and maturity has been emphasized by Bernice Neugarten and others (Neugarten, 1969; 1973). A psychoanalytic approach to adult development has been based upon the influential writings of Eric Erikson (1950). Prominent among the extenders of Erikson's ideas are Daniel Levinson (1978) and George Vaillant (1977) who have proposed various stages of adult life. Most groups studied, however, have been male.

Periods of transition from one developmental phase to another are periods of increased stress and distress, often with symptoms of depression and tension. From the epidemiologic point of view, these are periods when individuals are at risk for depression and suicide.

Developmental studies of adolescents, particularly the study by Offer and Petersen (1982), have questioned some of the conventional wisdom of mental health professionals that adolescence and young adulthood are periods of turmoil. According to Offer and Petersen (1982), adolescents in turmoil are in a minority; perhaps 25 percent of this population ". . . experience severe mood swings and rebelliousness, while the rest accomplish the transition from childhood to adulthood without the upheaval said to characterize teenage" (p. 86).

There was disagreement among the participants at the Research Workshop as to the validity of stage theories. Levinson's view generated considerable discussion. The stage theories, as put forward by Erikson, Levinson, and Vaillant, tend mainly to be derived from psychiatric and psychoanalytic backgrounds. These theories have been criticized by sociologists and social psychologists. An alternative view is a social history perspective.

Social History Perspectives

The life stage theory emphasized that the changing historical position, especially of women, has contributed to different social strains and expectations. Perun and Erkut have discussed these shifts in their chapter. They are reflected in the changing expectations of young women around timing and balance of marriage, family, child-rearing, career, economic independence, and other concerns.

Demographic Perspectives

A number of demographers, particularly Easterlin (1980), have drawn attention to the increased risk for a number of adverse eco-nomic and career consequences for individuals born during periods of large birth cohorts; that is, the "baby boom" generation. Only recently have these ideas been applied to mental health phenomena. Of particular interest are the analyses of suicide rates in the United States (Holinger and Offer, 1982), Alberta, Canada (Solomon and Hellon, 1980), and Australia (Goldney and Katsikitis, 1983).

Cultural Perspectives

There was universal agreement among members of the Work-shop that there needed to be understanding of the differences in etiology of depression and suicide among various ethnic groups, particularly blacks, Latinos, Asian Americans, and native Americans. This is emphasized in the chapter by Earls and Jemison.

Evidence for Increase in Depression and Suicide: Are We in an Epidemic?

The evidence for a rise in suicide through the 1970s has been well documented (Klerman et al., 1985). At issue is whether this rise is continuing, or whether it may well have reached its peak. Daniel Offer reports that the estimated rate for suicide in ages 15 to 24 for 1983 was 11.7 per 100,000, a decline from the 1982 levels. Based on Census Bureau projections of the population by age through the year 2000, Offer and Holinger are projecting a steady decrease in suicide in this age group to a rate of 9.0 by the year 2000. This is a considerable decrease from the peak of 1977, though it is still higher than the rate in 1956.

These trends in suicide have been paralleled by trends indicating a rise in depression among young adults, and earlier age of onset of samples through the 20th century (D. Offer, personal communication).

In the 1970s, a number of observers hypothesized the increase in rates of affective disorders. Among the observations leading to this hypothesis were the increasing attention devoted by the lay press and clinical literature to depression among young women. The average age of onset for depression in large series studies reported since World War II is considerably younger than the age of onset reported from series studies prior to World War II. Moreover, involutional melancholia, an important clinical condition in the period around World War II, is now almost nonexistent.

Verification of this hypothesis has been difficult because of a lack of large samples representative of the general population, and a lack of specific subpopulations such as families of affectively ill patients. In recent years, the situation has improved greatly. Standardized diagnostic techniques such as the Schedule of Affective Disorders and the Diagnostic Interview Schedule are now available and have been applied in large clinical, family, and epidemiologic studies.

There are now several studies reporting on research programs that have used large samples (Klerman, 1985). These include: the NIMH Collaborative Program on the Psychobiology of Depression– Clinical Studies (Katz and Klerman, 1979); the NIMH Epidemiologic Catchment Area (ECA) Study conducted in five cities (Regier et al., 1984); the 25-year follow-up study from Lunby, Sweden (Hagnell et al., 1982); the epidemiologic study of mental disorder in females from Gothenburg, Sweden (Hallstrom, 1984); and the Stirling County Study conducted in Nova Scotia, Canada, initiated by Leighton et al. (1963), and analyzed by Murphy et al. (1984).

Taken together, these studies indicate a rise in depression, particularly for young adults after World War II. This appears to have had its greatest impact in the early 1970s. It is not clear at this moment whether this trend will continue. One possibility is that the epidemic of depression and suicide has peaked and is gradually declining, as has been suggested by Offer. The other possibility is that the rates will continue and that this represents a sort of "learned behavior" that this cohort has experienced and will continue to experience as they mature. The "baby boom" generation seems to have been particularly vulnerable to rapid social change and environmental conditions, and within this group, young females seem most at risk.

There remains the problem of reconciling these epidemiologic data with the strong evidence of genetic contribution, as reported in this volume by Reich. The findings of progressive increases in the rate of depression, earlier age of onset, and shifts in the male–female ratio cannot be explained by a single-factor theory that affective illness is due only to genetic predisposition. Although depression is familial and may be genetically determined, current evidence does not support a specific mode of genetic transmission, whether the mode of transmission is a single locus or is polygenic. The demonstration of birth-cohort trends does not rule out genetic contribution to the vulnerability to depression. Environmental factors often must operate to make manifest a genetic vulnerability, as demonstrated for diabetes, phenylketonuria (PKU), and other genetic disorders.

Some complex form of gene–environment interaction is likely operating in the pathogenesis of clinical depression. The birth cohort trends and shifts in age of onset and in the male–female ratio require a multifactorial model that incorporates the role of environmental risk factors along with genetic factors. The nature of possible environmental risk factors is not established. The environmental risk factors could be biological, including changes in nutrition, the possible role of viruses, or the effects of an unknown depressogenic chemical agent in the water or air. Other environmental risk factors could be nonbiological: historical, cultural, and economic factors have been suggested. These include urbanization, demographic fluctuation, changes in family structure, alterations in the roles of women, an increased rate of women in the labor force, and shifts in occupational patterns.

Some form of temporal effect is operating to increase rates of depression among relatives of affectively ill probands in recent decades. A birth cohort effect for affective disorder, if substantiated by further research, has implications for theories of causation, particularly gene–environment interaction, and is important for those involved in planning health services and the clinical care and prevention of depression and related affective disorder.

Recommendations

The easiest recommendations are those that involve areas of further research. At the Conference, several areas of research were identified as meriting further attention. These included:

1. Familial and genetic studies to establish the role of social and genetic modes of transmission.
2. Increased neuroendocrine and physiological studies of puberty and adolescence. These aspects were not represented at the Workshop, but is an important area to be studied, particularly in adolescence, when endocrine changes related to puberty have great impact on psychological and physical development.
3. Studies of normal adolescents, as well as surveys of depressive symptoms in adolescence in young adulthood.
4. Clinical studies of suicide attempters. Having identified risk factors that are potentially modifiable by clinical intervention and/or social change, preventive trials should be planned. There is a need to identify areas of social change that might impact upon these conditions, such as reduction of unemployment (particularly among minority males) or gun control.
5. Research more directly related to prevention, particularly epidemiologic studies, to identify rates of symptoms in illness for these age groups in general, and by subgroups (blacks, whites, college bound, those not in college, military, males, females, and so forth). These could include special ECA-type studies, case control studies, and cohort longitudinal studies.

Far more difficult are recommendations regarding possible preventive interventions. Congressional attention to this matter has led to the formation of a task force on teenage suicide within the Department of Health and Human Services, and it is likely that increased federal attention will be given. Proposals have been made for federal support of hotlines and crisis intervention programs, specifically aimed at teenage populations. Other more clinically oriented recommendations would be that attention be given to casefinding of families in which one or both parents are depressed (Beardslee et al., 1983). Others, however, have denied that the relation between depression and suicide, so well established for adults, is operating in adolescents. Rather, they believe that the rise in suicide does not reflect a rise in clinical depression, but is rather a response of adolescents to the stress of modern living.

References

Beardslee WR, Bemporad J, Keller MB, et al: Children of parents with major affective disorder: a review. Am J Psychiatry 140:825–832, 1983

Easterlin RA: Birth and Fortune. New York, Basic Books, 1980

Erikson EH: Childhood and Society. New York, Norton, 1950

Goldney RD, Katsikitis M: Cohort analysis of suicide rates in Australia. Arch Gen Psychiatry 40:71–74, 1983

Hagnell O, Lanke J, Rorsman B, et al: Are we entering an age of melancholy? Depressive illnesses in a prospective epidemiological study over 25 years: the Lunby study, Sweden. Psychol Med 12:122–129, 1982

Hallstrom T: Point prevalence of major depressive disorder in a Swedish urban female population. Acta Psychiatr Scand 69:52–59, 1984

Holinger PC, Offer D: Prediction of adolescent suicide: a population model. Am J Psychiatry 139:302–306, 1982

Katz MM, Klerman GL: Introduction: overview of the clinical studies program of the NIMH, Clinical Research Branch Collaborative Study on the Psychobiology of Depression. Am J Psychiatry 136:49–51, 1979

Kety SS, Rosenthal D, Wender PH, et al: The types and prevalence of mental illness in the biological and adoptive families of adopted schizophrenics, in The Transmission of Schizophrenia. Edited by Rosenthal D, Kety SS. Oxford, Pergamon, 1968

Klerman GL: Evidence for increase in rates of depression in North America and Western Europe in recent decades. Paper presented at Conference on New Research in Depression at Murnau, Bavaria, West Germany, March 25–27, 1985

Klerman GL, Lavori PW, Rice J, et al: Birth-cohort trends in rates of major depressive disorder among relatives of patients with affective disorder. Arch Gen Psychiatry 42:689–693, 1985

Leighton D, Harding JS, Macklin DB, et al: Psychiatric findings of the Stirling County study. Am J Psychiatry 119:1021–1031, 1963

Levinson DJ: The Seasons of a Man's Life. New York, Knopf, 1978

Murphy JM, Sobol AM, Neff RK, et al: Stability of prevalence. Arch Gen Psychiatry 41:990–997, 1984

Neugarten BL: Continuities and discontinuities of psychological issues into adult life. Hum Dev 12:121–130, 1969

Neugarten BL, Datan N: Sociological perspectives on the life cycle, in Life Span Development Psychology: Personality and Socialization. Edited by Baltes PB, Schaie KW. New York, Academic Press, 1973

Offer D, Petersen AC. Child psychiatry perspectives. J Am Acad Child Psychiatry 21:86–87, 1982

Regier DA, Myers JK, Kramer M, et al: The NIMH Epidemiological Catchment Area Program. Arch Gen Psychiatry 41:934–941, 1984

Solomon MI, Hellon CP: Suicide and age in Alberta, Canada, 1951–1977. Arch Gen Psychiatry 137:511–513, 1980

Vaillant GE: Adaptation to Life. Boston, Little, Brown, 1977

Weissman MM, Klerman GL: Sex differences and the epidemiology of depression. Arch Gen Psychiatry 34:98–111, 1977

Wells VE, Deykin EY, Klerman GL: Risk factors for depression in adolescence. Psychiatr Dev 3:83–108, 1985

INDEX

community health worker, 285–
286
data collection and analysis of,
286–287
direct work with subjects, 290
educational component of, 286,
294–295
future work, 295–296
study review, 282–289
Involuntary commitment, 339
Involutional melancholia, 113
Isolation, 230–232

Juvenile delinquency. *See*
Delinquency

Leisure time, 202
Life dissatisfaction measures, 303
Life events, 139, 238, 261, 263
Life stress, 222, 230
Life Stress Inventory, 223
Life structure
concept of individual, 4–5
evolution of, 3–7
Lithium, 84, 351
Living alone, 241, 246
Loneliness
affective disorder link to, 188–189
chronic, 193
effects on adolescent
development, 206–208
existential, 192–193, 194
extent of, 196–197
fear of, 206–207
forms of, 189–193
moral, 195
predisposition to, 200–202
response to, 204–205
spiritual, 191–192, 195, 204
suicide link, 188–189, 206
temporary, 193
theories of, 197–204
LSD use, 302
Lymphoblastoid cell membranes, 84
Lymphocytes, 84

Macrocosm, 57–59
Maladjustment, 266
Manic behavior, 217, 351
Marijuana use, 154, 160, 163–165,
173, 302
Marriage
breakup of, 118

component of life structure, 5
marital status, 115–116
median age of, 262
quality of, 116–118
see also Unmarried individuals
Masked depression, 217
Maternal nutrition, 329
Measles, 320
Medical care utilization, 220
Medical professionals, 124
Medical technology, 323
Menarche, 260
Menopause, 112–113
Menstrual period
See Menarche; Menopause;
Premenstrual tension (PMT);
Puberty
Mental health, 150, 271
Mental health disorders, 29–37
physical disease relationship, 143
Mental health professionals, 73, 352
education for depression
treatment, 124
Mental retardation, 330
Metropolitan Readiness Test, 159
Mexican-Americans, 140
Middle adulthood development
period, 5–13
Migration of black Americans, 135
Minnesota Multiphasic Personality
Inventories (MMPIs), 229
Moodiness, 41
Moral development, 24–25, 38, 40
Morality, 192
Moral loneliness, 195
Moratorium identity phase, 26, 196,
207
Mortality, 192
Mother Symptom Inventory (MSI),
159, 171, 173
Moving, 70, 71, 119–120
MSI. *See* Mother Symptom Inventory
Muscarinic receptors, 84

Nail biting, 152
Narcissism, 61, 63
National Collaborative Study of
Depression—Clinical, 91
Nervous breakdown, 312
Neuroendocrine profiles, 354
Neuroendocrine variables, 84
Neurotic character, 246